Inflammatory Bowel Disease: Role of Nutrition

Inflammatory Bowel Disease: Role of Nutrition

Editor: Jack Marlow

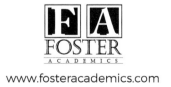

www.fosteracademics.com

www.fosteracademics.com

Cataloging-in-Publication Data

Inflammatory bowel disease : role of nutrition / edited by Jack Marlow.
   p. cm.
Includes bibliographical references and index.
ISBN 978-1-64646-568-2
1. Inflammatory bowel diseases. 2. Inflammatory bowel diseases--Nutritional aspects.
3. Inflammatory bowel diseases--Diet therapy. 4. Nutrition. I. Marlow, Jack.
RC862.I53 I54 2023
616.344--dc23

© Foster Academics, 2023

Foster Academics,
118-35 Queens Blvd., Suite 400,
Forest Hills, NY 11375, USA

ISBN 978-1-64646-568-2 (Hardback)

This book contains information obtained from authentic and highly regarded sources. Copyright for all individual chapters remain with the respective authors as indicated. All chapters are published with permission under the Creative Commons Attribution License or equivalent. A wide variety of references are listed. Permission and sources are indicated; for detailed attributions, please refer to the permissions page and list of contributors. Reasonable efforts have been made to publish reliable data and information, but the authors, editors and publisher cannot assume any responsibility for the validity of all materials or the consequences of their use.

Trademark Notice: Registered trademark of products or corporate names are used only for explanation and identification without intent to infringe.

Contents

Preface VII

Chapter 1   **Nutrition in Pediatric Inflammatory Bowel Disease: From Etiology to Treatment** 1
Francesca Penagini, Dario Dilillo, Barbara Borsani, Lucia Cococcioni, Erica Galli,
Giorgio Bedogni, Giovanna Zuin and Gian Vincenzo Zuccotti

Chapter 2   **An Examination of Diet for the Maintenance of Remission in
Inflammatory Bowel Disease** 28
Natasha Haskey and Deanna L. Gibson

Chapter 3   **Potential Impact of Diet on Treatment Effect from Anti-TNF Drugs in
Inflammatory Bowel Disease** 48
Vibeke Andersen, Axel Kornerup Hansen and Berit Lilienthal Heitmann

Chapter 4   **Intestinal Anti-Inflammatory Effect of a Peptide Derived from Gastrointestinal
Digestion of Buffalo (*Bubalus bubalis*) Mozzarella Cheese** 63
Gian Carlo Tenore, Ester Pagano, Stefania Lama, Daniela Vanacore,
Salvatore Di Maro, Maria Maisto, Raffaele Capasso, Francesco Merlino,
Francesca Borrelli, Paola Stiuso and Ettore Novellino

Chapter 5   **The Role of Vitamin D in Inflammatory Bowel Disease: Mechanism to
Management** 78
Jane Fletcher, Sheldon C. Cooper, Subrata Ghosh and Martin Hewison

Chapter 6   **Chemopreventive Effects of Strawberry and Black Raspberry on Colorectal
Cancer in Inflammatory Bowel Disease** 94
Tong Chen, Ni Shi and Anita Afzali

Chapter 7   **A Personalised Dietary Approach — A Way Forward to Manage Nutrient Deficiency,
Effects of the Western Diet and Food Intolerances in Inflammatory Bowel Disease** 114
Bobbi B Laing, Anecita Gigi Lim and Lynnette R Ferguson

Chapter 8   **Cross-Sectional Analysis of Overall Dietary Intake and Mediterranean
Dietary Pattern in Patients with Crohn's Disease** 142
Lorian Taylor, Abdulelah Almutairdi, Nusrat Shommu, Richard Fedorak,
Subrata Ghosh, Raylene A. Reimer, Remo Panaccione and Maitreyi Raman

Chapter 9   **Influence of Vitamin D Deficiency on Inflammatory Markers and Clinical Disease
Activity in IBD Patients** 156
Pedro López-Muñoz, Belén Beltrán, Esteban Sáez-González, Amparo Alba,
Pilar Nos and Marisa Iborra

VI   Contents

Chapter 10   **Dietary Protein Intake Level Modulates Mucosal Healing and Mucosa-Adherent Microbiota in Mouse Model of Colitis**..**172**
Sandra Vidal-Lletjós, Mireille Andriamihaja, Anne Blais, Marta Grauso,
Patricia Lepage, Anne-Marie Davila, Roselyne Viel, Claire Gaudichon,
Marion Leclerc, François Blachier and Annaïg Lan

Chapter 11   **Inflammatory Bowel Diseases and Food Additives: To Add Fuel on the Flames!**................................**188**
Rachel Marion-Letellier, Asma Amamou, Guillaume Savoye and Subrata Ghosh

Chapter 12   **Dietary Support in Elderly Patients with Inflammatory Bowel Disease**..**200**
Piotr Eder, Alina Niezgódka, Iwona Krela-Kaźmierczak, Kamila Stawczyk-Eder,
Estera Banasik and Agnieszka Dobrowolska

Chapter 13   **Dietary Factors in Sulfur Metabolism and Pathogenesis of Ulcerative Colitis**......................................**216**
Levi M. Teigen, Zhuo Geng, Michael J. Sadowsky, Byron P. Vaughn,
Matthew J. Hamilton and Alexander Khoruts

Permissions

List of Contributors

Index

Preface

Inflammatory bowel disease (IBD) refers to conditions that are characterized by chronic inflammation of the digestive tract. There are two common types of IBD, which include ulcerative colitis and Crohn's disease. Ulcerative colitis is a type of IBD that involves inflammation and sores along the superficial lining of the large intestine and rectum. Crohn's disease can affect any part of the gastrointestinal tract but commonly affects the small intestine and upper part of the large intestine. Some common symptoms of IBD are persistent diarrhea, abdominal pain, rectal bleeding, fatigue, reduced appetite, and unintended weight loss. Patients suffering from IBD are at the risk of malnutrition, and developing deficiencies of iron, vitamin B12, folic acid and several other macronutrients. Nutrition plays an important role in managing IBD. The Crohn's disease exclusion diet (CDED) can serve as an effective means to reduce possible nutrient deficiencies and improve dysbiosis. CDED consists of a reduced intake of animal and saturated fat, gluten-containing grains, and emulsifiers; and an increase in intake of fruits, vegetables, and resistant starch. This book outlines the role of nutrition in inflammatory bowel disease (IBD). It aims to serve as a resource guide for medical students and professionals.

The researches compiled throughout the book are authentic and of high quality, combining several disciplines and from very diverse regions from around the world. Drawing on the contributions of many researchers from diverse countries, the book's objective is to provide the readers with the latest achievements in the area of research. This book will surely be a source of knowledge to all interested and researching the field.

In the end, I would like to express my deep sense of gratitude to all the authors for meeting the set deadlines in completing and submitting their research chapters. I would also like to thank the publisher for the support offered to us throughout the course of the book. Finally, I extend my sincere thanks to my family for being a constant source of inspiration and encouragement.

Editor

Nutrition in Pediatric Inflammatory Bowel Disease: From Etiology to Treatment

Francesca Penagini [1,*], Dario Dilillo [1], Barbara Borsani [1], Lucia Cococcioni [1], Erica Galli [1], Giorgio Bedogni [2], Giovanna Zuin [1] and Gian Vincenzo Zuccotti [1]

[1] Pediatric Department, "V. Buzzi" Children's Hospital, University of Milan, Via Castelvetro 32, 20154 Milan, Italy; dario.dilillo@icp.mi.it (D.D.); barbara.borsani1@gmail.com (B.B.); lucia.cococcioni@gmail.com (L.C.); egsorridi@gmail.com (E.G.); giovanna.zuin@icp.mi.it (G.Z.); gianvincenzo.zuccotti@unimi.it (G.V.Z.)

[2] Clinical Epidemiology Unit, Liver Research Center, Basovizza, 34012 Trieste, Italy; giorgiobedogni@gmail.com

* Correspondence: Francesca.Penagini@unimi.it

Abstract: Nutrition is involved in several aspects of pediatric inflammatory bowel disease (IBD), ranging from disease etiology to induction and maintenance of disease. With regards to etiology, there are pediatric data, mainly from case-control studies, which suggest that some dietary habits (for example consumption of animal protein, fatty foods, high sugar intake) may predispose patients to IBD onset. As for disease treatment, exclusive enteral nutrition (EEN) is an extensively studied, well established, and valid approach to the remission of pediatric Crohn's disease (CD). Apart from EEN, several new nutritional approaches are emerging and have proved to be successful (specific carbohydrate diet and CD exclusion diet) but the available evidence is not strong enough to recommend this kind of intervention in clinical practice and new large experimental controlled studies are needed, especially in the pediatric population. Moreover, efforts are being made to identify foods with anti-inflammatory properties such as curcumin and long-chain polyunsaturated fatty acids n-3, which can possibly be effective in maintenance of disease. The present systematic review aims at reviewing the scientific literature on all aspects of nutrition in pediatric IBD, including the most recent advances on nutritional therapy.

Keywords: nutrition; inflammatory bowel disease; children; etiology; treatment

1. Introduction

Nutrition is involved in several aspects of pediatric inflammatory bowel disease (IBD), ranging from disease etiology to induction and maintenance of disease. The etiology of inflammatory bowel disease (IBD) is believed to be multifactorial, caused by an interplay of genetic, environmental, microbial, and immunological factors. Among the environmental risk factors, dietary elements have received considerable attention in recent years. Epidemiological studies have demonstrated a rising incidence of IBD in countries where the disease is more prevalent, such as Europe and North America, as well as in areas where IBD was previously thought to be uncommon [1]. This increase has occurred with the spread of the "Western" diet, which is high in fat and protein but low in fruit and vegetables [2,3]. Numerous studies, conducted mainly in adults, assessed whether there are associations between the development of IBD and diet and suggested that specific nutrients may play a role as risk factors or protective factors for the development of disease [3–8]. However, it must be noted that many of these studies rely on food frequency questionnaires, which have a poor accuracy due to recall bias. The hypothesis of dietary factors influencing gut inflammation may be explained through several biological mechanisms, including antigen presentation, change in prostaglandin balance, and alteration of the microflora [2,9]. Aside from etiology, nutrition plays a significant role in treatment of disease. Among the traditional nutritional approaches, exclusive enteral nutrition (EEN) is an extensively studied, well established, and valid approach to remission of pediatric Crohn's disease (CD). The latter nutritional therapy presents several advantages including control of inflammatory changes, mucosal healing, positive benefits to growth and overall nutritional status, and avoidance of other medical therapies. Aside from EEN, recently several new nutritional approaches are emerging and have seemed to be successful. The present systematic review aims at reviewing the scientific literature on all aspects of nutrition in pediatric IBD, including the most recent advances in nutritional therapy.

2. Methods

A structured literature search was performed by two investigators (Francesca Penagini and Barbara Borsani) independently, in PubMed, EMBASE, and Medline starting from January 1982 up to April 2016 using the following keywords: "Pediatric Inflammatory Bowel Disease", "Pediatric IBD", "Inflammatory Bowel Disease in children", "IBD in children" in any combination with "diet", "dietary intakes", "nutrition" and cross referenced with "etiology", "induction of remission", "relapse" and "treatment". The search was limited to full-text papers in English and resulted in a total of 8229 articles. By screening titles and abstracts, studies performed *in vitro*, in animals, uncontrolled studies, case reports, and reviews were excluded. Duplicate studies were removed. Eligible papers were cross-checked for references, which resulted in two additional papers. Figure 1 shows the flow-chart of our systematic review. For randomized clinical trials the absolute risk change with exact 95% confidence intervals (CI) was calculated. For cohort studies, the incidence rates with exact 95% CI were calculated.

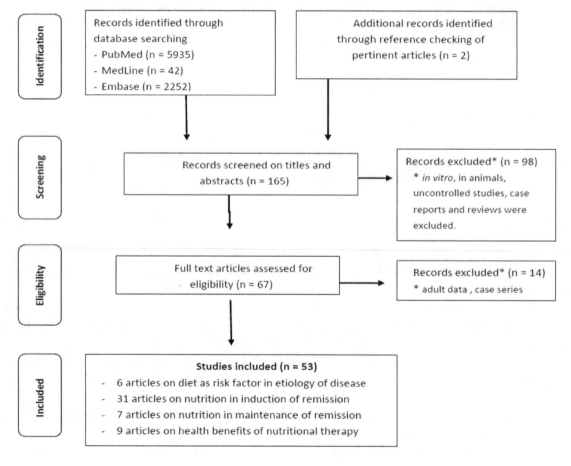

Figure 1. Flow-chart on the methods of the systematic review.

3. Nutrition in Etiology of Pediatric Inflammatory Bowel Disease

Data on diet as a risk factor for the onset of pediatric IBD are scarce. There are few studies in the literature apart from case-control studies, which have shown a potential role of some dietary elements as risk factors for disease onset in pediatric IBD. Nevertheless, these studies present methodological limitations such as the use of self-administered patient questionnaires, therefore recall bias. Table 1 summarizes the main studies on nutrition factors in etiology of pediatric IBD.

The Japanese Epidemiology Group of the Research Committee of IBD conducted a multisite, hospital-based, case-control study to examine the environmental risk factors for UC in 101 patients who were 10–39 years old at the time of disease onset [10]. Information was obtained from self-administered patient questionnaires. Combined consumption of Western foods (bread for breakfast, butter, margarine, cheese, meats, and ham and sausage) was significantly related to an increased risk of UC Relative risk (RR) for low consumption of Western foods 1.0 (CI not available), for intermediate consumption RR = 1.9; 95% CI 1.0 to 3.7, for high consumption RR = 2.1; 95% CI 1.0 to 4.1, $p = 0.04$. Margarine (as an individual Western food item) was positively associated with UC (RR for low consumption: 1.0 (CI not available), for intermediate consumption RR = 1.2; 95% CI 0.6 to 2.4, for high consumption RR = 2.6; 95% CI 1.4 to 5.2; trend, $p = 0.005$. There was also a tendency towards positive association of bread for breakfast with UC. For low consumption RR = 1.0, for intermediate consumption RR = 0.7; 95% CI 0.4 to 1.4, for high consumption RR = 2.1; 95% CI 1.0 to 4.3, $p = 0.07$. The'risk did not measurably vary with the consumption of typical Japanese foods, vegetables and fruits, confectioneries, or soft drinks (RR data not available) [10].

The group of Amre et al. [11] conducted a case-control study evaluating the pre-illness diet of new onset CD in Canadian children (age < 20 years, $n = 103$) using a validated food-frequency questionnaire (FFQ) in comparison to healthy controls matched for age and gender ($n = 202$). The FFQ was administered to the cases within one month of diagnosis and investigated dietary habits within the 12 months prior to disease diagnosis. Results showed negative associations with vegetables (OR = 0.69; 95% CI 0.33 to1.44, $p = 0.03$), fruits (OR = 0.49; 95% CI 0.25 to 0.96, $p = 0.02$), dietary fiber (OR = 0.12; 95%, CI 0.04 to 0.37, $p < 0.001$), and fish (OR 0,46, 95% CI 0.20–1.06, $p = 0.02$); consumption of long-chain ω-3 fatty acids was negatively associated with CD (OR = 0.44; 95%, CI 0.19 to 1.00, $p < 0.001$), whereas positive associations were evident for total fats (OR = 2.30; 95% CI 0.67 to 7.96, $p = 0.15$), monounsaturated (OR = 2.41; 95% CI 0.72 to 8.07, $p = 0.08$), and saturated (OR = 1.81; 95% CI 0.59 to 5.61, $p = 0.40$) fats, even though these associations were not statistically significant. The authors concluded that children who consumed higher amounts of fruits were at lower risk for CD ($p = 0.02$), as well as children who consumed higher amounts of fish and nuts, rich in long-chain ω-3 fatty acids such as docosahexaenoic acid (DHA), eicosapentaenoic acid (EPA) and docosapentaenoic acid (DPA) (OR = 0.44; 95% CI 0.19 to 1.0, $p = 0.03$). When the ratio of long chain ω-3/arachidonic acid was evaluated, a higher ratio was associated with a significantly reduced risk for CD (OR = 0.32; 95% CI 0.14 to 0.71, $p = 0.02$) [11]. In a similar case-control study, D'Souza et al. [12] investigated the role of specific dietary patterns in the risk for developing pediatric CD ($n = 149$, mean age at diagnosis 13.3 ± 2.6 years). They observed that dietary patterns characterized by meats, fatty foods, and desserts were positively associated with pediatric CD in both genders (OR = 4.7, 95% CI 1.6–14.2); on the contrary, dietary patterns characterized by vegetables, fruits, olive oil, fish, grains, and nuts were inversely associated with CD in both genders (girls OR = 0.3; 95% CI 0.1 to 0.9; boys OR = 0.2; 95% CI 0.1 to 0.5).

More recently, Jacobsen et al. [13] have investigated environmental risk factors for onset of IBD in children. The authors included 118 IBD patients aged < 15 years and 447 healthy controls. Risk factors were investigated by means of a questionnaire. Results showed that a high sugar intake was a risk factor for IBD (IBD OR = 2.5; 95% CI 1.0 to 6.2, CD OR = 2.9; 95% CI 1.0 to 8.5); while protective factors were daily vegetable consumption (CD OR = 0.3; 95% CI 0.1 to 1.0), UC OR = 0.3; 95% CI 0.1 to 0.8) and wholemeal bread consumption (IBD OR = 0.5; 95% CI 0.9 to 0.9), CD OR = 0.4; 95% 0.2 to 0.9) [13].

Table 1. Dietary factors and etiology in pediatric IBD. IBD = inflammatory bowel disease, UC = ulcerative colitis, CD = Crohn's disease, LC = long chain.

		Dietary Factors and Etiology in Pediatric IBD	
Author/Year	**Study Type**	**Population**	**Main Findings**
Gilat *et al.* 1987 [14]	Case-control study	Patients with IBD (*n* = 499; UC = 197, CD = 302) aged < 25 years with disease onset before 20 years of age. For each patient two age and sex matched health controls.	- Patients with CD and UC consumed significantly lower fruits and vegetables than controls (*p* < 0.01). For UC: low consumption (0 and <1/day) *vs.* high consumption (1–3 and >4/day) OR = 0.77; 95% CI 0.45 to 1.35. For CD: low consumption (0 and <1/day) *vs.* high consumption (1–3 and >4/day) OR = 0.58; 95% CI 0.37 to 0.91. - No significant differences were found between patients and controls in the frequency of breast feeding (*p* < 0.01), cereal consumption (*p* < 0.01) and sugar added to milk in infancy (*p* < 0.01).
Japanese Epidemiology Group of the Research Committee of IBD, 1994 [10]	Case-control study	Patients with UC (*n* = 101) who were aged 10–39 years at the time of disease onset. Healthy control subjects (*n* = 143).	- Combined consumption of Western foods (bread for breakfast, butter, margarine, cheese, meats, and ham and sausage) was significantly related to an increased risk of UC (Relative risk (RR) for low consumption 1.0, RR for intermediate consumption 1.9; 95% CI 1.0 to 3.7, RR for high consumption 2.1, 95% CI 1.0 to 4.1; trend, *p* = 0.04). - Margarine (as an individual Western food item) was positively associated with UC (trend, *p* = 0.005).
Baron *et al.* 2005 [15]	Case-control study	IBD patients (*n* = 282; CD 222, UC 60) with onset before 17 years of age and healthy controls matched for age, sex, and geographical location (*n* = 282).	- Breastfeeding either partially or exclusively was a risk factor for CD (CD OR = 2.1; 95% CI 1.3 to 3.4, *p* = 0.003). - Regular drinking of tap water was a protective factor for CD (CD = OR 0.6; 95% CI 0.3 to 1, *p* = 0.05).
Amre *et al.* 2007 [11]	Case-control study	Children and adolescents ≤20 years (*n* = 130), newly diagnosed with CD mean age at diagnosis (±SD) 14.2 ± 2.7 years. Healthy controls matched for age and sex (*n* = 202).	- Higher amounts of vegetables (OR = 0.69; 95% CI 0.33 to 1.44, *p* = 0.03), fruits (OR = 0.49; 95% CI 0.25–0.96, *p* = 0.02), fish (OR = 0.46; 95% CI 0.20 to 1.06, *p* = 0.02) and dietary fiber (OR = 0.12; 95% CI 0.04 to 0.37, *p* < 0.001) protected from CD. - Consumption of LC ω-3 (OR = 0.44; 95% CI 0.19 to 1.00, *p* < 0.001) were negatively associated with CD. - A higher ratio of LC ω-3/ω-6 fatty acids (OR = 0.32, 95% CI 0.14 to 0.71, *p* = 0.02) were significantly associated with lower risks for CD.
D'Souza *et al.* 2008 [12]	Case-control study	Children and adolescents ≤20 years (*n* = 149), newly diagnosed with CD mean age at diagnosis (±SD) 13.3 ± 2.6 years. Healthy controls matched for age and sex (*n* = 251).	- Meats, fatty foods and desserts (OR = 4.7; 95% CI 1.6 to 14.2) were positively associated with CD. - Vegetables, fruits, olive oil, fish, grains, and nuts were inversely associated with CD in both genders (girls: OR = 0.3; 95% CI 0.1 to 0.9; boys: OR = 0.2; 95% CI 0.1 to 0.5).
Jakobsen *et al.* 2012 [13]	Case-control study	Children and adolescents with IBD (*n* = 118; CD 59, UC 56, IBD-unclassified 3) aged <15 years. Healthy controls matched for age and sex (*n* = 477).	- High sugar intakes were a risk factor for IBD (IBD OR = 2.5; 95% CI 1.0 to 6.2, CD OR = 2.9; 95% CI 1.0 to 8.5). - Protective factors were daily *vs.* less than daily vegetable consumption (CD OR = 0.3; 95% CI 0.1 to 1.0, UC OR = 0.3; 95% CI 0.1 to 0.8) and whole-meal bread consumption (IBD OR = 0.5; 95% CI 0.3 to 0.9, CD OR = 0.4; 95% CI 0.2 to 0.9).

There are plausible biological mechanisms that can explain the abovementioned role of dietary factors in IBD pathogenesis. The n-3 polyunsaturated fatty acids (PUFAs) are present mainly in fish and can be synthesized in humans from alpha-linolenic acid, an essential fatty acid. EPA is a constituent of cell membranes and is metabolized to prostaglandin E3 and leukotriene B5, both of which are less pro-inflammatory than eicosanoids derived from n-6 PUFAs. A diet high in EPA may therefore protect the colonic mucosa against inflammation [7]. Plausible mechanisms exist to support the association between fiber intake and risk of CD. Anaerobic bacterial fermentation of undigested dietary carbohydrates and fiber polysaccharides produces short-chain fatty acids (SCAFs) like acetate, propionate, and butyrate, which are involved in the maintenance of colonic homeostasis. These molecules are utilized as fuel sources for colonocyte metabolism and seem to have an anti-inflammatory effect on epithelial cells, through inhibition of the production and release of inflammatory mediators. Consequently, a diet poor in fiber and lower in SCFAs may cause a disruption of the homeostasis between bacteria and colonocytes, leading to intestinal inflammation [16].

4. Nutrition in Induction of Remission in Pediatric Inflammatory Bowel Disease

The first reports on the successful use of enteral nutrition in induction of remission in pediatric CD date back to the 1980s [17,18]. Since then, exclusive enteral nutrition (EEN) with specific formulas has been thoroughly studied and has become a well-established nutritional approach shown to alleviate clinical symptoms, induce mucosal healing, improve nutritional status, and normalize laboratory parameters associated with active inflammation in pediatric CD. These data have been confirmed in two meta-analyses demonstrating that EEN is as effective as corticosteroids in inducing disease remission in pediatric CD [19,20], achieving normalization of inflammatory markers and clinical remission rates in >80% of subjects [21] irrespective of disease phenotype [22].

Studies on the efficacy of EEN in active CD are reported in Table 2, a comparison between two different nutritional regimens is given in Table 3, and studies comparing the efficacy of EEN on corticosteroids in active CD are reported in Table 4. As the included studies were significantly heterogeneous for study design, outcomes observed, and sample size, a meta-analysis was not performed.

Table 2. Clinical studies on efficacy of exclusive enteral nutrition in pediatric CD. CREN = constant rate enteral nutrition, PF = polymeric formula, ED = elemental diet, PCDAI = Pediatric Crohn Disease Activity Index, PEN = partial enteral nutrition, EEN = exclusive enteral nutrition, IFX = infliximab, anti-TNF = anti-tumor necrosis factor, TGFβ2 = transforming growth factor beta 2.

Clinical Studies on Efficacy of Exclusive Enteral Nutrition				
Author/Year	**Study Type**	**Population**	**Method**	**Main Findings**
Navarro *et al.* 1982 [17]	Clinical trial	Children with active CD ($n = 17$)	Exclusive constant rate enteral nutrition (CREN) using a combination of elemental diet and continuous alimentation for 2–7 months, subsequently CREN used to supplement oral alimentation from 12 to 22 months.	After 7 months of exclusive CREN: all children's symptoms improved; 100% of children presented moderate disease (Lloyd Still and Green scoring >50).
Fell *et al.* 2000 [23]	Clinical trial	Children with active CD ($n = 29$)	EEN with TGFβ2 enriched PF for 8 weeks.	- After 8 weeks 79% (23/29) of children were in clinical remission. - PCDAI declined with treatment. Median PCDAI at baseline 30 (range 12.5–72.5) declined with treatment by a median of 15 at 2 weeks and 25 at 8 weeks ($p < 0.00001$). - Macroscopic and histological healing in the terminal ileum and colon was associated with a decline in ileal and colonic interleukin-1β. (pre-treatment to post-treatment ratio 0.008 and 0.06: $p = 0.001$, $p = 0.006$).
Afzal *et al.* 2004 [24]	Clinical trial	Children and adolescents with active CD ($n = 26$), mean age 14 years	EEN with PF for 8 weeks.	88.6% achieved clinical remission.
Bannerjee *et al.* 2004 [25]	Clinical trial	Children with active CD ($n = 12$)	EEN with PF for 6 weeks.	Significant improvements in inflammatory markers by day 3 ($p < 0.05$) and in clinical activity index PCDAI by day 7.
Gavin *et al.* 2005 [26]	Retrospective cohort study	Children and adolescents with new onset CD ($n = 40$), aged 6–16 years	EEN with PF for 8 weeks.	All patients improved symptomatically and gained weight after 8 weeks of EEN.
Afzal *et al.* 2005 [27]	Prospective cohort study	Children and adolescents with active CD ($n = 65$), aged 8–17 years. Disease localization: ileal ($n = 12$), ileocolonic ($n = 39$), colonic ($n = 14$).	EEN with PF for 8 weeks.	77% remission rate. Remission rates: Colonic group: 50% (7/14), ileocolon group 82.1% (32/39), ileum group 91.7% (11/12), ($\chi 2$ test, $p = 0.021$)). The colonic disease group showed the least fall in PCDAI scores at completion of treatment with EEN ($p = 0.03$), with the lowest remission rate (50%).

Table 2. *Cont.*

| | Clinical Studies on Efficacy of Exclusive Enteral Nutrition | | | |
Author/Year	Study Type	Population	Method	Main Findings
Knight *et al.* 2005 [28]	Retrospective cohort study	Children with CD ($n = 44$)	Treatment with EEN as primary treatment for 6–8 weeks.	90% (40/44) of patients responded to EEN with a median time to remission of 6 weeks. Crohn's disease activity index (CDAI) decreased from pre-EEN to post-EEN, mean values of CDAI not available.
Day *et al.* 2006 [29]	Retrospective cohort study	Children with newly diagnosed CD (group 1, $n = 15$) and with active known long-standing CD (group 2, $n = 12$), mean age 11.8 years	- Group 1: EEN with PF for 6–8 weeks as sole initial therapy - Group 2: EEN with PF for 6–8 weeks in addition to any current medical therapy.	Twenty-four (89%) of 27 children completed their prescribed course of EEN. Nineteen (79%) of 24 children entered clinical remission (80% (12/15) in group 1 and 58% (7/12) in group 2). There was no clear relationship between disease location and response to treatment: 75% (3/4) with isolated small bowel, 72.5% (10/14) with ileocolonic and 67% (6/9) with pancolic disease attained remission ($p > 0.05$). In group 1 successful response to EEN was associated with positive weight gains (average weight gain 4.7 ± 3.5 kg) with mean PCDAI decreasing from 37.1 ± 10.8 to 6.7 ± 5.1 after 8 weeks ($p < 0.0001$). Also in group 2, despite a minor rate of remission, the overall average PCDAI scores significantly fell at 8 weeks ($p < 0.0001$) with an improvement of body weight and in at least one markers of inflammation.
De Bie *et al.* 2013 [30]	Retrospective cohort study	Children with newly diagnosed CD ($n = 77$), median age 13.9 years	Patients received EEN (as either hyperosmolar sip feeds or PF by nasogastric tube) for 6 weeks as remission induction therapy, combined with azathioprine maintenance treatment in 92%.	In patients completing a 6-week course of EEN (58) complete remission was achieved in 71% of patients, partial remission in 26%, and no response in 3%. Complete remission rates were higher in children presenting with isolated ileal/ileocaecal disease and malnutrition.
Grover *et al.* 2016 [31]	Clinical trial	Children with newly diagnosed predominantly luminal CD ($n = 54$), median age 12.4 years	EEN for 6–8 weeks in association with early thiopurine treatment (<3 months from diagnosis). Median duration between pre and post EEN assessments was 60.5 days (IQR 56–69.5)	Post EEN: remission rate (PCDAI < 10) 83% (45/54), biochemical remission (CRP < 5 mg/dL) 72% (39/54), complete mucosal healing 33% (18/54). Sustained remission was superior in those with complete mucosal healing *vs.* endoscopic disease 72% (13/18) *vs.* 28% (10/36), $p = 0.003$ at 1 year, 50% (8/16) *vs.* 8% (3/24), $p = 0.008$ at 2 years and 50% (8/16) *vs.* 6% (1/19), $p = 0.005$ at 3 years.

Table 3. Clinical studies comparing efficacy between two enteral nutrition regimens. PCDAI = Pediatric Crohn's Disease Activity Index, PF = polymeric formula, ED = elemental diet, PEN = partial enteral nutrition, EEN = exclusive enteral nutrition, IFX = infliximab, anti-TNF = anti-tumor necrosis factor, TGFβ2 = transforming growth factor beta 2, ARC = absolute risk change.

Clinical Studies Comparing Efficacy between Two Enteral Nutrition Regimens				
Author/Year	**Study Type**	**Population**	**Method**	**Main Findings**
Akobeng *et al.* 2000 [32]	Randomized controlled trial	Children with active CD ($n = 18$).	Standard PF with a low glutamine content (4% of amino-acid composition, group S) *vs.* glutamine enriched PF (42% of amino acid composition, group G) for 4 weeks.	- No difference in remission rates at week 4 between the two groups' remission 5/9 (55.5%) in group S, 4/9 (44.4%) in group G ($p = 0.5$). ARC −0.11 (exact 95% CI: −0.57 to 0.35). - Improvement in mean PCDAI was significantly more in group S ($p = 0.002$).
Ludvigsson *et al.* 2004 [33]	Randomized controlled trial	Children with active CD ($n = 33$) involving small bowel, colon and perianal region.	Exclusive EEN with ED ($n = 16$) *vs.* PF ($n = 17$) for 6 weeks.	- Similar remission rates at 6 weeks (ED 11/16 (69%), PF 14/17 (82%); $p = 0.438$). Patients on PF gained more weight compared to ED ($p = 0.004$). ARC 0.14 (exact 95% CI: −0.15 to 0.42).
Johnson *et al.* 2006 [34]	Randomized controlled trial	Children with active CD ($n = 50$) involving small bowel and/or colon.	Patients randomly assigned to receive: - 50% total energy requirements with ED (PEN, $n = 26$) for 6 weeks. - 100% energy requirements with ED (EEN, $n = 24$) for 6 weeks.	Remission rate with PEN was lower than with EEN (PEN 4/26 (15%), EEN 10/24 (42%) $p = 0.035$). Although PCDAI fell in both groups, the reduction was greater with EEN (PCDAI reduction PEN −13, 95% CI (−7 to −19) $p = 0.001$; EEN −26 95% CI (−19 to −33), $p = 0.001$) ($p = 0.005$). ARC = −0.26 (exact 95% CI −0.50 to −0.02).
Rodrigues *et al.* 2007 [35]	Retrospective cohort study	Children with active CD ($n = 98$) involving small bowel and/or colon.	Children received EEN at the time of first presentation either PF ($n = 45$, median age 12.2 years) or ED ($n = 53$, median age 11.8 years).	Remission rates were similar between children receiving PF and ED (ED 64%, 95% CI 51–77 *vs.* PF 51%, 95% CI 37–66, $p = 0.19$). ARC = −0.13 (exact 95% CI −0.32 to 0.06). The use of PF did not affect adherence to EEN but was significantly associated with reduced need for nasogastric tube administration.
Hartman *et al.* 2008 [36]	Retrospective cohort study	Children with CD ($n = 64$) involving small bowel, colon and upper GI tract.	Group 1 ($n = 28$, median age 14 years) and group 2 ($n = 18$, median age 12.7 years) received TGFβ2-enriched PF *vs.* standard PF, respectively, as a supplement to their regular nutrition (35%–50% of total caloric intake), for a median follow-up of 5.3 months for group 1 and 4.5 months for group 2. Group 3 ($n = 18$, median age 12.8 years) without formula supplementation, for a median follow-up of 5.5 months.	Supplementation of the diet with PF (both TGFβ enriched and standard) was associated with a decrease in PCDAI (in group 1 from 34.3 to 15.7, $p < 0.0001$; in group 2 from 35 to 22, $p = 0.02$). No significant decrease in PCDAI was recorded in group 3. Remission rates at follow-up: 57% (16/28, $p = 0.001$) in TGFβ2-enriched PF group, 22.2% (4/18, $p = 0.03$) in standard PF group. Remission rate in group 3 was 22.2 (4/18, $p = 0.03$). ARC = 0.35 (exact 95% CI 0.08 to 0.61). Significant improvements in body mass index ($p = 0.01$) and erythrocyte sedimentation rate ($p = 0.03$) were recorded at follow-up (median 3.4 months) only in the TGFβ2-enriched PF group.

Table 3. *Cont.*

Author/Year	Study Type	Population	Method	Main Findings
		Clinical Studies Comparing Efficacy between Two Enteral Nutrition Regimens		
Rubio *et al.* 2011 [37]	Retrospective cohort study	Children with newly diagnosed CD or with a first relapse of an established disease on stable medical treatment ($n = 106$).	Children received EEN with PF for 8 weeks as remission induction therapy either per os (group 1, $n = 45$, mean age 11.3 years) or by continuous enteral route via a nasogastric tube (group 2, $n = 61$, mean age 10.9 years).	Fractionated oral nutritional therapy (group 1) didn't significantly differ from continuous enteral administration (group 2) in inducing remission (75% *vs.* 85%, respectively, $p = 0.157$). All patients showed a significant decrease in disease severity assessed by PCDAI ($p < 0.0001$) and significant improvements in anthropometric measures and inflammatory indices.
Grogan *et al.* 2012 [38]	Double-blind randomized controlled trial	Children with newly diagnosed CD ($n = 34$).	Children were randomized to ED ($n = 15$, mean age 12.6 years) or PF ($n = 19$, mean age 11.7 years) for 6 weeks and were followed up for 2 years.	No significant difference was recorded between ED and PF in inducing remission (93% 14/15 *vs.* 79% 15/19, respectively). ARC = 0.14 (exact 95% CI −0.08 to 0.37). One-third of children maintained remission at 2 years.
Lee *et al.* 2015 [39]	Prospective study	Children with active CD ($n = 90$).	Children were treated with anti-TNF ($n = 52$), with EEN ($n = 22$), and with PEN plus ad lib diet ($n = 16$) for 8 weeks.	Clinical remission (final PCDAI $\leqslant 10$) was achieved by 50% on PEN, 76% EEN, and 73% anti-TNF ($p = 0.08$). ARC = −0.15 (exact 95% CI −0.47 to −0.16). Mucosal healing (estimated by fecal calprotectin $\leqslant 250$ μg/g) was achieved with PEN in 14%, EEN 45%, and anti-TNF 62% ($p = 0.001$). ARC = −0.25 (exact 95% CI −0.52 to 0.02).

Table 4. Clinical studies comparing exclusive enteral nutrition to corticosteroids. PCDAI = Pediatric Crohn's Disease Activity Index, ED = elemental diet, PEN = partial enteral nutrition, CS = corticosteroids, EEN = exclusive enteral nutrition, IFX = infliximab, anti-TNF = anti-tumor necrosis factor, TGFβ2 = transforming growth factor beta 2, ARC = absolute risk change.

Author/Year	Study Type	Population	Method	Main Findings
		Clinical Studies Comparing Exclusive Enteral Nutrition to Corticosteroids		
Sanderson *et al.* 1987 [18]	Randomized controlled trial	Children and adolescents with active CD aged 8.6–17.2 years ($n = 17$) involving the small bowel.	- 8 children treated with CS - 9 children treated with exclusive ED via nasogastric tube	- Disease activity (Lloyd–Still activity index) of the children improved significantly in both ED and PF groups after 6 weeks ($p < 0.01$). Growth velocity improved more in the ED group
Thomas *et al.* 1993 [40]	Randomized controlled trial	Children with active CD ($n = 24$): - 8% (2/24) confined to the small bowel - 29% (7/24) had ileal ± caecal involvement - 25% (6/24) ileocolic disease - 38% (9/24) disease confined to the colon	Children randomized to receive ED ($n = 12$) or CS ($n = 12$) for 4 weeks.	- Similar improvement in disease activity (PCDAI) and remission duration in both groups regardless of site of disease. In CS group activity index at baseline: 74, at week 4: 85, median change +11, ($p < 0.01$); in ED group activity index at baseline: 77, at week 4: 88, median change +11 ($p < 0.01$). - Growth velocity significantly better in ED group compared to CS group.

Table 4. *Cont.*

		Clinical Studies Comparing Exclusive Enteral Nutrition to Corticosteroids		
Author/Year	**Study Type**	**Population**	**Method**	**Main Findings**
Ruuska *et al.* 1994 [41]	Randomized controlled trial	Children with new onset or relapsing CD ($n = 19$). Ten children had widespread disease affecting both colon and small intestine; in three the disease was limited to the colon and rectum, and six children had only small bowel disease.	- 10 children treated with a whole-protein based formula through a nasogastric tube for 11 weeks -9 children received high dose CS for 11 weeks	- Similar improvements of PCDAI index, clinical symptoms and inflammatory markers within 2 weeks of treatment in both groups. After the end of the follow-up period 2 months after cessation of the treatment, PCDAI was still low in both groups (PCDAI 11.9 ± 7.9 in enteral diet group and 14.3 ± 9.6 in CS group) - During the routine follow-up after the trial (0.3–2.5 years, mean 1.3 years), five of the CS group 55.5% (5/9) whereas only one from the enteral group 10% (1/10) experienced a clinical relapse. ARC = -0.46 (exact 95% CI -0.8 to -0.08).
Terrin *et al.* 2002 [42]	Randomized controlled trial	Children with active CD ($n = 20$), aged 7–17 years, involving the terminal ileum and different areas of the colon; no fistulae or strictures were detected.	- Group A: CS and mesalazine ($n = 10$) - Group B: enteral nutrition group treated with extensively hydrolyzed formula for 8 weeks ($n = 10$)	- Clinical remission was achieved in 90% (9/10) of patients in group B but only in 50% (5/10) in corticosteroid group ($p < 0.01$). ARC = 0.40 (exact 95% CI 0.04 to 0.76). Both treatments were effective in reducing PCDAI scores (baseline group A 32.0 ± 4.7, group B 34.0 ± 4.3; at week 8 group A 13.0 ± 5.18, group B 7.2 ± 3.15, $p < 0.01$), endoscopic scores (baseline group A 3.7 ± 0.48, group B 3.8 ± 0.42; at week 8 group A 2.4 ± 0.96, group B 1.1 ± 0.87, $p < 0.01$) and histological scores (baseline group A 3.3 ± 0.67, group B 3.5 ± 0.52; at week 8 group A 2.5 ± 0.52, group B 1.3 ± 0.82, $p < 0.05$ for group A, $p < 0.01$ for group B). Group B had significantly lower post-trial PCDAI scores than the CS group (PCDAI scores change group B 14.6 ± 3.6, $p < 0.01$, group A 24.8 ± 4.4, not significant))
Borrelli *et al.* 2006 [43]	Randomized controlled trial	Children with active naïve CD ($n = 37$).	- 19 children received EEN with PF for 10 weeks - 18 children received oral CS for 10 weeks	At week 10 the remission rate was comparable between two groups: 15/19 (79%, 95% CI 56–92) in PF group and 12/18 (67%, 95% CI 44–84) in CS group ($p = 0.4$, not significant). ARC = 0.12 (exact 95% CI -0.16 to 0.40). The proportion of children showing mucosal healing was significantly higher in the PF (14/19, 74%; 95% CI 51 to 89) than the CS group (6/18, 33%; 95% CI 16 to 57; $p < 0.05$). ARC = 0.40, (exact 95% CI 0.11 to 0.70). At week 10 both endoscopic and histologic scores significantly decreased only in PF group.

Table 4. *Cont.*

		Clinical Studies Comparing Exclusive Enteral Nutrition to Corticosteroids		
Author/Year	Study Type	Population	Method	Main Findings
				For endoscopic score: in PF group pre-trial 12.9 ± 0.8, post-trial 5.9 ± 0.5, $p < 0.001$, in CS group pre-trial 12.9 ± 0.9, post-trial 9.8 ± 1.3, not significant. For histologic scores: in PF group ileum score pre-trial 10.4 ± 0.4, post-trial 3.8 ± 0.5, $p < 0.001$, in CS group pre-trial 11.0 ± 04, post-trial 9.6 ± 0.7, not significant.
Berni Canani *et al.* 2006 [44]	Retrospective cohort study	Children with newly diagnosed CD ($n = 47$), mean age 12.1 years.	Children received nutritional therapy (NT) for 8 weeks as - Polymeric formula ($n = 12$) - Semi-elemental diet ($n = 13$) - Elemental diet ($n = 12$) Ten subjects received oral CS for 8 weeks.	Similar clinical remission rates were observed after 8 weeks of treatment: 86.5% (32/37) receiving NT *vs.* 90% (9/10) treated with CS. ARC = −0.04 (exact 95% CI −0.25 to 0.18). Improvement in mucosal inflammation occurred in 64.8% (26/37) of patients on NT and 40% (4/10) of children on CS ($p < 0.05$).
Soo *et al.* 2013 [45]	Retrospective cohort study	Children with newly diagnosed CD ($n = 105$).	Children received either EEN ($n = 36$, mean age 12.9 years) or corticosteroids ($n = 69$, mean age 11.2 years) as induce remission therapy	Remission rate similar in two groups 88.9% (32/36) in the EEN group *vs.* 91.3% (63/69) in the CS group ($p = 0.73$) at 3 months). ARC= −0.02 (exact 95% CI −0.15 to 0.10). Relapse rate (40.6% *vs.* 28.6%), similar in both treatment groups ($p = 0.12$) over 12 months).
Luo *et al.* 2015 [46]	Retrospective cohort study	Children with newly diagnosed mild to moderate CD.	Children received either EEN ($n = 10$; median age 11.6 years) or CS ($n = 18$; median age 11.1 years) for 8 weeks.	The remission rate in EEN group was significantly higher than that in CS group (90.0% *vs.* 50.0%, respectively, $p < 0.05$).
Grover *et al.* 2015 [47]	Retrospective analysis of records	Children with newly diagnosed CD ($n = 89$) involving ileal, ileocolonic, and colonic sites.	Children received either EEN ($n = 43$; median age 13 years) or CS ($n = 46$; median age 11.5 years) as remission induction therapy together with an early use of thiopurines (within 6 months from diagnosis) as maintenance therapy. They were followed up for at least 2 years.	Choice of EEN over CS induction was associated with reduced linear growth failure (7% *vs.* 26%, $p = 0.02$), CS dependency (7% *vs.* 43%, $p = 0.002$), and improved primary sustained response to IFX (86% *vs.* 68%, $p = 0.02$).

More recently, novel nutritional approaches have been proposed and their efficacy has been proved in case series and dietary intervention studies [48–51]. Table 5 summarizes the main studies on the novel nutritional approaches for induction of remission in pediatric IBD. Among the novel approaches, the specific carbohydrate diet (SCD) has gained attention. It restricts complex carbohydrates and eliminates refined sugar from the diet, based on the rationale that the sugars and complex carbohydrates are malabsorbed and could cause alterations in microbiome composition, contributing to the intestinal inflammation of IBD. The clinical efficacy in inducing remission of symptoms and improvement of laboratory parameters has been demonstrated by reviewing medical records and in a prospective trial. Suskind *et al.* [49] reviewed medical records of children and adolescents with CD ($n = 10$) aged 7–16 years, treated with the SCD for a period of 5–30 months. Symptoms of all patients were resolved at a routine clinic visit three months after initiating the diet. Laboratory indices and fecal calprotectin either normalized or significantly improved at the follow-up clinic visits. It must be noted that the study was retrospective, hence the observed events (improvement of symptoms, laboratory parameters, and fecal calprotectin) could be due to chance. Cohen *et al.* conducted a trial evaluating clinical improvement and mucosal healing in children and adolescents with active CD, (mean age 13.6 years ($n = 9$)) after a 12–52 week trial of a SCD. The study showed at both the 12-week endpoint and the 52-week extension period clinical improvement assessed by PCDAI. In 6/10 patients (60%) remission was achieved by week 12. Mucosal healing (Lewis score < 135) was observed in 40% (4/10) of patients at week 12, 80% of patients showed significant mucosal improvement at week 12 when compared to baseline ($p = 0.012$) [50]. Aside from SCD, another novel dietary intervention has been proposed and studied in a prospective randomized trial by Sigall-Boneh *et al.* [51]. The new approach consists of 50% caloric intake with an exclusion diet specific for CD and 50% intake with a polymeric formula for a period of six weeks. The authors studied children and young adults ($n = 47, 34$ children) with active CD and with a mean age of 16.1 ± 5.6 years. The specific CD diet excludes many types of foods, including dairy products, margarine, gluten-containing cereals, smoked products (meat and fish), maize and potato flour, sauces, snacks, fruit juices, chocolate, coffee, and alcohol. Response and remission was obtained in 37 (78.7%) and 33 (70.2%), patients, respectively. Remission was obtained in 70% of children and 69% of adults.

The effect of a cow's milk protein (CMP) elimination diet on the induction and maintenance of remission in children with ulcerative colitis (UC) has been assessed in a randomized controlled trial by Strisciuglio *et al.* [52]. The authors randomized children to receive a CMP elimination diet or a free diet associated with concomitant steroid induction and mesalazine maintenance treatment. No significant differences were noted between the two groups in frequency of induction of remission and frequency of relapse.

Table 5. Novel nutritional approaches for induction of remission in pediatric IBD. SCD = Specific Carbohydrate Diet. CD = Crohn's Disease, PEN = partial enteral nutrition, PCDAI = Pediatric Crohn's Disease Activity Index, IR = incidence rate.

Novel Nutritional Approaches for Induction of Remission in Pediatric IBD				
Author/Year	Study Type	Population	Method	Main Findings
Gupta *et al.* 2013 [48]	Retrospective cohort study	Children with active CD (*n* = 23), mean age 12.8 years.	Enteral nutrition providing 80%–90% of caloric needs, remaining calories from normal diet	Induction of remission achieved in 65% of cases and response in 87% of cases at a mean follow-up of 2 months.
Suskind *et al.* 2014 [49]	Retrospective cohort study	Children and adolescents with active CD (*n* = 10), age range 7–16 years	SCD as treatment of active CD (either soon after diagnosis, or as second line therapy if steroid dependent or failure of mesalazine treatment). Duration of dietary therapy: 5–30 months.	Symptoms of all patients resolved at a routine clinic visit 3 months after initiating the diet. Laboratory indices and fecal calprotectin either normalized or significantly improved at the follow-up clinic visits.
Cohen *et al.* 2014 [50]	Clinical trial	Children and adolescents with active CD, mean age 13.6 years (*n* = 9).	SCD for 101% caloric needs, for 12 and 52 weeks.	At both: 12 week and 52-week endpoint s, there was clinical improvement assessed by PCDAI. In 6/10 patients (60%) remission was achieved by week 12. IR = 0.60 (exact 95% CI 0.26 to 0.88). Mucosal healing (Lewis score < 135) was observed in 40% (4/10) of patients at week 12. IR = 0.40 (exact 95% CI 0.12 to 0.74). 80% showed significant mucosal improvement at week 12 when compared to baseline (*p* = 0.012). IR = 0.80 (exact 95% CI 0.44 to 0.97).
Sigall-Boneh *et al.* 2014 [51]	Clinical trial	Children and young adults with active CD *n* = 47 (mean age 16.1 ± 5.6 years, children *n* = 34)	PEN with a CD exclusion diet + 50% polymeric formula for 6 weeks.	Response and remission was obtained in 37 (78.7%) and 33 (70.2%) patients respectively. IR = 0.79 (exact 95% CI 0.64 to 0.89). Remission was obtained in 70% of children and 69% of adults. IR = 0.70 (exact 95% CI 0.55 to 0.83).

5. Nutrition in Maintenance of Remission in Pediatric IBD

Exclusive Enteral Nutrition (EEN) is recommended as first line therapy to induce remission in pediatric CD [53], but only few studies analyzed the effect of dietary intervention for IBD maintenance of remission. New approaches recently proposed consider the elimination of foods thought to be noxious, through exclusion diets, or the supplementation of anti-inflammatory substances. Some data show that maintenance enteral nutrition (MEN) could reduce relapse rates. Table 6 summarizes the main studies focusing on enteral nutrition in maintenance of disease remission in pediatric IBD. In a study of Belli *et al.* [54], a small group of children continued intermittent EEN via nasogastric tube (NT) for one month out of four over the course of one year, showing improvement in CD clinical activity and growth [2]. Recently, in a retrospective study, Duncan *et al.* [55] analyzed 59 children with newly diagnosed CD, showing that the remission rate at one year was significantly higher in patients continuing MEN 60% (9/15), compared to 15% (2/13) in patients taking no treatment ($p = 0.001$) and with patients taking azathioprine ($p = 0.14$). Referring to Partial Enteral Nutrition (PEN), data about maintenance of remission in pediatric IBD are scarce. Evidences from adult population suggest that this kind of treatment could reduce the risk of relapse and improve the response to biological drugs [55–60]. A report of Wilschanski *et al.* [61] studied the effect of providing supplementary enteral nutrition, in addition to normal diet, in children and adolescents affected by CD after induction of remission with EEN. The study demonstrated fewer relapses and improvements of linear growth in children who continued supplementary feeding respect to control group [61]. Considering new nutritional interventions, a lacto-ovo vegetarian diet, also called a semi-vegetarian diet (SVD), has been evaluated in a prospective study on patients affected by CD, showing a significant effect on relapse prevention compared to an omnivorous diet (remission rate at two years 94% (15/16) for SVD *vs.* 33% (2/6), $p = 0.0003$) [62]. Another kind of exclusion diet has been attempted by Obih *et al.* [63] in a retrospective study including pediatric patients affected by CD or UC. A group of children followed the Specific Carbohydrate Diet (SCD) for a period between three and 48 months (mean of 9.6 ± 0.1 months); some of the patients were treated in conjunction with medical therapy, while the second group was treated only with standard medical therapy. The SCD group showed improvement of clinical and inflammatory markers, but the compliance to SCD was often poor and some of the patients who followed the SCD experienced weight loss [63].

Beyond nutritional therapy for maintenance of remission through exclusion diets, efforts are being made to evaluate the possible efficacy of supplementation of anti-inflammatory substances. One of the most studied is diferuloymethane, also known as curcumin. It is the most important component of the plant *Curcuma longa* or turmeric, belonging to the family Zingiberaceae. This kind of plant is typical of India, China, and Sri Lanka [64]. It is used in Indian and Chinese traditional medicine and it appears to have many properties such as anti-inflammatory, antioxidant, anti-tumor, antiplatelet, antibacterial, and antifungal effects [65,66]. Pathogenic mechanisms that explain all the curcumin properties are complex and partially known, but evidences suggest that the modulation of the NF-kB pathway has a pivotal role [67].The therapeutic use of curcumin is limited by its unfavorable pharmacokinetics, but oral administration of the drug reaches active levels in the gastrointestinal tract, so this natural substance could be useful for treating gut diseases [68]. Recent studies demonstrate that curcumin may be used as an adjunctive therapy for maintenance of remission in IBD, in particular in UC. Hanai *et al.* [69] evaluated the efficacy of curcumin as additional therapy for maintenance of remission in patients between 13 and 65 years with quiescent UC and consuming mesalazine or sulfasalazine. In this randomized, multicenter, double-blind, placebo-controlled trial, a group of patients receiving 2 g curcumin per day for six months has been compared with a group treated with a placebo. During the study period, relapses were lower in patients taking curcumin than in the placebo group (2/43 (4.65%) in curcumin group *vs.* 8/39 (20.51%) in placebo group, $p = 0.049$). Moreover, the authors noted improvements in the Clinical Activity Index (CAI) and the Endoscopic Index (EI) (secondary pre-specified outcomes) in patients receiving curcumin (CAI, $p = 0.038$ and EI, $p = 0.0001$) [69]. Finally, this natural anti-inflammatory agent seems to have high tolerability, without severe adverse effects in the pediatric population. The average intake of curcumin in countries where it is traditionally used in the diet, such as in India, is approximately 60–100 mg of curcumin daily in an adult individual [70]. Suskind *et al.* [71] enrolled 11 patients between 11 and 18 years affected by CD or UC in a tolerability study. During the trial, the curcumin dose was gradually increased from 500 mg twice a day to 2 g twice a day and continued for three weeks, without significant side effects [71].

Great interest has also been shown in *n*-3 PUFAs and their pleiotropic effects. The longer chain *n*-3 PUFAs, represented by EPA, DHA, and DPA, are mainly contained in fish oil and have numerous properties such as anti-inflammatory, anti-thrombotic, anti-arrhythmic, hypolipidemic, and vasodilatory activity [72,73]. Their anti-inflammatory effect, especially, seems to be due to *n*-3's role in the arachidonic acid pathway and the subsequent downregulation of proinflammatory cytokine synthesis, decreased leukocyte chemotaxis, and decreased T cell reactivity [74,75]. During the last decades, the idea that an *n*-3 rich diet could have positive effects in patients affected by IBD has been evaluated in numerous studies, particularly in the adult population, with conflicting results [76–78]. Meister *et al.* have studied *in vitro* the influence of a fish oil enriched enteral diet on intestinal tissues taken from CD, UC, and non-IBD control patients, showing that the anti-inflammatory effect of fish oil is significantly more marked in UC compared with CD [79]. Some evidence has shown clinical improvement after supplementation of *n*-3; however the most robust evidence is from two randomized double-blind, placebo-controlled studies on large adult populations affected by CD; these have not demonstrated any significant effects of *n*-3 supplementation in relapse prevention [80], and a recent Cochrane review has concluded that omega 3 fatty acids are probably ineffective for maintenance of remission in CD [81]. Concerning pediatric IBD, an Italian double-blind, randomized, placebo-controlled study showed a significant effect on reduction of relapse. The number of patients who relapsed at 12 months was significantly lower in the Omega-3 fatty acid group (group 1) compared to patients receiving a placebo (group 2) (relapse rate group 1 11/18 (61%), group 2 19/20 (95%); $p < 0.001$ [82]. In conclusion, although Omega-3 appears to be safe, except for mild gastrointestinal tract symptoms (diarrhea, unpleasant taste, bad breath, heartburn, and nausea), further studies are needed to confirm the real efficacy of *n*-3 for IBD treatment in pediatric population. Table 4 summarizes the main pediatric studies on nutrition in maintenance of disease remission.

Table 6. Nutrition in maintenance of disease remission. ED = elemental diet, MEN = maintenance enteral nutrition, EEN = exclusive enteral nutrition, SCD = specific carbohydrate diet, CR*P* = C-reactive protein, BMI = body mass index, 5-ASA = 5-aminosalycilates, ARC = risk change.

			Nutrition in Maintenance of Disease Remission in Pediatric IBD	
Author/Year	**Study Type**	**Population**	**Method**	**Main Findings**
			PEN	
Belli *et al.* 1988 [54]	Clinical trial	Children and adolescents with CD (*n* = 8) aged 9.8–14.2 years	- 8 children treated with chronic Intermittent ED for 1 month out of 4, over the course of 1 year - 4 children treated with conventional medical treatment	- CD activity index and prednisone intake decreased significantly in patients receiving ED therapy when compared with controls on conventional medical therapy ($p < 0.05$).
Duncan *et al.* 2014 [55]	Clinical trial	Children and adolescents newly diagnosed CD (*n* = 59) aged 2.5–16.33 years	Patients newly diagnosed CD who commenced EEN for 8 weeks, than followed up: - 11/59 poor response to EEN, switched to steroids. 48/59 completed 8 weeks with EEN and achieved remission - 15/48 continued MEN, post EEN completion. Duration of MEN ranged 4–14 months (mean 10.8 months)	- Remission rates at 1 year in patients continuing MEN were 60% (9/15), compared to 15% (2/13) in patients taking no treatment ($p = 0.001$) and 65% (13/20) in patients taking azathioprine ($p = 0.14$).
Wilschanski *et al.* 1996 [61]	Retrospective cohort study	Children and adolescents (*n* = 65) aged 7–17 years	After induction of remission of CD with EEN: - Group 1: patients (*n* = 28) continued nocturnal nasogastric supplementary feeding combined with a normal diet - Group 2: patients (*n* = 19) stopped nocturnal supplements after the remission	- Higher relapse rate in group 2 *vs.* group 2 at 6 and 12 months (At 6 months relapse rate of group 2: 78% (15/19) *vs.* 17.8% (5/28) of group 1, $p < 0.02$; at 12 months relapse rate of group 2 78.9% (15/19) *vs.* group 1 42.8% (12/28), $p < 0.02$). - Mean changes in height velocity was greater for group 1 (2.87 cm/year) compared to group 2 (0.4 cm/year), p =0.057.
Obih *et al.* 2015 [63]	Retrospective cohort study	Children affected by IBD (*n* = 26), CD (*n* = 20) or UC (*n* = 6) aged 1.5–19 years	- Group of patients (*n* = 26) who followed a SCD for more than 2 weeks (mean duration 9.6 ± 10.1 months). 15/26 patients were on concurrent medication with SCD; 11/26 were not on IBD-related drugs - Children with IBD (*n* = 10), CD (*n* = 7), UC (*n* = 3) who did not follow SCD but only standard medical therapy	- In SCD group PCDAI improved from 32.8 ± 13.2 at baseline to 20.8 ± 16.6 by week 4 ± 2 w and 8.8 ± 8.5 by month 6. - The mean Pediatric Ulcerative Colitis Index (PUCAI) decreased from baseline 28.3 ± 10.3 to 20.0 + 17.3 at week 4 ± 2 w and to 18.3 ± 31.7 at month 6. - Significant improvement of Crohn's disease activity index, CRP, and calprotectin in SCD group respect to control group ($p = 0.03$, 0.03, and 0.03, respectively) - lower BMI, height and weight in SCD group than in control ($p = 0.01$, 0.03, and 0.009, respectively)

Table 6. *Cont.*

		Nutrition in Maintenance of Disease Remission in Pediatric IBD		
Author/Year	**Study Type**	**Population**	**Method**	**Main Findings**
		PEN		
		Curcumin		
Hanai H *et al.* 2006 [69]	Randomized double-blind, placebo-controlled trial	Adolescents and adults with quiescent UC aged 13–65 years (*n* = 89)	- 43 patients received curcumin 2 g/day plus sulfasalazine or mesalazine; - 39 patients received placebo plus sulfasalazine or mesalazine	- Relapse rate at 6 months of therapy was lower for curcumin group compared to placebo group: - 2/43 (4.65%) in curcumin group *vs.* 8/39 (20.51%) in placebo group, *p* = 0.049. ARC = −0.16 (exact 95% CI −0.30 to −0.02). - Curcumin improved both clinical activity index (CAI, *p* = 0.038) and endoscopic index (EI, *p* = 0.0001). - High tolerability and no serious side effect associated to curcumin
Suskind *et al.* 2013 [71]	Clinical trial	Children and adolescents (*n* = 11) aged 11–18 years affective by CD (*n* = 6) or UC (*n* = 5).	All patients, in addition to their standard IBD therapy, received increasing doses of curcumin, up to 2 g twice daily for 3 weeks	- High tolerability of curcumin without side effects except for increase in gassiness which was consistently reported in two patients. Three patients had lowering of PUCAI/PCDAI scores. - No patients had IBD relapse or worsening of symptoms.
		n-3 PUFAs		
Romano *et al.* 2005 [82]	Double-blind, randomized, placebo-controlled study	Children and adolescents affected by CD (*n* = 38) in remission, aged 5–16 years and treated for 12 months.	- Group 1 (*n* = 18): patients treated with 5-ASA (50 mg/kg/day) and omega-3 fatty acids for 12 months. - Group 2 (*n* = 20): patients treated with 5-ASA (50 mg/kg/day) plus placebo (olive oil in capsules) for 12 months.	Number of patients who relapsed at 12 months was significantly lower in Omega-3 fatty acid group than in patients receiving placebo (relapse rate group 1 11/18 (61%), group 2 19/20 (95%); *p* < 0.001). ARC −0.34 (exact 95% CI −0.58 to −0.09).

6. Health Benefits of Nutritional Therapy in Pediatric IBD

With respect to adult forms, pediatric IBD have specific features, not only for severity and extension, but also because the disease involves growing individuals, with possible irreversible consequences in adult life. Weight loss and failure to thrive, delayed puberty, and low bone mineral density are frequent signs in children affected by IBD, in particular in CD, because of malabsorption and malnutrition. The etiology of poor nutritional status in children affected by IBD is complex and involves reduced dietary intake, increased gastrointestinal nutrient losses, increased energy requests due to inflammation, and altered metabolism [83,84]. Moreover, the linear growth and nutritional status of children affected by IBD are also compromised by immunosuppressant drugs, especially corticosteroids, used for the treatment of the disease [85]. All these reasons justify the particular importance of nutritional therapy in pediatric IBD. EEN is at least as efficacious as corticosteroids in inducing remission in pediatric CD, but it has minimal side effects and several advantages in terms of mucosal healing, restoration of nutritional status, bone health, and liner growth in children [53]. Multiple studies demonstrate that, with respect to conventional immunosuppressant drugs, nutritional therapy improves weight gain, height velocity, body composition, and insulin-like growth factor (IGF)-1 and IGF binding protein 3 (IGFBP-3) [18,54,61,86–90]. Table 5 illustrates the main studies on the health benefits of nutritional therapy in pediatric IBD. Berni Canani *et al.* [44], in a retrospective study on 47 children with active CD, compared the effect of EEN *versus* corticosteroid therapy. Children treated with EEN for eight weeks showed higher serum iron and albumin levels, and more pronounced linear growth than group treated with corticosteroids [44]. Moreover, bone health seems to benefit from nutritional therapy too. The pathogenesis of bone loss in pediatric IBD is complex: malnutrition, compromised linear growth, lean mass deficit, delayed puberty, menstrual irregularity, reduced physical activity, persistent inflammation, and prolonged use of corticoids are the major factors responsible [91–93]. Although the direct effect of EEN in increasing bone mineral density (BMD) has been poorly studied, Whitten *et al.* demonstrated that the normalization of bone turnover markers in children was affected by CD after eight weeks of treatment with EEN [6]. In addition, in the latest clinical guidelines about skeletal health issued by ESPGHAN and NASPGHAN, the authors affirm the benefits of enteral nutrition. In terms of linear growth and lean mass, EEN or supplemental enteral nutrition could induce improvement of bone health, and they recommend these tactics not only during the acute phase, but also during remission phases of IBD, particularly in children and adolescents with delayed linear growth [7]. Table 7 shows the main studies on the health benefits of nutritional therapy in pediatric IBD.

Table 7. Health benefits of nutritional therapy in pediatric IBD. ED = elemental diet, REE = resting energy expenditure, IGF-1 = insulin like growth factor 1, IGFBP-3 = insulin like growth factor binding protein, EEN = exclusive enteral nutrition, corticosteroids = CS.

	Health Benefits of Nutritional Therapy in Pediatric IBD			
Author/Year	Study Type	Population	Method	Main Findings
Azcue *et al.* 1997 [83]	Clinical trial	Children and adolescents affected by CD (n = 24); malnourished adolescents with anorexia nervosa (n = 19); healthy control subjects (n = 22)	- Group of patients (n = 12) treated with nocturnal enteral nutrition via nasogastric tube for 5–6 weeks, then 1 night a week for 2 months - Group of patients (n = 12) treated with prednisolone - control group (n = 22), healthy subjects - group of malnourished adolescents with anorexia nervosa (n = 19)	- All body compartments and REE increased significantly in enteral nutrition group compared to patients treated with corticosteroids. In enteral nutrition group REE (kcal/day) from 1153 ± 283 at baseline to 1415 ± 535 at 1 month post-treatment; in prednisolone group REE at baseline 1380 ± 308 to 1432 ± 265 at one month post-treatment. For lean body mass (LBM % weight) in enteral nutrition group 86.6 ± 8.9 at baseline to 88.8 + 9.9 at one month post-treatment, in prednisolone group 87.5 ± 9.4 at baseline to 79.1 ± 9.4 at one month post-treatment. - Significant height increase in enteral nutrition group compared with prednisolone group ($p < 0.01$).
Beattie *et al.* 1998 [86]	Clinical trial	Children and adolescents affected by CD (n = 23)	- Study A: 14 patients treated with EEN for 8 weeks, then gradual reduction of nutritional support over 2 months - Study B: 9 patients treated with intestinal resection	Study A - Significant weight gain for all patients treated with EEN after 8 and 16 weeks, compared to pre-treatment values (weight SDS at baseline= -0.9 (−1.3 to −0.5), weight SDS at week 8 = −0.5 (−0.9 to 0), at 16 weeks weight SDS = −0.6 (−1.1 to 0) ($p < 0.05$) - Significant increase of median IGF-1 and IGFBP-3 at 2, 8, and 16 weeks in EEN group compared to pre-treatment values ($p < 0.01$) Study B - No significant changes in auxological data, IGF-1 and IGFBP-3 in patients who had surgical resection compared to pre-treatment values

Table 7. *Cont.*

Health Benefits of Nutritional Therapy in Pediatric IBD				
Author/Year	**Study Type**	**Population**	**Method**	**Main Findings**
Wilschanski *et al.* 1996 [61]	Retrospective cohort study	Children and adolescents ($n = 65$) aged 7–17 years	After induction of remission of CD with EEN: - Group 1: patients ($n = 28$) continued nocturnal nasogastric supplementary feeding combined with a normal diet - Group 2: patients ($n = 19$) stopped nocturnal supplements after the remission	- Mean changes in height velocity was greater for group 1 (2.87 cm/year) compared to group 2 (0.4 cm/year), $p = 0.057$.
Belli *et al.* 1988 [54]	Clinical trial	Children and adolescents with CD ($n = 8$) aged 9.8–14.2 years	- 8 children treated with chronic intermittent enteral ED for 1 month out of 4, over the course of 1 year - 4 children treated with conventional medical treatment	- Significant height and weight gains in the ED group *vs.* controls. Weight gain for ED group 6.9 ± 1.5 kg; $209.8\% \pm 41.9\%$; weight gain for control group $-0.9 + 1.6$ kg; $-9.8\% \pm 52.6\%$ ($p < 0.01$). Height changes in ED group $7.0 + 0.8$ cm; $126.0\% \pm 11.8\%$ of ideal predicted. Height change in control group $1.7 + 0.8$ cm; $28.7\% \pm 13.1\%$ ($p < 0.01$).
Berni Canani *et al.* 2006 [44]	Retrospective study	Children and adolescents affected by active CD ($n = 47$)	Children received nutritional therapy (NT) for 8 weeks as - Polymeric formula ($n = 12$) - Semi-elemental diet ($n = 13$) - Elemental diet ($n = 12$) Ten subjects received oral CS for 8 weeks.	- Significant improvement of serum albumin and iron levels in NT compared to CS group. In NT group elemental: albumin at baseline 13.14 ± 0.47 to 3.98 ± 0.36 at 8 weeks, $p < 0.001$; NT group semi-elemental: albumin at baseline $3.13 + 0.40$ to $3.88 + 0.26$ at 8 weeks, $p < 0.001$; NT group polymeric: albumin at baseline $3.09 + 0.39$ to $3.86 + 0.38$ at 8 weeks, $p < 0.001$)). In CS group: albumin at baseline 3.37 ± 0.24 to 3.40 ± 0.22 after 8 weeks, $p = 0.28$). In NT group elemental: iron at baseline 31.25 ± 20.4 to 72.17 ± 20.4 at 8 weeks, $p = 0.001$; NT group semi-elemental: iron at baseline $29.46 + 23.7$ to $66.69 + 19.8$ at 8 weeks, $p = 0.002$; NT group polymeric: iron at baseline $32.58 + 24.0$ to $69.25 + 29.6$ at 8 weeks, $p = 0.004$)). In CS group: iron at baseline 20.80 ± 15.5 to 35.80 ± 16.0 after 8 weeks, $p = 0.01$). Linear growth recovery was superior in nutritional group compared to CS group ($p < 0.05$).

Table 7. *Cont.*

		Health Benefits of Nutritional Therapy in Pediatric IBD		
Author/Year	Study Type	Population	Method	Main Findings
Motil *et al.* 1982 [87]	Clinical trial	Adolescents affected by CD	- 6 patients affected by CD received nutritional supplements for 7 months - 5 healthy control subjects	Increase of linear and ponderal growth velocities in patients treated with nutritional support (Height gain cm/month pre-supplements 0.10 ± 0.08, post-supplements $0.50 + 0.16$; weight gain kg/month pre-supplements 0.21 ± 0.09, post-supplements 1.22 ± 0.25). Achievement of weight and height gain similar to control group levels after the 7 months treatment with nutritional supplements (height gain cm/month 0.38 ± 0.12, weight gain kg/month $0.40 + 0.17$).
O'Morain *et al.* 1983 [88]	Clinical trial	Children and adolescents affected by CD ($n = 15$) aged 6–20 years	14 patients received ED as the main energy source for 4 weeks; 1 received corticosteroids.	Improvement of nutritional status, weight, and height gain in children receiving ED.
Whitten *et al.* 2010 [94]	Clinical trial	Children newly diagnosed CD ($n = 23$) compared to a healthy control group ($n = 20$)	Children newly diagnosed with CD received 8 weeks EEN for induction of remission	Normalization of serum markers of bone turnover after EEN therapy. CTX levels at diagnosis 2.967 ± 0.881 ng/mL and after EEN 2.260 ± 0.547 ng/mL, $p = 0.002$. BAP levels at diagnosis 51.24 ± 31.31 microg/L and after EEN 64.82 ± 30.51 microg/L, $p = 0.02$.
Polk *et al.* 1992 [89]	Clinical trial	Adolescents affected by CD ($n = 6$)	All patients received enteral nutrition via nasogastric tube during night 1 out of 4 months for 1 year. Then the patients received a 2-week exclusion diet and a 2-week low-residue diet for 2 months, before re-starting a normal diet.	Significant increase of weight, height, IGF-1, and albumin; decrease of steroid use and disease activity compared to pretreatment values

7. Strengths and Limitations

The main strength of the present systematic review is the rigorous methodological assessment and analysis of the literature using pre-specified criteria. The methods we used helped to reduce the risk of bias (thorough literature research performed by two researchers independently and duplicate data abstraction). Nevertheless, some limitations should be pointed out. In the first instance, the methodological quality of included trials was not high and some trials had small sample sizes. Moreover, a significant limitation lies in the lack of standardization of outcome measures, clinical heterogeneity of subjects enrolled, variation in the length of follow-up and in the duration of interventions, and the use of concomitant medications.

8. Conclusions

Nutrition has a significant role in pediatric IBD. With regards to etiology, the available pediatric data suggest that dietary patterns characterized by consumption of meats, fatty foods, desserts, and a high sugar intake are associated with an increased risk of disease. Likely protective factors are represented by consumption of vegetables, fruits, fish, olive oil, and wholemeal bread. Large scale randomized controlled clinical trials are needed to confirm these data.

For treatment of disease, EEN is the only nutritional approach with robust evidence of effectiveness in induction of remission; PEN is known to be advantageous in reducing relapse rates. Besides the known elemental, semi-elemental, and polymeric formulas, the scientific community is currently looking into modifying dietary habits to maintain disease remission mainly through exclusion diets: the Specific Carbohydrate Diet and the Crohn's Disease exclusion diet are now in the spotlight. Nevertheless, the poor compliance to nutritional intervention and the risk of nutritional deficits when exclusion diets are too strict are factors that have to be considered when these kinds of treatments are proposed. Despite the promising results of the novel nutritional approaches, the available data are not strong enough to recommend these interventions in clinical practice and new large controlled studies are needed, especially in pediatric population, to confirm these data.

Acknowledgments: This systematic review would not have been possible without the excellent collaboration of all the participants. We would like to thank Barbara Borsani, Lucia Cococcioni, Erica Galli for the effort in the literature research, selection of manuscripts, interpretation of results and writing of our systematic review. We would like to thank Giorgio Bedogni for his fundamental help for the statistical analyses. We would like to thank Dario Dilillo, Giovanna Zuin and Gian Vincenzo Zuccotti for their involvement in the study coordination and for mentoring us during the preparation of the manuscript.

Author Contributions: All authors actively contributed to the conceptual development of this review paper. All authors have primary responsibility for the final content.

References

1. Thia, K.T.; Loftus, E.V., Jr.; Sandborn, W.J.; Yang, S.K. An update on the epidemiology of inflammatory bowel disease in Asia. *Am. J. Gastroenterol.* **2008**, *103*, 3167–3182. [CrossRef] [PubMed]
2. Hou, J.K.; Abraham, B.; El-Serag, H. Dietary intake and risk of developing inflammatory bowel disease: A systematic review of the literature. *Am. J. Gastroenterol.* **2011**, *106*, 563–573. [CrossRef] [PubMed]
3. Ananthakrishnan, A.N.; Khalili, H.; Konijeti, G.G.; Higuchi, L.M.; de Silva, P.; Fuchs, C.S.; Willett, W.C.; Richter, J.M.; Chan, A.T. Long term intake of dietary fat and risk of ulcerative colitis and Crohn's disease. *Gut* **2014**, *63*, 776–784. [CrossRef] [PubMed]
4. Jantchou, P.; Morois, S.; Clavel-Chapelon, F.; Boutron-Ruault, M.C.; Carbonnel, F. Animal protein intake and risk of inflammatory bowel disease: The E3N prospective study. *Am. J. Gastroenterol.* **2010**, *105*, 2195–2201. [CrossRef] [PubMed]
5. Tjonneland, A.; Overvad, K.; Bergmann, M.M.; Nagel, G.; Linseisen, J.; Hallmans, G.; Palmqvist, R.; Sjodin, H.; Hagglund, G.; Berglund, G.; *et al.* IBD in EPIC Study Investigators. Linoleic acid, a dietary *n*-6 polyunsaturated fatty acid, and the aetiology of ulcerative colitis: A nested case-control study within a European prospective cohort study. *Gut* **2009**, *58*, 1606–1611. [PubMed]

6. De Silva, P.S.; Luben, R.; Shrestha, S.S.; Khaw, K.T.; Hart, A.R. Dietary arachidonic and oleic acid intake in ulcerative colitis etiology: A prospective cohort study using 7-day food diaries. *Eur. J. Gastroenterol. Hepatol.* **2014**, *26*, 11–18. [CrossRef] [PubMed]

7. John, S.; Luben, R.; Shrestha, S.S.; Welch, A.; Khaw, K.T.; Hart, A.R. Dietary *n*-3 polyunsaturated fatty acids and the aetiology of ulcerative colitis: A UK prospective cohort study. *Eur. J. Gastroenterol. Hepatol.* **2010**, *22*, 602–606. [CrossRef] [PubMed]

8. Ananthakrishnan, A.N.; Khalili, H.; Konijeti, G.G.; Higuchi, L.M.; de Silva, P.; Korzenik, J.R.; Fuchs, C.S.; Willett, W.C.; Richter, J.M.; Chan, A.T. A prospective study of long term intake of dietary fiber and risk of Crohn's disease and ulcerative colitis. *Gastroenterology* **2013**, *145*, 970–977. [CrossRef] [PubMed]

9. Lee, D.; Albenberg, L.; Compher, C.; Baldassano, R.; Piccoli, D.; Lewis, J.D.; Wu, G.D. Diet in the pathogenesis and treatment of inflammatory bowel diseases. *Gastroenterology* **2015**, *148*, 1087–1106. [CrossRef] [PubMed]

10. Epidemiology Group of the Research Committee of Inflammatory Bowel Disease in Japan. Dietary and other risk factors of ulcerative colitis. A case-control study in Japan. *J. Clin. Gastroenterol.* **1994**, *19*, 166–171.

11. Amre, D.K.; D'Souza, S.; Morgan, K.; Seidman, G.; Lambrette, P.; Grimard, G.; Israel, D.; Mack, D.; Ghadirian, P.; Deslandres, C.; *et al.* Imbalances in dietary consumption of fatty acids, vegetables, and fruits are associated with risk for Crohn's disease in children. *Am. J. Gastroenterol.* **2007**, *102*, 2016–2025. [CrossRef] [PubMed]

12. D'Souza, S.; Levy, E.; Mack, D.; Israel, D.; Lambrette, P.; Ghadirian, P.; Deslandres, C.; Morgan, K.; Seidman, E.G.; Amre, D.K. Dietary patterns and risk for Crohn's disease in children. *Inflamm. Bowel Dis.* **2008**, *14*, 367–373. [CrossRef] [PubMed]

13. Jakobsen, C.; Paerregaard, A.; Munkholm, P.; Wewer, V. Environmental factors and risk of developing paediatric inflammatory bowel disease—A population based study 2007–2009. *J. Crohn's Colitis* **2013**, *7*, 79–88. [CrossRef] [PubMed]

14. Gilat, T.; Hacohen, D.; Lilos, P.; Langman, M.J. Childhood factors in ulcerative colitis and Crohn's disease. An international cooperative study. *Scand. J. Gastroenterol.* **1987**, *22*, 1009–1024. [CrossRef] [PubMed]

15. Baron, S.; Turck, D.; Leplat, C.; Merle, V.; Gower-Rousseau, C.; Marti, R.; Yzet, T.; Lerebours, E.; Dupas, J.L.; Debeugny, S.; *et al.* Environmental risk factors in paediatric inflammatory bowel diseases: A population based case control study. *Gut* **2005**, *54*, 357–363. [CrossRef] [PubMed]

16. Galvez, J.; Rodríguez-Cabezas, M.E.; Zarzuelo, A. Effects of dietary fiber on inflammatory bowel disease. *Mol. Nutr. Food Res.* **2005**, *49*, 601–608. [CrossRef] [PubMed]

17. Navarro, J.; Vargas, J.; Cezard, J.P.; Charritat, J.L.; Polonovski, C. Prolonged constant rate elemental enteral nutrition in Crohn's disease. *J. Pediatr. Gastroenterol. Nutr.* **1982**, *1*, 541–546. [CrossRef] [PubMed]

18. Sanderson, I.R.; Udeen, S.; Davies, P.S.; Savage, M.O.; Walker-Smith, J.A. Remission induced by an elemental diet in small bowel Crohn's disease. *Arch. Dis. Child.* **1987**, *62*, 123–127. [CrossRef] [PubMed]

19. Heuschkel, R.B.; Menache, C.C.; Megerian, J.T.; Baird, A.E. Enteral nutrition and corticosteroids in the treatment of acute Crohn's disease in children. *J. Pediatr. Gastroenterol. Nutr.* **2000**, *31*, 8–15. [CrossRef] [PubMed]

20. Dziechciarz, P.; Horvath, A.; Shamir, R.; Szajewska, H. Meta-analysis: enteral nutrition in active Crohn's disease in children. *Aliment. Pharmacol. Ther.* **2007**, *26*, 795–806. [CrossRef] [PubMed]

21. Zachos, M.; Tondeur, M.; Griffiths, A.M. Enteral nutritional therapy for induction of remission in Crohn's disease. *Cochrane Database Syst. Rev.* **2007**, *1*, CD000542. [CrossRef] [PubMed]

22. Buchanan, E.; Gaunt, W.W.; Cardigan, T.; Garrick, V.; McGrogan, P.; Russell, R.K. The use of exclusive enteral nutrition for induction of remission in children with Crohn's disease demonstrates that disease phenotype does not influence clinical remission. *Aliment. Pharmacol. Ther.* **2009**, *30*, 501–507. [CrossRef] [PubMed]

23. Fell, J.M.; Paintin, M.; Arnaud-Battandier, F.; Beattie, R.M.; Hollis, A.; Kitching, P.; Donnet-Hughes, A.; MacDonald, T.T.; Walker-Smith, J.A. Mucosal healing and a fall in mucosal pro-inflammatory cytokine mRNA induced by a specific oral polymeric diet in paediatric Crohn's disease. *Aliment. Pharmacol. Ther.* **2000**, *14*, 281–289. [CrossRef] [PubMed]

24. Afzal, N.A.; Van Der Zaag-Loonen, H.J.; Arnaud-Battandier, F.; Davies, S.; Murch, S.; Derkx, B.; Heuschkel, R.; Fell, J.M. Improvement in quality of life of children with acute Crohn's disease does not parallel mucosal healing after treatment with exclusive enteral nutrition. *Aliment. Pharmacol. Ther.* **2004**, *20*, 167–172. [CrossRef] [PubMed]

25. Bannerjee, K.; Camacho-Hübner, C.; Babinska, K.; Dryhurst, K.M.; Edwards, R.; Savage, M.O.; Sanderson, I.R.; Croft, N.M. Anti-inflammatory and growth-stimulating effects precede nutritional restitution during enteral feeding in Crohn disease. *J. Pediatr. Gastroenterol. Nutr.* **2004**, *38*, 270–275. [CrossRef] [PubMed]

26. Gavin, J.; Anderson, C.E.; Bremner, A.R.; Beattie, R.M. Energy intakes of children with Crohn's disease treated with enteral nutrition as primary therapy. *J. Hum. Nutr. Diet.* **2005**, *18*, 337–342. [CrossRef] [PubMed]

27. Afzal, N.A.; Davies, S.; Paintin, M.; Arnaud-Battandier, F.; Walker-Smith, J.A.; Murch, S.; Heuschkel, R.; Fell, J. Colonic Crohn's disease in children does not respond well to treatment with enteral nutrition if the ileum is not involved. *Dig. Dis. Sci.* **2005**, *50*, 1471–1475. [CrossRef] [PubMed]

28. Knight, C.; El-Matary, W.; Spray, C.; Sandhu, B.K. Long-term outcome of nutritional therapy in paediatric Crohn's disease. *Clin. Nutr.* **2005**, *24*, 775–779. [CrossRef] [PubMed]

29. Day, A.S.; Whitten, K.E.; Lemberg, D.A.; Clarkson, C.; Vitug-Sales, M.; Jackson, R.; Bohane, T.D. Exclusive enteral feeding as primary therapy for Crohn's disease in Australian children and adolescents: A feasible and effective approach. *J. Gastroenterol. Hepatol.* **2006**, *21*, 1609–1614. [CrossRef] [PubMed]

30. De Bie, C.; Kindermann, A.; Escher, J. Use of exclusive enteral nutrition in paediatric Crohn's disease in The Netherlands. *J. Crohns Colitis* **2013**, *7*, 263–270. [CrossRef] [PubMed]

31. Grover, Z.; Burgess, C.; Muir, R.; Reilly, C.; Lewindon, P.J. Early Mucosal Healing with Exclusive Enteral Nutrition is Associated with Improved Outcomes in Newly Diagnosed Children with Luminal Crohn's disease. *J. Crohn's Colitis* **2016**, 1–6. [CrossRef] [PubMed]

32. Akobeng, A.K.; Miller, V.; Stanton, J.; Elbadri, A.M.; Thomas, A.G. Double-blind randomized controlled trial of glutamine-enriched polymeric diet in the treatment of active Crohn's disease. *J. Pediatr. Gastroenterol. Nutr.* **2000**, *30*, 78–84. [CrossRef] [PubMed]

33. Ludvigsson, J.F.; Krantz, M.; Bodin, L.; Stenhammar, L.; Lindquist, B. Elemental *versus* polymeric enteral nutrition in paediatric Crohn's disease: A multicentre randomized controlled trial. *Acta Paediatr.* **2004**, *93*, 327–335. [CrossRef] [PubMed]

34. Johnson, T.; Macdonald, S.; Hill, S.M.; Thomas, A.; Murphy, M.S. Treatment of active Crohn's disease in children using partial enteral nutrition with liquid formula: A randomised controlled trial. *Gut* **2006**, *55*, 356–361. [CrossRef] [PubMed]

35. Rodrigues, A.F.; Johnson, T.; Davies, P.; Murphy, M.S. Does polymeric formula improve adherence to liquid diet therapy in children with active Crohn's disease? *Arch. Dis. Child.* **2007**, *92*, 767–770. [CrossRef] [PubMed]

36. Hartman, C.; Berkowitz, D.; Weiss, B.; Shaoul, R.; Levine, A.; Adiv, O.E.; Shapira, R.; Fradkin, A.; Wilschanski, M.; Tamir, A.; *et al.* Nutritional supplementation with polymeric diet enriched with transforming growth factor-beta 2 for children with Crohn's disease. *Isr. Med. Assoc. J.* **2008**, *10*, 503–507. [PubMed]

37. Rubio, A.; Pigneur, B.; Garnier-Lengliné, H.; Talbotec, C.; Schmitz, J.; Canioni, D.; Goulet, O.; Ruemmele, F.M. The efficacy of exclusive nutritional therapy in paediatric Crohn's disease, comparing fractionated oral *vs.* continuous enteral feeding. *Aliment. Pharmacol. Ther.* **2011**, *33*, 1332–1339. [CrossRef] [PubMed]

38. Grogan, J.L.; Casson, D.H.; Terry, A.; Burdge, G.C.; El-Matary, W.; Dalzell, A.M. Enteral feeding therapy for newly diagnosed pediatric Crohn's disease: A double-blind randomized controlled trial with two years follow-up. *Inflamm. Bowel Dis.* **2012**, *18*, 246–253. [CrossRef] [PubMed]

39. Lee, D.; Baldassano, R.N.; Otley, A.R.; Albenberg, L.; Griffiths, A.M.; Compher, C.; Chen, E.Z.; Li, H.; Gilroy, E.; Nessel, L.; *et al.* Comparative Effectiveness of Nutritional and Biological Therapy in North American Children with Active Crohn's Disease. *Inflamm. Bowel Dis.* **2015**, *21*, 1786–1793. [CrossRef] [PubMed]

40. Thomas, A.G.; Taylor, F.; Miller, V. Dietary intake and nutritional treatment in childhood Crohn's disease. *J. Pediatr. Gastroenterol. Nutr.* **1993**, *17*, 75–78. [CrossRef] [PubMed]

41. Ruuska, T.; Savilahti, E.; Mäki, M.; Ormälä, T.; Visakorpi, J.K. Exclusive whole protein enteral diet *versus* prednisolone in the treatment of acute Crohn's disease in children. *J. Pediatr. Gastroenterol. Nutr.* **1994**, *19*, 175–180. [CrossRef] [PubMed]

42. Terrin, G.; Canani, R.B.; Ambrosini, A.; Viola, F.; De Mesquita, M.B.; Di Nardo, G.; Dito, L.; Cucchiara, S. A semielemental diet (Pregomin) as primary therapy for inducing remission in children with active Crohn's disease. *Ital. J. Pediatr.* **2002**, *28*, 401–405.

43. Borrelli, O.; Cordischi, L.; Cirulli, M.; Paganelli, M.; Labalestra, V.; Uccini, S.; Russo, P.M.; Cucchiara, S. Polymeric diet alone *versus* corticosteroids in the treatment of active pediatric Crohn's disease: A randomized controlled open-label trial. *Clin. Gastroenterol. Hepatol.* **2006**, *4*, 744–753. [CrossRef] [PubMed]

44. Berni Canani, R.; Terrin, G.; Borrelli, O.; Romano, M.T.; Manguso, F.; Coruzzo, A.; D'Armiento, F.; Romeo, E.F.; Cucchiara, S. Short- and long-term therapeutic efficacy of nutritional therapy and corticosteroids in paediatric Crohn's disease. *Dig. Liver. Dis.* **2006**, *38*, 381–387. [CrossRef] [PubMed]

45. Soo, J.; Malik, B.A.; Turner, J.M.; Persad, R.; Wine, E.; Siminoski, K.; Huynh, H.Q. Use of exclusive enteral nutrition is just as effective as corticosteroids in newly diagnosed pediatric Crohn's disease. *Dig. Dis. Sci.* **2013**, *58*, 3584–3591. [CrossRef] [PubMed]
46. Luo, Y.; Yu, J.; Zhao, H.; Lou, J.; Chen, F.; Peng, K.; Chen, J. Short-Term Efficacy of Exclusive Enteral Nutrition in Pediatric Crohn's Disease: Practice in China. *Gastroenterol. Res. Pract.* **2015**, *2015*, 428354. [CrossRef] [PubMed]
47. Grover, Z.; Muir, R.; Lewindon, P. Exclusive enteral nutrition induces early clinical, mucosal and transmural remission in paediatric Crohn's disease. *J. Gastroenterol.* **2014**, *49*, 638–645. [CrossRef] [PubMed]
48. Gupta, K.; Noble, A.; Kachelries, K.E.; Albenberg, L.; Kelsen, J.R.; Grossman, A.B.; Baldassano, R.N. A novel enteral nutrition protocol for the treatment of pediatric Crohn's disease. *Inflamm. Bowel Dis.* **2013**, *19*, 1374–1378. [CrossRef] [PubMed]
49. Suskind, D.L.; Wahbeh, G.; Gregory, N.; Vendettuoli, H.; Christie, D. Nutritional therapy in pediatric Crohn disease: The specific carbohydrate diet. *J. Pediatr. Gastroenterol. Nutr.* **2014**, *58*, 87–91. [CrossRef] [PubMed]
50. Cohen, S.A.; Gold, B.D.; Oliva, S.; Lewis, J.; Stallworth, A.; Koch, B.; Eshee, L.; Mason, D. Clinical and mucosal improvement with specific carbohydrate diet in pediatric Crohn disease. *J. Pediatr. Gastroenterol. Nutr.* **2014**, *59*, 516–521. [CrossRef] [PubMed]
51. Sigall-Boneh, R.; Pfeffer-Gik, T.; Segal, L.; Zangen, T.; Boaz, M.; Levine, A. Partial enteral nutrition with a Crohn's disease exclusion diet is effective for induction of remission in children and young adults with Crohn's disease. *Inflamm. Bowel Dis.* **2014**, *20*, 1353–1360. [CrossRef] [PubMed]
52. Strisciuglio, C.; Giannetti, E.; Martinelli, M.; Sciorio, E.; Staiano, A.; Miele, E. Does cow's milk protein elimination diet have a role on induction and maintenance of remission in children with ulcerative colitis? *Acta Paediatr.* **2013**, *102*, e273–e278. [CrossRef] [PubMed]
53. Ruemmele, F.M.; Veres, G.; Kolho, K.L.; Griffiths, A.; Levine, A.; Escher, J.C.; Amil Dias, J.; Barabino, A.; Braegger, C.P.; Bronsky, J.; *et al.* Consensus guidelines of ecco/espghan on the medical management of pediatric Crohn's disease. *J. Crohn's Colitis* **2014**, *8*, 1179–1207. [CrossRef] [PubMed]
54. Belli, D.C.; Seidman, E.; Bouthillier, L.; Weber, A.M.; Roy, C.C.; Pletincx, M.; Beaulieu, M.; Morin, C.L. Chronic intermittent elemental diet improves growth failure in children with Crohn's disease. *Gastroenterology* **1988**, *94*, 603–610. [PubMed]
55. Duncan, H.; Buchanan, E.; Cardigan, T.; Garrick, V.; Curtis, L.; McGrogan, P.; Barclay, A.; Russell, R.K. A retrospective study showing maintenance treatment options for paediatric CD in the first year following diagnosis after induction of remission with EEN: Supplemental enteral nutrition is better than nothing! *BMC Gastroenterol.* **2014**, *14*, 50. [CrossRef] [PubMed]
56. Takagi, S.; Utsunomiya, K.; Kuriyama, S.; Yokoyama, H.; Takahashi, S.; Iwabuchi, M.; Takahashi, H.; Takahashi, S.; Kinouchi, Y.; Hiwatashi, N.; *et al.* Effectiveness of an 'half elemental diet' as maintenance therapy for Crohn's disease: A randomized-controlled trial. *Aliment. Pharmacol. Ther.* **2006**, *24*, 1333–1340. [CrossRef] [PubMed]
57. Yamamoto, T.; Nakahigashi, M.; Umegae, S.; Kitagawa, T.; Matsumoto, K. Impact of long-term enteral nutrition on clinical and endoscopic recurrence after resection for Crohn's disease: A prospective, non-randomized, parallel, controlled study. *Aliment. Pharmacol. Ther.* **2007**, *25*, 67–72. [CrossRef] [PubMed]
58. Yamamoto, T.; Shiraki, M.; Nakahigashi, M.; Umegae, S.; Matsumoto, K. Enteral nutrition to suppress postoperative Crohn's disease recurrence: A five-year prospective cohort study. *Int. J. Colorectal Dis.* **2013**, *28*, 335–340. [CrossRef] [PubMed]
59. Hirai, F.; Ishihara, H.; Yada, S.; Esaki, M.; Ohwan, T.; Nozaki, R.; Ashizuka, S.; Inatsu, H.; Ohi, H.; Aoyagi, K.; *et al.* Effectiveness of concomitant enteral nutrition therapy and infliximab for maintenance treatment of Crohn's disease in adults. *Dig. Dis. Sci.* **2013**, *58*, 1329–1334. [CrossRef] [PubMed]
60. Yamamoto, T.; Nakahigashi, M.; Umegae, S.; Matsumoto, K. Prospective clinical trial: Enteral nutrition during maintenance infliximab in Crohn's disease. *J. Gastroenterol.* **2010**, *45*, 24–29. [CrossRef] [PubMed]
61. Wilschanski, M.; Sherman, P.; Pencharz, P.; Davis, L.; Corey, M.; Griffiths, A. Supplementary enteral nutrition maintains remission in paediatric Crohn's disease. *Gut* **1996**, *38*, 543–548. [CrossRef] [PubMed]
62. Chiba, M.; Abe, T.; Tsuda, H.; Sugawara, T.; Tsuda, S.; Tozawa, H.; Fujiwara, K.; Imai, H. Lifestyle-related disease in Crohn's disease: Relapse prevention by a semi-vegetarian diet. *World J. Gastroenterol.* **2010**, *16*, 2484–2495. [CrossRef] [PubMed]

63. Obih, C.; Wahbeh, G.; Lee, D.; Braly, K.; Giefer, M.; Shaffer, M.L.; Nielson, H.; Suskind, D.L. Specific carbohydrate diet for pediatric inflammatory bowel disease in clinical practice within an academic ibd center. *Nutrition* **2015**, *32*, 418–425. [CrossRef] [PubMed]

64. Goel, A.; Kunnumakkara, A.B.; Aggarwal, B.B. Curcumin as "curcumin": From kitchen to clinic. *Biochem. Pharmacol.* **2008**, *75*, 787–809. [CrossRef] [PubMed]

65. Basile, V.; Ferrari, E.; Lazzari, S.; Belluti, S.; Pignedoli, F.; Imbriano, C. Curcumin derivatives: Molecular basis of their anti-cancer activity. *Biochem. Pharmacol.* **2009**, *78*, 1305–1315. [CrossRef] [PubMed]

66. O'Sullivan-Coyne, G.; O'Sullivan, G.C.; O'Donovan, T.R.; Piwocka, K.; McKenna, S.L. Curcumin induces apoptosis-independent death in oesophageal cancer cells. *Br. J. Cancer* **2009**, *101*, 1585–1595. [CrossRef] [PubMed]

67. Lawrence, T.; Fong, C. The resolution of inflammation: Anti-inflammatory roles for nf-kappab. *Int. J. Biochem. Cell Biol.* **2010**, *42*, 519–523. [CrossRef] [PubMed]

68. Hanai, H.; Sugimoto, K. Curcumin has bright prospects for the treatment of inflammatory bowel disease. *Curr. Pharm. Des.* **2009**, *15*, 2087–2094. [CrossRef] [PubMed]

69. Hanai, H.; Iida, T.; Takeuchi, K.; Watanabe, F.; Maruyama, Y.; Andoh, A.; Tsujikawa, T.; Fujiyama, Y.; Mitsuyama, K.; Sata, M.; *et al.* Curcumin maintenance therapy for ulcerative colitis: Randomized, multicenter, double-blind, placebo-controlled trial. *Clin. Gastroenterol. Hepatol.* **2006**, *4*, 1502–1506. [CrossRef] [PubMed]

70. Shah, B.H.; Nawaz, Z.; Pertani, S.A.; Roomi, A.; Mahmood, H.; Saeed, S.A.; Gilani, A.H. Inhibitory effect of curcumin, a food spice from turmeric, on platelet-activating factor- and arachidonic acid-mediated platelet aggregation through inhibition of thromboxane formation and Ca^{2+} signaling. *Biochem. Pharmacol.* **1999**, *58*, 1167–1172. [CrossRef]

71. Suskind, D.L.; Wahbeh, G.; Burpee, T.; Cohen, M.; Christie, D.; Weber, W. Tolerability of curcumin in pediatric inflammatory bowel disease: A forced-dose titration study. *J. Pediatr. Gastroenterol. Nutr.* **2013**, *56*, 277–279. [CrossRef] [PubMed]

72. Akabas, S.R.; Deckelbaum, R.J. Summary of a workshop on *n*-3 fatty acids: Current status of recommendations and future directions. *Am. J. Clin. Nutr.* **2006**, *83*, 1536S–1538S. [PubMed]

73. Ergas, D.; Eilat, E.; Mendlovic, S.; Sthoeger, Z.M. *N*-3 fatty acids and the immune system in autoimmunity. *Isr. Med. Assoc. J.* **2002**, *4*, 34–38. [PubMed]

74. Calder, P.C. *N*-3 polyunsaturated fatty acids, inflammation, and inflammatory diseases. *Am. J. Clin. Nutr.* **2006**, *83*, 1505S–1519S. [PubMed]

75. Calder, P.C. Fatty acids and immune function: Relevance to inflammatory bowel diseases. *Int. Rev. Immunol.* **2009**, *28*, 506–534. [CrossRef] [PubMed]

76. Belluzzi, A.; Brignola, C.; Campieri, M.; Pera, A.; Boschi, S.; Miglioli, M. Effect of an enteric-coated fish-oil preparation on relapses in Crohn's disease. *N. Engl. J. Med.* **1996**, *334*, 1557–1560. [CrossRef] [PubMed]

77. Lorenz-Meyer, H.; Bauer, P.; Nicolay, C.; Schulz, B.; Purrmann, J.; Fleig, W.E.; Scheurlen, C.; Koop, I.; Pudel, V.; Carr, L. Omega-3 fatty acids and low carbohydrate diet for maintenance of remission in Crohn's disease. A randomized controlled multicenter trial. Study group members (german Crohn's disease study group). *Scand. J. Gastroenterol.* **1996**, *31*, 778–785. [CrossRef] [PubMed]

78. Seidner, D.L.; Lashner, B.A.; Brzezinski, A.; Banks, P.L.; Goldblum, J.; Fiocchi, C.; Katz, J.; Lichtenstein, G.R.; Anton, P.A.; Kam, L.Y.; *et al.* An oral supplement enriched with fish oil, soluble fiber, and antioxidants for corticosteroid sparing in ulcerative colitis: A randomized, controlled trial. *Clin. Gastroenterol. Hepatol.* **2005**, *3*, 358–369. [CrossRef]

79. Meister, D.; Ghosh, S. Effect of fish oil enriched enteral diet on inflammatory bowel disease tissues in organ culture: Differential effects on ulcerative colitis and Crohn's disease. *World J. Gastroenterol.* **2005**, *11*, 7466–7472. [CrossRef] [PubMed]

80. Feagan, B.G.; Sandborn, W.J.; Mittmann, U.; Bar-Meir, S.; D'Haens, G.; Bradette, M.; Cohen, A.; Dallaire, C.; Ponich, T.P.; McDonald, J.W.; *et al.* Omega-3 free fatty acids for the maintenance of remission in Crohn disease: The epic randomized controlled trials. *J. Am. Med. Assoc.* **2008**, *299*, 1690–1697. [CrossRef] [PubMed]

81. Lev-Tzion, R.; Griffiths, A.M.; Leder, O.; Turner, D. Omega 3 fatty acids (fish oil) for maintenance of remission in Crohn's disease. *Cochrane Database Syst. Rev.* **2014**, *2*, CD006320. [CrossRef] [PubMed]

82. Romano, C.; Cucchiara, S.; Barabino, A.; Annese, V.; Sferlazzas, C. Usefulness of omega-3 fatty acid supplementation in addition to mesalazine in maintaining remission in pediatric Crohn's disease: A double-blind, randomized, placebo-controlled study. *World J. Gastroenterol.* **2005**, *11*, 7118–7121. [CrossRef] [PubMed]

83. Azcue, M.; Rashid, M.; Griffiths, A.; Pencharz, P.B. Energy expenditure and body composition in children with Crohn's disease: Effect of enteral nutrition and treatment with prednisolone. *Gut* **1997**, *41*, 203–208. [CrossRef] [PubMed]

84. Bannerman, E.; Davidson, I.; Conway, C.; Culley, D.; Aldhous, M.C.; Ghosh, S. Altered subjective appetite parameters in Crohn's disease patients. *Clin. Nutr.* **2001**, *20*, 399–405. [CrossRef] [PubMed]

85. Gerasimidis, K.; McGrogan, P.; Edwards, C.A. The aetiology and impact of malnutrition in paediatric inflammatory bowel disease. *J. Hum. Nutr. Diet.* **2011**, *24*, 313–326. [CrossRef] [PubMed]

86. Beattie, R.M.; Camacho-Hubner, C.; Wacharasindhu, S.; Cotterill, A.M.; Walker-Smith, J.A.; Savage, M.O. Responsiveness of IGF-1 and IGFBP-3 to therapeutic intervention in children and adolescents with Crohn's disease. *Clin. Endocrinol.* **1998**, *49*, 483–489. [CrossRef]

87. Motil, K.J.; Grand, R.J.; Maletskos, C.J.; Young, V.R. The effect of disease, drug, and diet on whole body protein metabolism in adolescents with Crohn's disease and growth failure. *J. Pediatr.* **1982**, *101*, 345–351. [CrossRef]

88. O'Morain, C.; Segal, A.M.; Levi, A.J.; Valman, H.B. Elemental diet in acute Crohn's disease. *Arch. Dis. Child.* **1983**, *58*, 44–47. [CrossRef] [PubMed]

89. Polk, D.B.; Hattner, J.A.; Kerner, J.A., Jr. Improved growth and disease activity after intermittent administration of a defined formula diet in children with Crohn's disease. *J. Parenter. Enteral. Nutr.* **1992**, *16*, 499–504. [CrossRef]

90. Cosgrove, M.; Jenkins, H.R. Experience of percutaneous endoscopic gastrostomy in children with Crohn's disease. *Arch. Dis. Child.* **1997**, *76*, 141–143. [CrossRef] [PubMed]

91. Sylvester, F.A.; Leopold, S.; Lincoln, M.; Hyams, J.S.; Griffiths, A.M.; Lerer, T. A two-year longitudinal study of persistent lean tissue deficits in children with Crohn's disease. *Clin. Gastroenterol. Hepatol.* **2009**, *7*, 452–455. [CrossRef] [PubMed]

92. Finkelstein, J.S.; Klibanski, A.; Neer, R.M. A longitudinal evaluation of bone mineral density in adult men with histories of delayed puberty. *J. Clin. Endocrinol. Metab.* **1996**, *81*, 1152–1155. [CrossRef] [PubMed]

93. Lopes, L.H.; Sdepanian, V.L.; Szejnfeld, V.L.; de Morais, M.B.; Fagundes-Neto, U. Risk factors for low bone mineral density in children and adolescents with inflammatory bowel disease. *Dig. Dis. Sci.* **2008**, *53*, 2746–2753. [CrossRef] [PubMed]

94. Whitten, K.E.; Leach, S.T.; Bohane, T.D.; Woodhead, H.J.; Day, A.S. Effect of exclusive enteral nutrition on bone turnover in children with Crohn's disease. *J. Gastroenterol.* **2010**, *45*, 399–405. [CrossRef] [PubMed]

An Examination of Diet for the Maintenance of Remission in Inflammatory Bowel Disease

Natasha Haskey and Deanna L. Gibson *

Department of Biology, The Irving K. Barber School of Arts and Sciences, University of British Columbia, Room, ASC 368, 3187 University Way, Okanagan campus, Kelowna, BC V1V 1V7, Canada; natasha.haskey@gmail.com
* Correspondence: deanna.gibson@ubc.ca

Abstract: Diet has been speculated to be a factor in the pathogenesis of inflammatory bowel disease and may be an important factor in managing disease symptoms. Patients manipulate their diet in attempt to control symptoms, often leading to the adoption of inappropriately restrictive diets, which places them at risk for nutritional complications. Health professionals struggle to provide evidence-based nutrition guidance to patients due to an overall lack of uniformity or clarity amongst research studies. Well-designed diet studies are urgently needed to create an enhanced understanding of the role diet plays in the management of inflammatory bowel disease. The aim of this review is to summarize the current data available on dietary management of inflammatory bowel disease and to demonstrate that dietary modulation may be an important consideration in managing disease. By addressing the relevance of diet in inflammatory bowel disease, health professionals are able to better support patients and collaborate with dietitians to improve nutrition therapy.

Keywords: diet; diet therapy; nutrition; nutrition therapy; inflammatory bowel disease; ulcerative colitis; Crohn's disease

---

1. Introduction

Inflammatory Bowel Disease (IBD) is a chronic inflammatory condition that includes ulcerative colitis (UC) and Crohn's disease (CD). CD is a transmural inflammatory disease of the gastrointestinal mucosa that can affect any component of the gastrointestinal tract including the small and/or large intestine, the mouth, esophagus, stomach and anus. UC is non-transmural and primarily involves only the colonic mucosa. Patients with IBD experience periods of relapse (active disease) and clinical remission [1]. Clinical symptoms of IBD are diarrhea and/or constipation, passage of blood or mucus in the stool and abdominal cramping. In addition, CD patients may also experience bowel obstruction, strictures and abscesses.

Medications are the first-line of therapy in the management of IBD. Surgery is generally reserved for those patients who are intolerant to medications or have refractory disease. The main classes of drugs used in the treatment of IBD include 5-aminosalicylates (5-ASA) (e.g., sulphasalazine, and mesalamine), corticosteroids (e.g., hydrocortisone, prednisone, and prednisolone), immunomodulators (e.g., azathioprine, 6-mercaptopurine, methotrexate and cyclosporine) and biologics (e.g., infliximab, adalimumab, and vedolizumab). Although many patients have a good response to pharmacotherapy, medications can have severe adverse side effects. Drug hypersensitivity, nephrotoxicity, fever, rash, lymphadenopathy, hepatitis, pancreatitis, diarrhea exacerbation, nausea, vomiting, abdominal pain, myalgia and an increased risk for lymphoma with the use of immunomodulators are some of the reported side effects. In addition, medication adherence is a concern, as a recent study reported that approximately one quarter of patients with IBD attending at a tertiary care practice did not use the prescribed IBD-specific medications [2]. It is clear the adoption of novel strategies and preventative medicine is crucial to the well-being of patients with IBD to avoid complications and side-effects related to both the disease, as well as the treatments.

Exclusive enteral nutrition is a nutritional therapy where 100% of a patient's nutritional requirements are met via a liquid nutrition formula and administered orally or through a feeding tube. Exclusive enteral nutrition is provided for 6–8 weeks and then an oral diet is gradually reintroduced [3]. In children with active CD, exclusive enteral nutrition can be used in place of corticosteroid therapy and has been shown to improve time to relapse [4]. This approach has also been shown to positively impact inflammatory changes, mucosal healing, enhance growth and overall nutritional status in children [4]. Outside of Japan, exclusive enteral nutrition is not routinely used as first-line therapy in adults. There is some evidence to support the use of exclusive enteral nutrition as a treatment modality in a select group of adult patients with CD, specifically those with a new diagnosis of CD, those with ileal involvement and those that are motivated to adhere to the exclusive enteral nutrition regimen [5].

IBD is associated with nutritional complications during both relapse and clinical remission. Some of the nutritional complications include reduced dietary intake, nutrient malabsorption, macro- or micronutrient deficiencies, weight loss and osteoporosis [6–10]. IBD patients are concerned about food and diet [11,12] and use various dietary strategies in attempt to control or minimize gastrointestinal distress [13], as well as improve overall health. Up to 71% of patients with IBD believe diet affects their disease symptoms, with 90% of CD patients and 71% of UC patients employing elimination diets while in remission [14,15]. Dietary modification can be of concern if patients drastically reduce or completely avoid nutritionally important foods/food groups, as this may place them at increased risk for developing nutritional deficiencies [16], as well as poorer quality of life. Up to 77.1% of patients with IBD report avoidance of particular foods [14]. A case-control study found significantly lower mean daily intakes of carbohydrates, monounsaturated fat, fiber, calcium, and vitamins C, D, E, and K compared to controls, as a result of the exclusion of dairy products, vegetables and fruit [17].

There is a plethora of information on the internet that assert that certain diets improve or exacerbate symptoms, yet few rigorous nutrition studies have examined specific dietary factor(s) as being detrimental or protective against UC or CD. Implementation of diet strategies and approaches into clinical practice are slow and limited. Common barriers to implementation into practice include issues relating to knowledge management, such as access to research evidence sources, time to review evidence-based sources and a lack of skills to appraise and understand research evidence [18]. In addition to knowledge management, financial barriers, inappropriate skill mix and problems working with and across professional disciplines contribute to the lag in knowledge translation [18]. This review attempts to consolidate the existing evidence on diet/pharmoconutrition and maintenance of remission in IBD, including studies that evaluate the association between pre-illness intake of nutrients and food groups and the risk of a subsequent diagnosis of IBD, diet intervention studies in maintaining remission in IBD, as well as existing guidelines [19–21], in light of the most current limitations in evidence and practice. Evidence-based dietary recommendations for IBD patients are summarized in Tables 1 and 2 and Figure 1.

Table 1. Evidence-based diet recommendations for the maintenance of remission in IBD.

Statement	Recommendation
Encourage high dietary fiber intake from foods, especially from fruits and vegetables [22–25]	Strongly Recommend *
Avoid n-6 PUFA (safflower oils, corn oils, margarine) and trans-unsaturated fatty acid consumption [23,24,26,27]	Strongly Recommend
Encourage consumption of dairy products [28,29]	Recommend † (if tolerated)
Limit/avoid refined carbohydrates, especially sweetened beverages and soft drinks [30]	Recommend

Table 1. *Cont.*

Statement	Recommendation
Limit red meat consumption, especially from beef, pork, lamb and processed meats [22,31]	Recommend
FODMAP Diet [32–34]	Optional ‡ (for the management of IBS-overlay)
Mediterranean Diet Pattern [35–37]	Optional
Specific Carbohydrate Diet [38–41] Low Residue Diet [42] Semi-vegetarian Diet [43] IgG4-guided Elimination Diet [44] IBD-AID [45]	No Recommendation β
Paleo Diet	No Recommendation

Evidence graded according to the American Academy of Pediatrics, Steering Committee on Quality Improvement and Management—"Classifying recommendations for clinical practice guidelines" [46]. * Strongly Recommend: The quality of the supporting evidence is excellent, based on well-designed randomized control trials (RCTs) and/or consistent evidence from observational studies. Benefit clearly outweighs harm. † Recommend: The quality of the supporting evidence is good, but RCTs and/or evidence from case-control/cohort studies has limitations. Anticipated benefits outweigh harm. ‡ Optional: The quality of evidence is suspect, further well-performed studies needed. May be of limited advantage, however there is still unclear balance between benefit and harm. β No recommendation: There is a lack of or poor evidence. Unclear balance between benefit and harm.

Table 2. Evidence-based nutrition recommendations for supplements in the maintenance of remission in IBD.

Statement	Type of IBD	Recommendation
Vitamin D (minimum 1200 IU/day) [47–51]	Both	Strongly Recommend * (aim for levels of serum 25 (OHD) >75 nmol/L
Psyllium (minimum 4 grams/day) [52,53]	UC	Recommend †
Curcumin (1-gram bid) [54–56]	UC	Optional ‡
Oat bran supplementation (20 grams/day) [57]	UC	Optional
Germinated Barley Foodstuff (minimum 20 grams/day) [58–60]	UC	Optional
Wheat bran (1/2 cup daily) [61]	CD	Optional

Evidence graded according to the American Academy of Pediatrics, Steering Committee on Quality Improvement and Management—"Classifying recommendations for clinical practice guidelines" [46]. * Strongly Recommend: The quality of the supporting evidence is excellent, based on well-designed randomized control trials (RCTs) and/or consistent evidence from observational studies. Benefit clearly outweighs harm. † Recommend: The quality of the supporting evidence is good, but RCTs and/or evidence from case-control/cohort studies has limitations. Anticipated benefits outweigh harm. ‡ Optional: The quality of evidence is suspect, further well-performed studies needed. May be of limited advantage, however there is still unclear balance between benefit and harm. β No recommendation: There is a lack of or poor evidence. Unclear balance between benefit and harm.

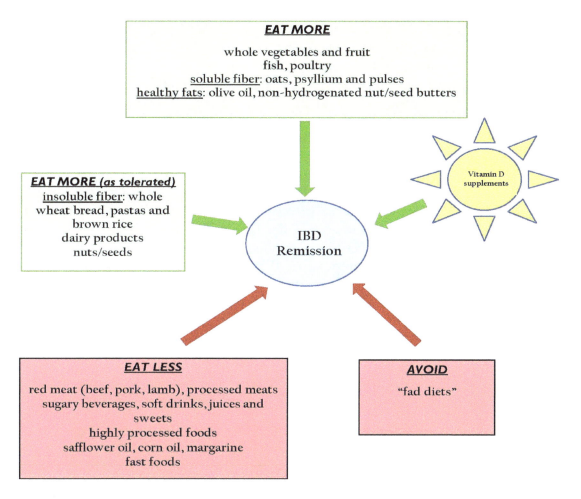

Figure 1. Summary of practical dietary recommendations for maintenance of remission in IBD.

2. Literature Search

A systematic literature search was conducted using PubMed, EMBASE and Medline from 1966 to October 2016 using the medical subject heading (MeSH) terms "inflammatory bowel disease", "Crohn's disease", "ulcerative colitis", "nutrition", "nutrition therapy", "diet" and "diet therapy". Searches containing relevant synonyms and combinations of the above terms were also utilized. We reviewed intervention studies, systematic reviews, as well as relevant review articles that contained practice guidelines with a focus on adults. Studies covering active IBD, enteral/parenteral nutrition and IBD with colectomy/ostomy were excluded from the review.

3. Diet in the Etiology of IBD

IBD has traditionally been thought of as a disease of the Western hemisphere, however there is an increasing incidence in Japan, Hong Kong, Korea and Eastern Europe [62,63]. Although still rarer, an increasing incidence of IBD is also being identified in South Africa, South America and Saudi Arabia [64–66]. The dramatic rise in incidence of IBD, particularly in South Asia, India and Japan, where traditionally there was a low incidence, suggests that environmental factors, such as the Western diet pattern, play an important role in disease pathogenesis [67–69]. This hypothesis is further confirmed by the increasing incidence of the disease in immigrants to the Western hemisphere. Migration from a country with a history of low-incidence to a country of a higher incidence increases the risk of developing IBD, particularly in the first generation children [70]. Diet composition has long been suspected to contribute to IBD. Thus, dietary patterns and nutrients are important environmental factors to consider in the etiology of IBD [22,71].

3.1. The Western Diet Pattern

The diet of today is considerably different from the traditional diet of previous generations, when the prevalence of IBD was considerably lower. The Western diet pattern is dominated by increased consumption of refined sugar, omega-6 polyunsaturated fats and fast food, combined with a diet deficient in fruit, vegetables, and fiber [72]. Much of today's food supply has been processed, modified, stored and transported great distances, in contrast to the traditional diet, where food that was produced locally was consumed shortly after harvest. This shift to the Western diet pattern is hypothesized to increase pro-inflammatory cytokines, modulate intestinal permeability, and alter the intestinal microbiota promoting a low-grade chronic inflammation in the gut [73]. A diet that contains pro-inflammatory foods is an important risk factor in the development of UC. A case-control study completed in Iran with newly diagnosed UC patients (n = 62 UC patients, 124 controls) found that subjects that had a higher dietary inflammatory index (pro-inflammatory diet) had an increased risk of developing UC (Odds Ratio (OR): 1.55, 95% Confidence Interval (CI): 1.04–2.32) [23]. The authors concluded that encouraging intake of more anti-inflammatory dietary factors, such as plant-based foods rich in fiber and phytochemicals, and reducing intake of pro-inflammatory factors, such as fried or processed foods rich in trans-fatty acids, could be a potential strategy for reducing risk of UC. This was one of the first studies that has examined dietary inflammatory index as an outcome for developing UC. Several large scale studies have attempted to elucidate the dietary components that are associated with IBD risk [22,24,26,27]. Overall, this suggests that the Western diet pattern is a risk factor for IBD.

3.2. Carbohydrate Intake as a Risk Factor for IBD

A systematic review (n = 19 studies with 2609 IBD subjects) reported a negative association between dietary fiber (OR 0.12, 95% CI: 0.04–0.37) and fruit intake (OR: 0.2, 95% CI: 0.1–0.9) and CD risk [22]. Soluble fiber from fruit may have a protective effect on CD [24]. High vegetable intake may be associated with decreased risk of UC (OR range 0.32–0.75) [22]. The European Investigation into Cancer and Nutrition study (n = 366,351 with 256 incident cases of UC and 117 of CD, and four matched controls per case) reported that an increased consumption of sugar and soft drinks with low vegetable intake was positively associated with UC risk (OR 1.31, 95% CI: 0.85–2.02; p = 0.05) [25]. Increased consumption of sweets is positively associated with CD (OR: 2.83, 95% CI: 1.38–5.83) and UC (OR: 2.86, 95% CI: 1.24–6.57) [30]. Overall, this suggests that while refined and processed carbohydrates and intake of sweetened beverages are risk factors for IBD, complex carbohydrates including fruit, vegetables and fiber should be included in the diet to manage IBD.

3.3. Protein Intake as a Risk Factor for IBD

A large prospective cohort study (n = 67,581) completed over a 10.5-year period found that high protein intake, specifically animal protein (meat, not dairy products) was positively associated with an increased risk of IBD [31]. A systematic review (n = 2609 IBD patients; 19 studies) reported an association with high total protein intake with the development of UC (OR range 0.2–3.7) and CD (OR range 0.45–3.34) [22]. High protein intake was associated with a 3.3-fold increased risk of IBD, suggesting a diet high in animal protein is a major risk factor for the development of IBD.

3.4. Dairy Intake as Risk Factor for IBD

The European Investigation into Cancer and Nutrition study found that individuals that consumed milk had significantly reduced odds of developing CD (OR: 0.30, 95% CI: 0.13–0.65), suggesting a protective effect with dairy product consumption [28]. Individual dairy products consisted of milk, yogurt, and cheese with varying fat content (e.g., full fat, skimmed, semi-skimmed, and unspecified). This is supported by a case-control study in children (n = 130 CD patients and n = 202 controls) that demonstrated that consumption of dairy products was not associated with CD

(OR: 0.86, 95% CI: 0.42–1.76, p = 0.65) [29]. Overall, the consumption of dairy products is not a risk factor for IBD.

3.5. Dietary Fat Intake as a Risk Factor for IBD

There have been conflicting data on the association between dietary fat intake and the development of IBD, as many of the studies are retrospective and use small sample sizes. However, a very large, long-term, prospective study (n = 170,805) completed over 26 years did not observe a significant association with increased risk of developing CD or UC with total dietary fat intake, saturated fatty acids (SFA) and monounsaturated fatty acids (MUFA) [26], which has been well supported by other research studies [74–76]. A growing body of scientific evidence indicates that the Mediterranean diet pattern has been associated with significant improvements in health status [77,78] and decreases in inflammatory markers in humans [79]. The protective effect is hypothesized to be derived from the balance in fats, which includes incorporating MUFA, SFA and fish intake [80]. While a few studies do show that MUFAs are beneficial during colitis, studies on the effects of SFA and PUFAs on gut health are controversial.

Dietary n-6 PUFA, in particular linoleic acid, have been implicated in the etiology of IBD. Dietary n-6 PUFAs are essential fatty acids present in high amounts in red meat, cooking oils (safflower and corn oil) and margarines. A prospective cohort study (n = 203,193) conducted over four years found that intake of linoleic acid was associated with an increased risk of UC (OR: 2.49, 95% CI: 1.23 to 5.07, p = 0.01) [27]. Further analysis of the European Investigation into Cancer and Nutrition study (n = 260,686) over five years found an increased risk of UC with a higher total PUFA intake (trend across quartiles OR = 1.19 (95% CI: 0.99–1.43) p = 0.07) [74], which was also supported by a systematic review (n = 2609 patients with IBD) that examined pre-illness intake of nutrients and subsequent development of UC [22]. A case-control study in CD found that increased total PUFA consumption was positively associated with CD risk (OR: 2.31, 95% CI: 1.12–4.79) [30].

The Nurses' Health Study cohorts (n = 170,805 women with 269 incident cases of CD and 338 incident cases of UC) reported high, long-term intake of trans-unsaturated fatty acids was associated with a trend towards an increased incidence of UC (HR 1.34, 95% CI: 0.94–1.92) but not CD [26]. An increased relative risk of developing IBD has also been associated with frequent intake of fast foods (fast foods are high in trans-unsaturated fatty acids) [81,82]. The relative risk associated with the consumption of fast foods at least two times a week was estimated at 3.4 (95% CI: 1.3–9.3) for CD and 3.9 (95% CI: 1.4–10.6) for UC [82]. Frequent fast food intake, defined as more than once a week, was significantly associated with a risk of UC (43%, OR: 5.78, 95% CI: 2.38–14.03) and CD (27%, OR: 2.84, 95% CI: 1.21–6.64) [81].

It has been speculated that the intake of long-chain n-3 PUFAs (docosapentaenoic acid, eicosapentaenoic acid, docosahexaenoic acid), known as omega-3s, may be of benefit to patients with IBD. The beneficial effects are believe to be derived from the anti-inflammatory properties of n-3 PUFAs; however, clinical and experimental studies have shown conflicting results [83]. Meta-analyses have failed to show benefit with supplementation with fish oils in the maintenance of remission in CD and UC [84–86]. Dietary intake of n-3 PUFAs were inversely associated with risk of UC, whereas no association has been found with CD [26]. The European Investigation into Cancer and Nutrition study (n = 203,193) found a negative association with the development of UC with increasing dietary intake of the n-3 PUFA, specifically docosahexaenoic acid (OR: 0.23, 95% CI: 0.06 to 0.97) [27], and is supported by the European Investigation into Cancer and Nutrition -Norfolk study (n = 26,639) (OR: 0.43, 95% CI: 0.22–0.86) [57]. Two case-control studies in CD report that a diet with regular consumption of fish had a protective effect on the development of CD (OR 0.52, 95% CI: 0.33–0.80, p = 0.003) and (OR 0.46, 95% CI: 0.20–1.06, p = 0.02) [29,69].

The total ratio of n-3 PUFA: n-6 PUFA found in the diet has been hypothesized to be an important consideration. One prospective cohort [87] and one case-control study [29] report that a high n-3PUFA: n-6 PUFA ratio in the diet is inversely associated with the risk of IBD. In support of this explanation, a dietary intervention trial that focused on increasing the n-3 PUFA: n-6 PUFA ratio was found to be effective in maintaining disease remission in patients with both UC and CD, through increasing n-3 PUFA intake [88]. Overall, it does not appear that full fat diets should be avoided, however fat including diets rich in olive oil, dairy products and fish but not fish oil pills should be consumed while avoiding large intakes of vegetable oils rich in n-6 PUFA.

In summary, several epidemiological studies provide compelling evidence for the role of food in IBD pathogenesis. Furthermore, the rise in incidence of IBD in countries that previously have had a very low incidence suggests that industrialization and adoption of the westernized diet may be a risk factor in the development of IBD. Reduced consumption of fruits and possibly vegetables, resulting in a reduced overall intake of fiber, with high intake of meats, fast foods and trans-fatty acids appears to be associated with an overall increase in the risk of developing IBD [71].

4. Diet Interventions and IBD

Diet interventions have been studied in IBD in attempt to manage active disease or to maintain remission. A number have been shown to be efficacious, however, the precise components that are important for each diet are not clearly delineated or often contradict one another. With no gold standard, nutrition guidance provided at this time by health professionals is based on the "best available evidence".

4.1. Low Residue Diet

A low-residue diet is often recommended for the management of an acute flare of IBD, especially in patients that have intestinal strictures or narrowing. Although the low-residue diet is prescribed for short-term use, in clinical practice, patients often follow the diet long-term. The primary purpose of a low residue diet is to reduce the frequency and volume of stools and reduce the risk for intestinal obstruction [89]. In the literature, there have been discrepancies as to the actual composition of low-fiber and/or low-residue diets. A low-residue diet requires the elimination of whole grains, legumes and all fruits and vegetables (except for bananas and skinless potatoes), dairy and fibrous meats [89]. This is not the same as a low-fiber diet which excludes only insoluble fiber. A prospective study in subjects with active CD ($n = 70$) that compared a low-residue diet to an unrestricted diet found no differences in outcome including symptoms, need for hospitalization, need for surgery, new complications, nutritional status, or postoperative recurrence [42]. Due to lack of evidence, there appears to be no reason to restrict residue from the diet, however anecdotally CD patients with obstructive symptoms and strictures report improvement in symptoms when following a diet reduced in fiber (total daily fiber intake < 10 g) [89,90].

Research is still in its infancy, however there is growing evidence for an association between IBD and an alteration in the gut microbiota. The Westernized diet, characterized by increased consumption of PUFA, animal protein, and sugar as well as decreased consumption of fiber has been implicated as factor contributing to dysbiosis [91–93]. A small pilot study in CD ($n = 6$), reported a marked decrease in microbial diversity with a low-residue diet [94]. This is concerning considering that low diversity of the microbiota has been linked to a variety of chronic diseases [95]. Furthermore, improvements in inflammatory markers have not been demonstrated with a low-residue diet in CD [96]. More research is required; however, a low-residue diet could potentially have negative consequences on IBD, therefore prolonged avoidance of fiber is discouraged [90].

4.2. Semi-Vegetarian Diet

A prospective trial conducted in Japan in hospitalized subjects with CD ($n = 22$) examined the effect of a semi-vegetarian diet on maintaining remission [43]. The diet was lacto-ovo vegetarian, in which eggs and milk were allowed with small portions of meat offered once every two weeks and fish weekly. Remission rate achieved with the semi-vegetarian diet was 100% after one year and 92% after two years. A semi-vegetarian diet showed significant prevention of relapse compared to that of individuals following an omnivorous diet ($p = 0.003$ log rank test). Based on these observations, the semi-vegetarian diet may be a highly effective way to maintain remission CD. While this study is promising, large, randomized control studies are required to validate the efficacy of this type of diet for IBD patients.

4.3. FODMAPs Diet

The low Fermentable Oligosaccharide, Disaccharide, Monosaccharide, and Polyol diet (FODMAPs) consists of eliminating foods high in fermentable but poorly absorbed carbohydrates and polyols for six to eight weeks [97]. FODMAPs comprise fructose, lactose, fructo- and galacto-oligosaccharides (fructans and galactans), and polyols (sorbitol, mannitol, xylitol and maltitol) [97]. Common food sources of foods containing FODMAPS are as follows: (1) fructans: onion, garlic and wheat; (2) fructose: fruits and fruit products, honey, and foods with added high-fructose sweeteners; (3) lactose: mainly dairy products; (4) oligosaccharides: legumes, nuts, seeds, some grains; and (5) polyols: fruits and vegetables, and sugar-free products. After symptom resolution, patients are guided by a dietitian on how to gradually reintroduce foods high in fermentable carbohydrates to determine individual tolerance to specific FODMAPs.

Fair evidence supports the effectiveness of a low-FODMAP diet for the symptom management of irritable bowel syndrome (IBS), especially a reduction in abdominal bloating, pain, and diarrhea [98,99]. IBS-like symptoms are common in IBD and have been reported in 57% of patients with CD, and 33% of patients with UC [100], therefore a low-FODMAP diet has been proposed for the management of patients with IBD with IBS-overlay. There have been three retrospective studies evaluating the low-FODMAP diet in IBD [32–34]. A retrospective study of 72 IBD patients who received dietary intervention focusing on low-FODMAP diet, reported one in two patients reported a significant improvement in abdominal symptoms, abdominal pain, bloating, wind and diarrhea ($p < 0.02$ for all symptoms) [32]. Second, a case-note review of electronic medical records of 88 IBD patients with functional gut symptoms who received low-FODMAP diet advice found a significant reduction in symptoms of any severity (mild, moderate, or severe) for abdominal pain ($p < 0.001$), bloating ($p < 0.001$), flatulence ($p = 0.041$), belching ($p = 0.001$), incomplete evacuation ($p = 0.012$), nausea ($p = 0.011$), and heartburn ($p = 0.035$) [33]. Improvements in stool consistency and frequency were observed, including an increase in "normal" stool form ($p = 0.002$) and "normal" stool frequency ($p < 0.001$) [33]. A retrospective, cross-sectional study ($n = 49$) was conducted to investigate long-term adherence and effect on disease course in IBD patients treated with the low-FODMAP diet [34]. Forty-three percent of the IBD patients reported full efficacy ($p = 0.08$) with greatest improvements seen in abdominal pain (63%) and bloating (83%) while on the low-FODMAP diet. The proportion of patients having normal stools increased by 66% in the IBD group ($p < 0.001$). Twenty-four percent of IBD patients became asymptomatic while following the diet. In summary, while there have been no prospective intervention trials completed in IBD, retrospective data suggests that a low FODMAP diet may be a strategy to manage concurrent functional gut symptoms in this population.

4.4. Exclusion Diets

Enteral feeding is often used as an adjunctive therapy for maintenance of remission in CD, particularly in Japan. In a randomized control trial, subjects were provided half of the nutrition requirements by an elemental formula (taken orally ($n = 21$) or by nasogastric tube ($n = 5$)), with the remaining 50% of the nutrition requirements met by consuming an unrestricted diet [101]. The relapse rates in the half elemental diet group were significantly lower (34.6% vs. 64.0%; multivariate hazard ratio 0.40 (95% CI: 0.16–0.98)) than the control group after a mean follow-up of 11.9 months. A follow-up report on this study stated that the elemental diet as a maintenance therapy for CD contributed to keeping subjects in a clinically stable state, without affecting their quality of life, nor leading to additional medical expenses [102].

Exclusion diets can be unpalatable and difficult to follow, therefore in a double blind, randomized control trial, the efficacy of a IgG4-guided exclusion diet in subjects with CD was evaluated [44]. The objective of the study was to identify which components of the diet are most important to avoid due to the induction of IgG4, an antibody produced in response to chronic exposure to an antigenic stimulus like a food antigen. It is hypothesized that dietary protein antigens might perpetuate inflammation in CD as a result of previous sensitization. IgG4 titers were tested against 16 common food types. Subjects in the treatment group removed the four food types with the highest antibody titer for four weeks, whereas controls removed the four food types with the lowest antibody titer. The researchers found significant improvements in quality of life, measured by the short inflammatory bowel disease questionnaire (3.05 (0.01–6.11) $p < 0.05$) and disease activity scores, measured by Crohns Disease Activity Index (41 (10.4–71.5) $p = 0.009$). Forty-one percent of subjects receiving the treatment experienced an improvement in Crohns Disease Activity Index score of >100, whereas 16% of controls experienced an improvement. The exclusion of milk, pork, beef and egg was most strongly associated with improvement. This study was underpowered, however, it did demonstrate clinical improvement and this novel approach to dietary management of IBD does warrant further investigation.

4.5. Novel Anti-Inflammatory Diet Therapies

While the exact etiology of IBD remains unclear, increasing evidence suggests that the gastrointestinal microbiome plays a critical role in disease pathogenesis [103,104]. Manipulation of the gastrointestinal microbiome through diet interventions, in attempt to reduce systemic inflammation, is increasingly recommended as adjuncts to ongoing medical therapy. The Anti-Inflammatory Diet (IBD-AID) is a nutritional approach designed to address nutrient adequacy, malabsorption and symptoms [45]. IBD-AID restricts the intake of particular carbohydrates (lactose, refined and processed complex carbohydrates), includes the ingestion of pre- and probiotic foods, and modifies dietary fatty acid intake specifically decreasing the total fat, saturated fats, the elimination of hydrogenated oils, and encouraging the increased intake of foods rich in n-3 PUFA. A retrospective case series using IBD-AID found that subjects who attempted the diet ($n = 40$), 60% reported reduced symptoms, including reduced stool frequency (patient self-report). A small subset of the subjects ($n = 7$) was able to discontinue at least one of their IBD medications. An intervention trial with a rigorous study design that examines both biomarkers of inflammation, as well as histological changes is needed to further assess efficacy.

4.6. Fiber Supplements

The benefits of fiber in IBD are more commonly seen for the use of supplements rather than diet interventions and for the management of UC and CD [105]. Although the evidence is still not clear, interventions with fiber have the potential to relieve symptoms and/or to maintain disease remission in IBD patients. The type of fiber may be an important consideration.

4.6.1. Oat Bran

A controlled intervention study adding 60 grams/day of oat bran (equivalent to 20 grams oat fiber/day) to the diet of subjects ($n = 22$) with quiescent UC reported no signs or symptoms of colitis relapse after 12 weeks [57]. A subgroup of subjects noted a decrease in abdominal pain, reflux and diarrhea ($p < 0.05$). The greatest impact of the oat bran intervention was seen on the fecal short chain fatty acid (SCFA) concentrations found in the stool. Fifteen subjects demonstrated a 36% increase in fecal butyrate concentrations within four weeks ($p < 0.01$) of intervention which was maintained throughout the 12-week intervention. This finding is important as increasing evidence suggests SCFAs play an essential role in maintaining the health of colonic mucosa as butyrate is the main energy substrate for colonocytes [106]. Butyrate also plays an important role in the prevention and treatment of distal UC [107]. Supplementation with oat bran in this population warrants further investigation with a larger sample size, over a longer-term to determine the overall benefit as a maintenance therapy for UC.

4.6.2. Wheat Bran

A randomized control trial completed in CD ($n = 7$) where subjects were instructed to consume a high fiber diet, including consumption of whole wheat bran cereal (1/2 cup daily) and restrict refined carbohydrates, reported improved health-related quality of life as measured by the Inflammatory Bowel Disease Questionnaire ($p = 0.028$) [61]. Significant improvements were seen in the clinical disease activity scores, as measured by partial Harvey-Bradshaw index ($p = 0.008$). This was a feasibility study with a very small sample size ($n = 4$ receiving intervention) that did not include subjects receiving biologic therapies. A much larger sample size, over a longer term, including subjects receiving a variety of medications, is needed to verify the results of this study.

4.6.3. Psyllium

A randomized control trial in subjects with UC in remission ($n = 105$) comparing psyllium fiber (10 g bid) versus mesalamine (500 mg tid) versus psyllium fiber plus mesalamine (10 g bid + 500 mg tid) reported continued remission at 12 months and slightly lower relapse rates in the mesalamine plus psyllium fiber group [52]. Probability of continued remission was similar between all three groups (Mantel-Cox test, $p = 0.67$; intent-to-treat analysis). Hallert et al. (1991) conducted a randomized control trial with UC in remission over four months ($n = 29$) found psyllium (7 g/day testa ispaghula) to be superior to placebo in relieving gastrointestinal symptoms ($p < 0.001$), especially for diarrhea and constipation [53]. Although the dosage of psyllium needs to be elucidated, weak evidence suggests that psyllium fiber may be efficacious in maintaining remission in UC.

4.6.4. Germinated Barley Foodstuff

Germinated barley foodstuff is an insoluble dietary fiber made by milling and sieving brewer's spent grain [108]. Germinated barley foodstuff has prebiotic properties, containing glutamine-rich protein and hemicellulose-rich fiber which has been shown to reduce clinical activity and prolong remission in UC [58–60]. An open-label trial with 41 patients (21 controls, 20 germinated barley foodstuff intervention) with UC in remission received 30 grams (three times daily) of germinated barley foodstuff in addition to conventional medication for two months [59]. A statistically significant reduction in mean CRP was seen in the germinated barley foodstuff intervention group ($p = 0.017$), as well as a significant reduction in abdominal pain and cramping ($p = 0.017$). A similar designed study found that 20 grams of germinated barley foodstuff ($n = 41$) reduced levels of TNF-α, IL-6 and IL-8, with significant reductions in IL-6 ($p = 0.034$) and IL-8 ($p = 0.013$) [60]. Length of remission has also been prolonged with long-term administration (12 months) of 20 grams of germinated barley foodstuff [58]. Germinated barley foodstuff appears to be a safe and effective maintenance therapy to prolong remission in patients with UC.

4.7. Role of Fat in the Diet

Systematic reviews of the efficacy of n-3 PUFA supplementation in maintaining remission in IBD have shown no clear evidence of their efficacy [84,85,109]. However, it may be the type of fatty acids consumed in the diet that are important in maintaining remission. Uchiyama et al. implemented a diet therapy in IBD subjects ($n = 230$) that involved the use of an "n-3 PUFA food exchange table" (n-3 PUFA diet plan)) to achieve a dietary n-3/n-6 ratio of [almost equal to]1 [88]. In this regimen, to achieve an n-3/n-6 ratio of ~1, the n-6 PUFA intake was restricted to 50% of the mean intake, and the n-3 PUFA intake was increased. The subjects were prohibited from consuming the main sources of dietary n-6 PUFA, i.e., vegetable oil; seasonings such as margarine, dressings, and mayonnaise; food cooked in vegetable oil; and snacks. In a subset of subjects, the mean n-3/n-6 ratio significantly increased after intervention. The mean n-3/n-6 ratios in the remission were significantly higher than relapse groups (0.65 ± 0.28 and 0.53 ± 0.18, $p < 0.001$) and increase in the n-3/n-6 ratio was seen in the erythrocyte membrane of IBD subjects. This study concluded that n-3/n-6 ratio may influence disease activity in IBD subjects.

The Mediterranean diet pattern may have a protective effect on IBD, as the incidence of IBD in the south of Europe is lower than in northern Europe [110]. The Mediterranean diet pattern is a diet that is high in fiber-rich plant-based foods (e.g., cereals, fruits, vegetables, legumes, nuts, seeds and olives), with olive oil as the principle source of added fat, along with high to moderate intakes of fish and seafood, moderate consumption of eggs, poultry, dairy products (cheese and yogurt), wine and low consumption of red meat [111]. A growing body of scientific evidence indicates that the Mediterranean diet pattern has been associated with significant improvements in health status and [77,78] decreases in inflammatory markers [79]. The protective effect is hypothesized to be derived from the balance in the omega-6/omega-3 ratio of the Mediterranean diet pattern (35% total fat: 15% MUFA (mainly from olive oil), 13% SFA, and 6% PUFA [80]. The mechanisms of how MUFA might be beneficial in colitis are unknown, although adherence to the Mediterranean diet pattern has been shown to beneficially affect the gut microbiome and gut metabolites (metabolome) [35]. A recent case-control study (n = 264 IBD subjects and 203 controls) found that low adherence to the Mediterranean diet pattern was a significant risk factor in the development of pediatric UC (OR: 2.3; 1.2–4.5) [36]. An intervention study examining the impact of the Mediterranean diet pattern in CD (n = 8) demonstrated a trend for reduction in inflammatory biomarkers (p = 0.39) and a tendency for "normalization" of the gut microbiota [37]. The challenge of this study was the lack of statistically significant results and the small sample size. Although a clearer understanding of the role of the Mediterranean Diet Pattern and its impact on IBD is needed, the Mediterranean Diet Pattern may offer a promising approach to reducing markers of inflammation and normalizing the microbiota, but this will need to be confirmed in future clinical trials.

4.8. Popular Diet Plans with Patients

The Specific Carbohydrate Diet™ is one of the most popular diets in the lay literature used by patients with IBD. Unfortunately, there is a lack of evidence-based published data on this diet. To date, the evidence for this diet is based on retrospective surveys and case reports. Based on the book "Breaking the Viscous Cycle", the diet is a strict grain free, sugar-free and complex carbohydrate free diet regimen [112]. An Internet survey (n = 451) that examined the IBD patient's perceptions of the Specific Carbohydrate Diet™, reported that symptoms decreased (abdominal pain, diarrhea, and blood in stool) [38]. Forty-two percent of patients believed the diet helped them achieve remission. A smaller internet survey (n = 51) of patients that had used the Specific Carbohydrate Diet™ for management of IBD reported 84% improved on the diet with 75% reporting improved symptoms [113]. Fifty-four percent reported that they maintained remission through use of the Specific Carbohydrate Diet™. In a case-series report (n = 50), thirty-three subjects (66%) noted complete symptom resolution at a mean of 9.9 months (range 1 to 60 months) after starting the Specific Carbohydrate Diet™ [41]. Patients' self-report of the effectiveness of the Specific Carbohydrate Diet™ was rated as a mean of 91.3% effective in controlling acute flare symptoms (range = 30% to 100%) and a mean of 92.1% effective at maintaining remission (range = 53% to 100%). There are two retrospective studies conducted in pediatric subjects that have examined the outcomes of the Specific Carbohydrate Diet™ on clinical outcomes and laboratory parameters in IBD [39,40]. Twenty six patients with IBD (n = 20 with CD, 6 with UC) plus 10 controls were analyzed [39]. A comparative analysis of the subjects on the Specific Carbohydrate Diet™ versus controls, revealed significant improvement in Pediatric Crohn's Disease Activity Index, CRP, and fecal calprotectin over time for both groups (p = 0.03, 0.03 and 0.03, respectively). Successful maintenance of remission with the Specific Carbohydrate Diet™ allowed some subjects to discontinue medications and maintain disease control on the Specific Carbohydrate Diet™ alone. A small retrospective chart review (n = 11) where pediatric patients followed the Specific Carbohydrate Diet™ for one year found significant improvements in hematocrit, albumin and ESR (p = 0.006, 0.002, 0.002, respectively) [40]. Ten children had improvements in weight percentile and nine children had increases in height percentile while following a strict Specific Carbohydrate Diet™.

Rigorous prospective, RCTs in pediatrics and adults are needed to determine the merits of this diet for management of IBD.

The Paleo Diet is another popular diet amongst patients with IBD. It recommends avoidance of processed food, refined sugars, legumes, dairy, grains and cereals, and instead it advocates for grass-fed meat, wild fish, fruit, vegetables, nuts and "healthy" saturated fat [114]. While it makes sense that a diet that promotes avoidance of refined and extra sugars and processed energy dense food would have health effects, there are no clinical trials that have examined the efficacy of this diet for IBD. Randomized controlled studies are required to determine whether the Paleo diet has beneficial effects over other diet advice.

5. Pharmaconutrition

5.1. Curcumin (Turmeric)

Curcumin is the active ingredient found in turmeric, a common Indian spice. Turmeric is commonly used in Ayurvedic medicine for managing a variety of inflammatory diseases. The yellow pigment (curcumin) present in turmeric has been shown to exhibit numerous anti-inflammatory properties [115]. Curcumin is mainly administered orally in the form of capsules filled with its powder. A randomized controlled trial of 82 subjects with UC demonstrated that curcumin at a dose of 2 g/day (1 g/day following breakfast and 1 g/day following supper), when added to standard therapy, significantly reduced relapse rates [54]. Two subjects relapsed during 6 months of therapy with concurrent curcumin therapy (4.65%), whereas 8 of 39 subjects (20.51%) in the placebo group relapsed ($p = 0.040$). Clinical Activity Index and Endoscopic Activity Indices in the curcumin group significantly improved at six months in subjects with UC in remission (Clinical Activity Index: $p = 0.038$ and Endoscopic Activity Indices: $p = 0.0001$). A systematic review [55] and one Cochrane review [56] conclude that curcumin may be an effective and safe therapy for maintaining remission in UC for up to six months when provided with standard therapy (sulfasalazine and mesalamine). More extensive, well-controlled clinical trials are needed to confirm the benefits of curcumin, at present it appears to be a safe, low cost option for maintenance of remission in UC when added to standard medical therapy.

5.2. Probiotics

The use of probiotics in the maintenance of remission in IBD has been investigated in several clinical trials, however results are inconsistent. The clinical studies have significant heterogeneity, including a variety of different genera, species, strains and doses of probiotics that have been examined, which makes it difficult to draw firm conclusions about efficacy. A meta-analysis of the probiotic strain *Escherichia coli* Nissle 1917 in maintenance of remission in UC found that *E.coli* Nissle 1917 maintained remission as well as standard therapy with mesalazine (OR = 1.07, 95% CI: 0.70–1.64) [116]. Similarly, another meta-analysis showed that probiotics could prevent relapse of UC as effectively as mesalazine ($n = 638$; 316 probiotic group, 322 mesalazine group; RR = 1.0, 95% CI: 0.79–1.26) [117]. The strains shown to be effective were *E. coli* Nissle 1917, *E. coli* (serotype O6:K5:H1), *Lactobacillus* GG and Probio-Tec AB-25 (*L.s acidophilus* La-5 and *Bifidobacterium animalis* subsp. lactis BB-1). Shen et al., (2013) also found that probiotics were comparable to 5-ASA in maintaining therapy in UC ($p = 0.69$, RR = 0.96) [118]. In contrast, a Cochrane collaboration found no difference between probiotics and mesalazine for maintenance of remission in UC (3 studies; 555 patients: OR 1.33; 95% CI: 0.94–1.90) [119]. Supplementation with probiotics in the maintenance of remission in CD is also unfavorable. Two meta-analyses found that the probiotic strains *Lactobacillus* GG and *Lactobacillus johnsonii* LA1 could not prevent relapse in CD (RR = 1.18, 95% CI: 0.81–1.70) [118,120] and concluded that probiotics had no significant benefit in CD with probiotic supplementation ($p = 0.71$, RR = 1.09) [120]. The probiotic strain *Lactobacillus* GG was shown to have significantly benefit in favor of relapse versus the placebo (RR 1.68, 95% CI: 1.07 to 2.64) [118]. Future studies examining probiotics in the maintenance of remission in IBD need to focus on the effects of different probiotic strains and different dosages, together with the homogeneous patient populations to determine which patients are most likely to benefit from probiotic treatment.

5.3. Vitamin D

Vitamin D deficiency is common in IBD patients with a frequency ranging from 16% to 95% [121]. One study reports that patients with UC had more than double the odds of vitamin D deficiency when compared with normal controls (OR = 2.28; 95% CI: 1.18–4.41; I = 41%; p = 0.01) [47]. There is also evidence to suggest that vitamin D deficiency may influence the severity of inflammation in IBD [48–50]. A cross-sectional study revealed that subjects with active disease had more frequent low vitamin D levels (80% vs. 50.4%, p = 0.005) when compared to subjects in remission [49]. A large prospectively collected cohort of 230 subjects demonstrated an inverse association between serum 25(OH)D concentrations and mucosal inflammation, as assessed by the Mayo endoscopy score (p = 0.01), disease activity as indicated by the total Mayo score (p = 0.001), and histologic activity (p = 0.02) in subjects with UC [48]. Serum 25(OH)D concentrations have been found to be inversely correlated with fecal calprotectin (r = −0.207, p = 0.030), particularly among CD subjects in clinical remission (r = −0.242, p = 0.022) [50]. Furthermore, a large cohort of over 3200 IBD patients demonstrated that low plasma 25(OH)D level (<50 nmol/L) was independently associated with an increased risk of subsequent surgery (OR: 1.76; 95% CI: 1.24–2.51) and hospitalization (OR: 2.07; 95% CI: 1.59–2.68) in CD with similar results found in UC [51]. A study that followed IBD patients for five years (n = 965) found that patients with low mean vitamin D levels (<50 nmol/L) had worse pain, disease activity scores, health care utilization and quality of life (p < 0.05) compared with subjects with normal mean vitamin D levels (>75 nmol/mL) [122]. A large-multi-institutional cohort of IBD patients found that patients with vitamin D deficiency (<50 nmol/L) had an increased risk of cancer (OR: 1.82; 95% CI: 1.25–2.65) compared to those patients that had sufficient levels [123].

Given that vitamin D status appears to be an independent risk factor for potential poorer outcomes in IBD, supplementation of vitamin D in this population is judicious. Patients with CD who were deficient in vitamin D (<75 nmol/L) and normalized their 25(OH)D had a reduced likelihood of surgery (OR: 0.56; 95% CI: 0.32–0.98) compared with those who remained deficient [51]. A prospective study in UC (n = 70) demonstrated that low vitamin D levels (<88 nmol/L) increased the risk of clinical relapse over 12 months, as well as was associated with increased presence of endoscopic inflammation (OR: 1.29; 95% CI: 1.07–1.85; p < 0.01) or histologic inflammation (OR: 1.46; 95% CI: 1.13–1.88; p = 0.005) [124]. The optimal concentration for patients with IBD remains unknown, but targeting serum 25(OH)D concentrations above 75 nmol/L appears safe and may have benefits for IBD disease activity, improving bone health, preventing colo-rectal cancer, and alleviating depression [125]. Daily doses of 1800–10,000 IU of vitamin D3 (cholecalciferol) are probably necessary, depending on the baseline vitamin D serum concentration, ileal involvement in CD and body mass index [125]. In a clinical trial by Jorgensen et al. (2010) (n = 108), in CD, oral vitamin D3 treatment with 1200 IU daily increased serum 25(OH)D from mean 69 nmol/L to mean 96 nmol/L after three months of treatment (p < 0.001) [126].

6. Challenges in Creating Evidence-Based Guidelines

Although there are diet intervention trials that show promise in maintaining remission, their efficacy remains in question. The short duration of the interventions (less than 12 weeks), the lack of a proper control group in some instances, and the small sample sizes (less than 20 individuals) make it very challenging for clinicians to draw firm conclusions from existing data. There is an overall lack of objective clinical and endoscopic disease markers. For example, many studies are completed retrospectively and they rely on patient questionnaires regarding disease symptoms, such as pain and stool frequency. Well-designed clinical trials in IBD are urgently required to define the precise role of each of these diets in the prevention or management of IBD. Up until now, the role of diet in IBD is highly undermined by lay and anecdotal reports without sufficient scientific proof.

High quality diet intervention studies for the treatment of IBD need to include the following: (1) quantification of baseline intake of the habitual diet; (2) monitoring of diet adherence through food recalls; (3) large prospective, control trials over a longer-term; (4) use of a control diet to determine the specificity of observed effects to the intervention; (5) use of a variety of endpoints (symptoms, quality of life, clinical biomarkers, endoscopic indices, diet and fecal assessment) to monitor response to diet interventions; and (6) consider the use of IBD animal models (e.g., gnotobiotic mouse model) to discover the mechanisms of pathogenesis.

As research in this field moves forward, a personalized approach to nutrition for individuals or for subsets of patients may be the next frontier. A personalized approach may not only be useful for primary prevention of IBD but also treating disease. We must be mindful that a generalized diet treatment for all patients may not work. Certainly, we are seeing emerging research to suggest that microbiota-targeted approaches have demonstrated some promise for managing chronic disease [127].

7. Conclusions

As our knowledge of the associations between a disrupted intestinal microbiota (dysbiosis) and chronic inflammatory diseases expands, the influence of diet becomes increasingly important. Clearly, diet and nutrition are of major interest for patients with IBD. Patients use a variety of diet strategies in attempt to manage underlying disease, as well as to provide relief from symptoms. Diet plays a key role in IBD pathogenesis, and there is a growing appreciation that the interaction between diet and microbes in a susceptible person contributes significantly to the onset of disease [128]. Several lines of evidence point to aspects of the typical Western diet that may promote the development of IBD. A low-residue diet is frequently recommended for IBD by health professionals [19] to reduce symptoms may be adding further insult. A diet that lacks dietary fiber may accelerate dysbiosis in IBD [94,95].

Pre-illness studies in IBD and intervention trials provide convincing evidence that a plant-based diet, with increased consumption of fruit/vegetables and less red meat intake could be suggested to patients with IBD in remission. Several of the diets/supplements discussed in this review appear to hold promise for in the maintenance of remission in IBD, especially when provided in addition to standard medical therapy.

Acknowledgments: Grant funding from the Canadian Foundation for Dietetic Research to NH and DLG support this work. Grant funding to DLG through the Crohn's and Colitis Canada support this research.

Author Contributions: Both authors actively contributed to the conceptual development of this review paper. Both authors have primary responsibility for the final content.

References

1. Baumgart, D.C.; Sandborn, W.J. Inflammatory bowel disease: Clinical aspects and established and evolving therapies. *Lancet* **2007**, *369*, 1641–1657. [CrossRef]
2. Bhasin, S.; Singh, H.; Targownik, L.E.; Israeli, E.; Bernstein, C.N. Rates and reasons for nonuse of prescription medication for inflammatory bowel disease in a referral clinic. *Inflamm. Bowel Dis.* **2016**, *22*, 919–924. [CrossRef] [PubMed]
3. Whitten, K.E.; Rogers, P.; Ooi, C.K.Y.; Day, A.S. International survey of enteral nutrition protocols used in children with Crohn's disease. *J. Dig. Dis.* **2012**, *13*, 107–112. [CrossRef] [PubMed]
4. Day, A.S.; Whitten, K.E.; Sidler, M.; Lemberg, D.A. Systematic review: Nutritional therapy in paediatric Crohn's disease. *Aliment. Pharmacol. Ther.* **2008**, *27*, 293–307. [CrossRef] [PubMed]
5. Wall, C.L.; Day, A.S.; Gearry, R.B. Use of exclusive enteral nutrition in adults with Crohn's disease: A review. *World J. Gastroenterol.* **2013**, *19*, 7652–7660. [CrossRef] [PubMed]
6. Vidarsdottir, J.B.; Johannsdottir, S.E.; Thorsdottir, I.; Bjornsson, E.; Ramel, A. A cross-sectional study on nutrient intake and -status in inflammatory bowel disease patients. *Nutr. J.* **2016**, *15*, 61. [CrossRef] [PubMed]
7. Piodi, L.P.; Poloni, A.; Ulivieri, F.M. Managing osteoporosis in ulcerative colitis: Something new? *World J. Gastroenterol.* **2014**, *20*, 14087–14098. [CrossRef] [PubMed]
8. Qin, J.; Li, Y.; Cai, Z.; Li, S.; Zhu, J.; Zhang, F.; Peng, Y. A metagenome-wide association study of gut microbiota in type 2 diabetes. *Nature* **2012**, *490*, 55–60. [CrossRef] [PubMed]

9. Weisshof, R.; Chermesh, I. Micronutrient deficiencies in inflammatory bowel disease. *Curr. Opin. Clin. Nutr. Metab. Care* **2015**, *18*, 1. [CrossRef] [PubMed]

10. Filippi, J.; Al-Jaouni, R.; Wiroth, J.; Hébuterne, X.; Schneider, S.M. Nutritional deficiencies in patients with Crohn's disease in remission. *Inflamm. Bowel Dis.* **2006**, *12*, 185–191. [CrossRef] [PubMed]

11. Ballegaard, M.; Bjergstrøm, A.; Brøndum, S.; Hylander, E.; Jensen, L.; Ladefoged, K. Self-reported food intolerance in chronic inflammatory bowel disease. *Scand. J. Gastroenterol.* **1997**, *32*, 569–571. [CrossRef] [PubMed]

12. Kinsey, L.; Burden, S. A survey of people with inflammatory bowel disease to investigate their views of food and nutritional issues. *Eur. J. Clin. Nutr.* **2016**, *70*, 852–854. [CrossRef] [PubMed]

13. Cohen, A.B.; Lee, D.; Long, M.D.; Kappelman, M.D.; Martin, C.F.; Sandler, R.S.; Lewis, J.D. Dietary patterns and self-reported associations of diet with symptoms of inflammatory bowel disease. *Dig. Dis. Sci.* **2013**, *58*, 1322–1328. [CrossRef] [PubMed]

14. Holt, D.Q.; Strauss, B.J.; Moore, G.T. Patients with inflammatory bowel disease and their treating clinicians have different views regarding diet. *J. Hum. Nutr. Diet.* **2016**, *30*, 66–72. [CrossRef] [PubMed]

15. Owczarek, D.; Rodacki, T.; Domagała-Rodacka, R.; Cibor, D.; Mach, T. Diet and nutritional factors in inflammatory bowel diseases. *World J. Gastroenterol.* **2016**, *22*, 895–905. [CrossRef] [PubMed]

16. Walton, M.; Alaunyte, I. Do patients living with ulcerative colitis adhere to healthy eating guidelines? A cross-sectional study. *Br. J. Nutr.* **2014**, *112*, 1628–1635. [CrossRef] [PubMed]

17. Sousa Guerreiro, C.; Cravo, M.; Costa, A.R.; Miranda, A.; Tavares, L.; Moura-Santos, P.; Leitão, C.N. A comprehensive approach to evaluate nutritional status in Crohn's patients in the era of biologic therapy: A case-control study. *Am. J. Gastroenterol.* **2007**, *102*, 2551–2556. [CrossRef] [PubMed]

18. Grimshaw, J.M.; Eccles, M.P.; Lavis, J.N.; Hill, S.J.; Squires, J.E. Knowledge translation of research findings. *Implement. Sci.* **2012**, *7*, 50. [CrossRef] [PubMed]

19. Brown, A.C.; Rampertab, S.D.; Mullin, G.E. Existing dietary guidelines for Crohn's disease and ulcerative colitis. *Expert Rev. Gastroenterol. Hepatol.* **2011**, *5*, 411–425. [CrossRef] [PubMed]

20. Richman, E.; Rhodes, J.M. Review article: Evidence-based dietary advice for patients with inflammatory bowel disease. *Aliment. Pharmacol. Ther.* **2013**, *38*, 1156–1171. [CrossRef] [PubMed]

21. Lee, J.; Allen, R.; Ashley, S.; Becker, S.; Cummins, P.; Gbadamosi, A.; Wilson, S. British Dietetic Association evidence-based guidelines for the dietary management of Crohn's disease in adults. *J. Hum. Nutr. Diet.* **2014**, *27*, 207–218. [CrossRef] [PubMed]

22. Hou, J.K.; Abraham, B.; El-Serag, H. Dietary intake and risk of developing inflammatory bowel disease: A systematic review of the literature. *Am. J. Gastroenterol.* **2011**, *106*, 563–573. [CrossRef] [PubMed]

23. Shivappa, N.; Hebert, J.R.; Rashvand, S.; Rashidkhani, B.; Hekmatdoost, A. Inflammatory Potential of Diet and Risk of Ulcerative Colitis in a Case-Control Study from Iran. *Nutr. Cancer* **2016**, *68*, 404–409. [CrossRef] [PubMed]

24. Ananthakrishnan, A.N.; Khalili, H.; Konijeti, G.G.; Higuchi, L.M.; De Silva, P.; Korzenik, J.R.; Chan, A.T. A prospective study of long-term intake of dietary fiber and risk of Crohn's disease and ulcerative colitis. *Gastroenterology* **2013**, *145*, 970–977. [CrossRef] [PubMed]

25. Racine, A.; Carbonnel, F.; Chan, S.S.M.; Hart, A.R.; Bueno-de-Mesquita, H.B.; Oldenburg, B.; Key, T. Dietary patterns and risk of inflammatory bowel disease in Europe. *Inflamm. Bowel Dis.* **2016**, *22*, 345–354. [CrossRef] [PubMed]

26. Ananthakrishnan, A.N.; Khalili, H.; Konijeti, G.G.; Higuchi, L.M.; de Silva, P.; Fuchs, C.S.; Chan, A.T. Long-term intake of dietary fat and risk of ulcerative colitis and Crohn's disease. *Gut* **2014**, *63*, 776–784. [CrossRef] [PubMed]

27. Tjonneland, A.; Overvad, K.; Bergmann, M.M.; Nagel, G.; Linseisen, J.; Hallmans, G.; Palmqvist, R.; Sjodin, H.; Hagglund, G.; Berglund, G.; et al. Linoleic acid, a dietary *n*-6 polyunsaturated fatty acid, and the aetiology of ulcerative colitis: A nested case-control study within a European prospective cohort study. *Gut* **2009**, *58*, 1606–1611. [PubMed]

28. Opstelten, J.L.; Leenders, M.; Dik, V.K.; Chan, S.S.M.; van Schaik, F.D.M.; Khaw, K.-T.; Grip, O. Dairy Products, Dietary Calcium, and Risk of Inflammatory Bowel Disease: Results From a European Prospective Cohort Investigation. *Inflamm. Bowel Dis.* **2016**, *22*, 1403–1411. [CrossRef] [PubMed]

29. Amre, D.K.; D'Souza, S.; Morgan, K.; Seidman, G.; Lambrette, P.; Grimard, G.; Chotard, V. Imbalances in dietary consumption of fatty acids, vegetables, and fruits are associated with risk for crohn's disease in children. *Am. J. Gastroenterol.* **2007**, *102*, 2016–2025. [CrossRef] [PubMed]

30. Sakamoto, N.; Kono, S.; Wakai, K.; Fukuda, Y.; Satomi, M.; Shimoyama, T.; Kobashi, G. Dietary risk factors for inflammatory bowel disease: A multicenter case-control study in Japan. *Inflamm. Bowel Dis.* **2005**, *11*, 154–163. [CrossRef] [PubMed]

31. Jantchou, P.; Morois, S.; Clavel-Chapelon, F.; Boutron-Ruault, M.-C.; Carbonnel, F. Animal protein intake and risk of inflammatory bowel disease: The E3N prospective study. *Am. J. Gastroenterol.* **2010**, *105*, 2195–2201. [CrossRef] [PubMed]

32. Gearry, R.B.; Irving, P.M.; Barrett, J.S.; Nathan, D.M.; Shepherd, S.J.; Gibson, P.R. Reduction of dietary poorly absorbed short-chain carbohydrates (FODMAPs) improves abdominal symptoms in patients with inflammatory bowel disease-a pilot study. *J. Crohn's Colitis* **2009**, *3*, 8–14. [CrossRef] [PubMed]

33. Prince, A.C.; Myers, C.E.; Joyce, T.; Irving, P.; Lomer, M.C.E.; Whelan, K. Fermentable Carbohydrate Restriction (Low FODMAP Diet) in Clinical Practice Improves Functional Gastrointestinal Symptoms in Patients with Inflammatory Bowel Disease. *Inflamm. Bowel Dis.* **2016**, *22*, 1129–1136. [CrossRef] [PubMed]

34. Maagaard, L.; Ankersen, D.V.; Vegh, Z.; Burisch, J.; Jensen, L.; Pedersen, N.; Munkholm, P. Follow-up of patients with functional bowel symptoms treated with a low FODMAP diet. *World J. Gastroenterol.* **2016**, *22*, 4009–4019. [CrossRef] [PubMed]

35. De Filippis, F.; Pellegrini, N.; Vannini, L.; Jeffery, I.B.; La Storia, A.; Laghi, L.; Turroni, S. High-level adherence to a Mediterranean diet beneficially impacts the gut microbiota and associated metabolome. *Gut* **2015**. [CrossRef] [PubMed]

36. Strisciuglio, C.; Giugliano, F.P.; Martinelli, M.; Cenni, S.; Greco, L.; Staiano, A.; Miele, E. Impact of Environmental and Familial Factors in a Cohort of Pediatric Patients with Inflammatory Bowel Disease. *J. Pediatr. Gastroenterol. Nutr.* **2016**. [CrossRef] [PubMed]

37. Marlow, G.; Ellett, S.; Ferguson, I.R.; Zhu, S.; Karunasinghe, N.; Jesuthasan, A.C.; Ferguson, L.R. Transcriptomics to study the effect of a Mediterranean-inspired diet on inflammation in Crohn's disease patients. *Hum. Genom.* **2013**, *7*, 24. [CrossRef] [PubMed]

38. Suskind, D.L.; Wahbeh, G.; Cohen, S.A.; Damman, C.J.; Klein, J.; Braly, K.; Lee, D. Patients Perceive Clinical Benefit with the Specific Carbohydrate Diet for Inflammatory Bowel Disease. *Dig. Dis. Sci.* **2016**, *61*, 3255–3260. [CrossRef] [PubMed]

39. Obih, C.; Wahbeh, G.; Lee, D.; Braly, K.; Giefer, M.; Shaffer, M.L.; Suskind, D.L. Specific carbohydrate diet for pediatric inflammatory bowel disease in clinical practice within an academic IBD center. *Nutrition* **2015**, *32*, 418–425. [CrossRef] [PubMed]

40. Burgis, J.C.; Nguyen, K.; Park, K.T.; Cox, K. Response to strict and liberalized specific carbohydrate diet in pediatric Crohn's disease. *World J. Gastroenterol.* **2016**, *22*, 2111–2117. [CrossRef] [PubMed]

41. Kakodkar, S.; Farooqui, A.J.; Mikolaitis, S.L.; Mutlu, E.A. The Specific Carbohydrate Diet for Inflammatory Bowel Disease: A Case Series. *J. Acad. Nutr. Diet.* **2015**, *115*, 1226–1232. [CrossRef] [PubMed]

42. Levenstein, S.; Prantera, C.; Luzi, C.; D'Ubaldi, A. Low residue or normal diet in Crohn's disease: A prospective controlled study in Italian patients. *Gut* **1985**, *26*, 989–993. [CrossRef] [PubMed]

43. Chiba, M.; Abe, T.; Tsuda, H.; Sugawara, T.; Tsuda, S.; Tozawa, H.; Imai, H. Lifestyle-related disease in Crohn's disease: Relapse prevention by a semi-vegetarian diet. *World. J. Gastroenterol.* **2010**, *16*, 2484–2495. [CrossRef] [PubMed]

44. Gunasekeera, V.; Mendall, M.A.; Chan, D.; Kumar, D. Treatment of Crohn's Disease with an IgG4-Guided Exclusion Diet: A Randomized Controlled Trial. *Dig. Dis. Sci.* **2016**, *61*, 1148–1157. [CrossRef] [PubMed]

45. Olendzki, B.C.; Silverstein, T.D.; Persuitte, G.M.; Ma, Y.; Baldwin, K.R.; Cave, D. An anti-inflammatory diet as treatment for inflammatory bowel disease: A case series report. *Nutr. J.* **2014**, *13*, 5. [CrossRef] [PubMed]

46. Academy, A.; Pediatrics, O.F.; Recommendations, C.; Guidelines, C.P. Classifying recommendations for clinical practice guidelines. *Pediatrics* **2004**, *114*, 874–877.

47. Del Pinto, R.; Pietropaoli, D.; Chandar, A.K.; Ferri, C.; Cominelli, F. Association Between Inflammatory Bowel Disease and Vitamin D Deficiency: A Systematic Review and Meta-analysis. *Inflamm. Bowel Dis.* **2015**, *21*, 2708–2717. [CrossRef] [PubMed]

48. Meckel, K.; Li, Y.C.; Lim, J.; Kocherginsky, M.; Weber, C.; Almoghrabi, A.; Cohen, R.D. Serum 25-hydroxyvitamin D concentration is inversely associated with mucosal inflammation in patients with ulcerative colitis. *Am. J. Clin. Nutr.* **2016**, *104*, 113–120. [CrossRef] [PubMed]

49. Torki, M.; Gholamrezaei, A.; Mirbagher, L.; Danesh, M.; Kheiri, S.; Emami, M.H. Vitamin D Deficiency Associated with Disease Activity in Patients with Inflammatory Bowel Diseases. *Dig. Dis. Sci.* **2015**, *60*, 3085–3091. [CrossRef] [PubMed]

50. Raftery, T.; Merrick, M.; Healy, M.; Mahmud, N.; O'Morain, C.; Smith, S.; O'Sullivan, M. Vitamin D Status Is Associated with Intestinal Inflammation as Measured by Fecal Calprotectin in Crohn's Disease in Clinical Remission. *Dig. Dis. Sci.* **2015**, *60*, 2427–2435. [CrossRef] [PubMed]

51. Ananthakrishnan, A.N.; Cagan, A.; Gainer, V.S.; Cai, T.; Cheng, S.-C.; Savova, G.; Shaw, S.Y. Normalization of plasma 25-hydroxy vitamin D is associated with reduced risk of surgery in Crohn's disease. *Inflamm. Bowel Dis.* **2013**, *19*, 1921–1927. [CrossRef] [PubMed]

52. Fernandez-Banares, F.; Hinojosa, J.; Sanchez-Lombrana, J.L.; Navarro, E.; Martinez-Salmeron, J.F.; Garcia-Puges, A.; Gine, J.J. Randomized clinical trial of Plantago ovata seeds (dietary fiber) as compared with mesalamine in maintaining remission in ulcerative colitis. Spanish Group for the Study of Crohn's Disease and Ulcerative Colitis (GETECCU). *Am. J. Gastroenterol.* **1999**, *94*, 427–433. [CrossRef] [PubMed]

53. Hallert, C.; Kaldma, M.; Petersson, B.G. Ispaghula husk may relieve gastrointestinal symptoms in ulcerative colitis in remission. *Scand. J. Gastroenterol.* **1991**, *26*, 747–750. [CrossRef] [PubMed]

54. Hanai, H.; Iida, T.; Takeuchi, K.; Watanabe, F.; Maruyama, Y.; Andoh, A.; Yamada, M. Curcumin maintenance therapy for ulcerative colitis: Randomized, multicenter, double-blind, placebo-controlled trial. *Clin. Gastroenterol. Hepatol.* **2006**, *4*, 1502–1506. [CrossRef] [PubMed]

55. Taylor, R.A.; Leonard, M.C. Curcumin for inflammatory bowel disease: A review of human studies. *Altern. Med. Rev.* **2011**, *16*, 152. [PubMed]

56. Kumar, S.; Ahuja, V.; Sankar, M.J.; Kumar, A.; Moss, A.C. Curcumin for maintenance of remission in ulcerative colitis. *Cochrane Database Syst. Rev.* **2012**. [CrossRef]

57. Hallert, C.; Bjorck, I.; Nyman, M.; Pousette, A.; Granno, C.; Svensson, H. Increasing fecal butyrate in ulcerative colitis patients by diet: Controlled pilot study. *Inflamm. Bowel Dis.* **2003**, *9*, 116–121. [CrossRef] [PubMed]

58. Hanai, H.; Kanauchi, O.; Mitsuyama, K.; Andoh, A.; Takeuchi, K.; Takayuki, I.; Bamba, T. Germinated barley foodstuff prolongs remission in patients with ulcerative colitis. *Int. J. Mol. Med.* **2004**, *13*, 643–647. [CrossRef] [PubMed]

59. Faghfoori, Z.; Shakerhosseini, R.; Navai, L.; Somi, M.H.; Nikniaz, Z.; Abadi, A. Effects of an Oral Supplementation of Germinated Barley Foodstuff on Serum CRP Level and Clinical Signs in Patients with Ulcerative Colitis. *Health Promot. Perspect.* **2014**, *4*, 116–121. [PubMed]

60. Faghfoori, Z.; Navai, L.; Shakerhosseini, R.; Somi, M.H.; Nikniaz, Z.; Norouzi, M.F. Effects of an oral supplementation of germinated barley foodstuff on serum tumour necrosis factor-alpha, interleukin-6 and -8 in patients with ulcerative colitis. *Ann. Clin. Biochem.* **2011**, *48*, 233–237. [CrossRef] [PubMed]

61. Brotherton, C.S.; Taylor, A.G.; Bourguignon, C.; Anderson, J.G. A high-fiber diet may improve bowel function and health-related quality of life in patients with Crohn disease. *Gastroenterol. Nurs.* **2014**, *37*, 206–216. [CrossRef] [PubMed]

62. Ng, S.C.; Tang, W.; Ching, J.Y.; Wong, M.; Chow, C.M.; Hui, A.J.; Li, M.F. Incidence and phenotype of inflammatory bowel disease based on results from the Asia-pacific Crohn's and colitis epidemiology study. *Gastroenterology* **2013**, *145*, 158 e2–165 e2. [CrossRef] [PubMed]

63. Lovasz, B.D.; Golovics, P.A.; Vegh, Z.; Lakatos, P.L. New trends in inflammatory bowel disease epidemiology and disease course in Eastern Europe. *Dig. Liver Dis.* **2013**, *45*, 269–276. [CrossRef] [PubMed]

64. Ukwenya, A.Y.; Ahmed, A.; Odigie, V.I.; Mohammed, A. Inflammatory bowel disease in Nigerians: Still a rare diagnosis? *Ann. Afr. Med.* **2011**, *10*, 175–179. [CrossRef] [PubMed]

65. Al-Mofarreh, M.A.; Al-Mofleh, I.A. Emerging inflammatory bowel disease in saudi outpatients: A report of 693 cases. *Saudi J. Gastroenterol.* **2013**, *19*, 16–22. [CrossRef] [PubMed]

66. Archampong, T.N.; Nkrumah, K.N. Inflammatory bowel disease in Accra: What new trends. *West Afr. J. Med.* **2013**, *32*, 40–44. [PubMed]

67. Ng, S.C. Emerging leadership lecture: Inflammatory bowel disease in Asia: Emergence of a "Western" disease. *J. Gastroenterol. Hepatol.* **2015**, *30*, 440–445. [CrossRef] [PubMed]

68. Holmboe-Ottesen, G.; Wandel, M. Changes in dietary habits after migration and consequences for health: A focus on South Asians in Europe. *Food Nutr. Res.* **2012**, *56*, 1–13. [CrossRef] [PubMed]

69. Pugazhendhi, S.; Sahu, M.K.; Subramanian, V.; Pulimood, A.; Ramakrishna, B.S. Environmental factors associated with Crohn's disease in India. *Indian J. Gastroenterol.* **2011**, *30*, 264–269. [CrossRef] [PubMed]

70. Legaki, E.; Gazouli, M. Influence of environmental factors in the development of inflammatory bowel diseases. *World J. Gastrointest. Pharmacol. Ther.* **2016**, *7*, 112–125. [CrossRef] [PubMed]

71. Lee, D.; Albenberg, L.; Compher, C.; Baldassano, R.; Piccoli, D.; Lewis, J.D.; Wu, G.D. Diet in the pathogenesis and treatment of inflammatory bowel diseases. *Gastroenterology* **2015**, *148*, 1087–1106. [CrossRef] [PubMed]

72. Devereux, G. The increase in the prevalence of asthma and allergy: Food for thought. *Nat. Rev. Immunol.* **2006**, *6*, 869–874. [CrossRef] [PubMed]

73. Huang, E.Y.; Devkota, S.; Moscoso, D.; Chang, E.B.; Leone, V.A. The role of diet in triggering human inflammatory disorders in the modern age. *Microbes Infect.* **2013**, *15*, 765–774. [CrossRef] [PubMed]

74. Hart, A.R.; Luben, R.; Olsen, A.; Tjonneland, A.; Linseisen, J.; Nagel, G.; Appleby, P. Diet in the aetiology of ulcerative colitis: A European prospective cohort study. *Digestion* **2008**, *77*, 57–64. [CrossRef] [PubMed]

75. Geerling, B.J.; Dagnelie, P.C.; Badart-Smook, A.; Russel, M.G.; Stockbrugger, R.W.; Brummer, R.J. Diet as a risk factor for the development of ulcerative colitis. *Am. J. Gastroenterol.* **2000**, *95*, 1008–1013. [CrossRef] [PubMed]

76. Reif, S.; Klein, I.; Lubin, F.; Farbstein, M.; Hallak, A.; Gilat, T. Pre-illness dietary factors in inflammatory bowel disease. *Gut* **1997**, *40*, 754–760. [CrossRef] [PubMed]

77. Schwingshackl, L.; Hoffmann, G. Adherence to Mediterranean diet and risk of cancer: A systematic review and meta-analysis of observational studies. *Int. J. Cancer* **2014**, *135*, 1884–1897. [CrossRef] [PubMed]

78. Schwingshackl, L.; Missbach, B.; König, J.; Hoffmann, G. Adherence to a Mediterranean diet and risk of diabetes: A systematic review and meta-analysis. *Public Health Nutr.* **2015**, *18*, 1292–1299. [CrossRef] [PubMed]

79. Estruch, R. Anti-inflammatory effects of the Mediterranean diet: The experience of the PREDIMED study. *Proc. Nutr. Soc.* **2010**, *69*, 333–340. [CrossRef] [PubMed]

80. Serra-Majem, L.; Bes-Rastrollo, M.; Román-Viñas, B.; Pfrimer, K.; Sánchez-Villegas, A.; Martínez-González, M.A. Dietary patterns and nutritional adequacy in a Mediterranean country. *Br. J. Nutr.* **2009**, *101*, S21–S28. [CrossRef] [PubMed]

81. Niewiadomski, O.; Studd, C.; Wilson, J.; Williams, J.; Hair, C.; Knight, R.; Dowling, D. Influence of food and lifestyle on the risk of developing inflammatory bowel disease. *Intern. Med. J.* **2016**, *46*, 669–676. [CrossRef] [PubMed]

82. Persson, P.G.; Ahlbom, A.; Hellers, G. Diet and inflammatory bowel disease: A case-control study. *Epidemiology* **1992**, *3*, 47–52. [CrossRef] [PubMed]

83. Feagan, B.G.; Sandborn, W.J.; Mittmann, U.; Bar-Meir, S.; D'Haens, G.; Bradette, M.; Hébuterne, X. Omega-3 free fatty acids for the maintenance of remission in Crohn disease: The EPIC Randomized Controlled Trials. *JAMA* **2008**, *299*, 1690–1697. [CrossRef] [PubMed]

84. Lev-Tzion, R.; Griffiths, A.M.; Leder, O.; Turner, D. Omega 3 fatty acids (fish oil) for maintenance of remission in Crohn's disease. *Cochrane Database Syst. Rev.* **2014**, *2*, CD006320.

85. Turner, D.; Shah, P.S.; Steinhart, A.H.; Zlotkin, S.; Griffiths, A.M. Maintenance of remission in inflammatory bowel disease using omega-3 fatty acids (fish oil): A systematic review and meta-analyses. *Inflamm. Bowel Dis.* **2011**, *17*, 336–345. [CrossRef] [PubMed]

86. Cabré, E.; Domènech, E. Impact of environmental and dietary factors on the course of inflammatory bowel disease. *World J. Gastroenterol.* **2012**, *18*, 3814–3822. [CrossRef] [PubMed]

87. John, S.; Luben, R.; Shrestha, S.S.; Welch, A.; Khaw, K.-T.; Hart, A.R. Dietary *n*-3 polyunsaturated fatty acids and the aetiology of ulcerative colitis: A UK prospective cohort study. *Eur. J. Gastroenterol. Hepatol.* **2010**, *22*, 602–606. [CrossRef] [PubMed]

88. Uchiyama, K.; Nakamura, M.; Odahara, S.; Koido, S.; Katahira, K.; Shiraishi, H.; Tajiri, H. *N*-3 polyunsaturated fatty acid diet therapy for patients with inflammatory bowel disease. *Inflamm. Bowel Dis.* **2010**, *16*, 1696–1707. [CrossRef] [PubMed]

89. Vanhauwaert, E.; Matthys, C.; Verdonck, L.; De Preter, V. Low-Residue and Low-Fiber Diets in Gastrointestinal Disease Management. *Adv. Nutr.* **2015**, *6*, 820–827. [CrossRef] [PubMed]

90. Hwang, C.; Ross, V.; Mahadevan, U. Popular exclusionary diets for inflammatory bowel disease: The search for a dietary culprit. *Inflamm. Bowel Dis.* **2014**, *20*, 732–741. [CrossRef] [PubMed]

91. Asakura, H.; Suzuki, K.; Kitahora, T.; Morizane, T. Is there a link between food and intestinal microbes and the occurrence of Crohn's disease and ulcerative colitis? *J. Gastroenterol. Hepatol.* **2008**, *23*, 1794–1801. [CrossRef] [PubMed]

92. Packey, C.D.; Sartor, R.B. Commensal bacteria, traditional and opportunistic pathogens, dysbiosis and bacterial killing in inflammatory bowel diseases. *Curr. Opin. Infect. Dis.* **2009**, *22*, 292–301. [CrossRef] [PubMed]

93. Sartor, R.B. Microbial Influences in Inflammatory Bowel Diseases. *Gastroenterology* **2008**, *134*, 577–594. [CrossRef] [PubMed]

94. Walters, S.S.; Quiros, A.; Rolston, M.; Grishina, I.; Li, J.; Fenton, A.; Nieves, R. Analysis of Gut Microbiome and Diet Modification in Patients with Crohn's Disease. *SOJ Microbiol. Infect. Dis.* **2014**, *2*, 1–13. [CrossRef]

95. Zhang, Y.-J.; Li, S.; Gan, R.-Y.; Zhou, T.; Xu, D.-P.; Li, H.-B. Impacts of gut bacteria on human health and diseases. *Int. J. Mol. Sci.* **2015**, *16*, 7493–7519. [CrossRef] [PubMed]

96. Bartel, G.; Weiss, I.; Turetschek, K.; Schima, W.; Puspok, A.; Waldhoer, T.; Gasche, C. Ingested matter affects intestinal lesions in Crohn's disease. *Inflamm. Bowel Dis.* **2008**, *14*, 374–382. [CrossRef] [PubMed]

97. Gibson, P.R.; Shepherd, S.J. Evidence-based dietary management of functional gastrointestinal symptoms: The FODMAP approach. *J. Gastroenterol. Hepatol.* **2010**, *25*, 252–258. [CrossRef] [PubMed]

98. Rao, S.S.C.; Yu, S.; Fedewa, A. Systematic review: Dietary fibre and FODMAP-restricted diet in the management of constipation and irritable bowel syndrome. *Aliment. Pharmacol. Ther.* **2015**, *41*, 1256–1270. [CrossRef] [PubMed]

99. Marsh, A.; Eslick, E.M.; Eslick, G.D. Does a diet low in FODMAPs reduce symptoms associated with functional gastrointestinal disorders? A comprehensive systematic review and meta-analysis. *Eur. J. Nutr.* **2016**, *55*, 897–906. [CrossRef] [PubMed]

100. Simrén, M.; Axelsson, J.; Gillberg, R.; Abrahamsson, H.; Svedlund, J.; Björnsson, E.S. Quality of life in inflammatory bowel disease in remission: The impact of IBS-like symptoms and associated psychological factors. *Am. J. Gastroenterol.* **2002**, *97*, 389–396. [CrossRef]

101. Takagi, S.; Utsunomiya, K.; Kuriyama, S.; Yokoyama, H.; Takahashi, S.; Iwabuchi, M.; Sasaki, I. Effectiveness of an "half elemental diet" as maintenance therapy for Crohn's disease: A randomized-controlled trial. *Aliment. Pharmacol. Ther.* **2006**, *24*, 1333–1340. [CrossRef] [PubMed]

102. Takagi, S.; Utsunomiya, K.; Kuriyama, S.; Yokoyama, H.; Takahashi, S.; Umemura, K.; Funayama, Y. Quality of life of patients and medical cost of "half elemental diet" as maintenance therapy for Crohn's disease: Secondary outcomes of a randomised controlled trial. *Dig. Liver Dis.* **2009**, *41*, 390–394. [CrossRef] [PubMed]

103. Gophna, U.; Sommerfeld, K.; Gophna, S.; Doolittle, W.F.; Van Zanten, S.J.O. Differences between tissue-associated intestinal microfloras of patients with Crohn's disease and ulcerative colitis. *J. Clin. Microbiol.* **2006**, *44*, 4136–4141. [CrossRef] [PubMed]

104. Ott, S.J.; Musfeldt, M.; Wenderoth, D.F.; Hampe, J.; Brant, O.; Fölsch, U.R.; Schreiber, S. Reduction in diversity of the colonic mucosa associated bacterial microflora in patients with active inflammatory bowel disease. *Gut* **2004**, *53*, 685–693. [CrossRef] [PubMed]

105. Wedlake, L.; Slack, N.; Andreyev, H.J.; Whelan, K. Fiber in the treatment and maintenance of inflammatory bowel disease: A systematic review of randomized controlled trials. *Inflamm. Bowel Dis.* **2014**, *20*, 576–586. [CrossRef] [PubMed]

106. Roediger, W.E. Utilization of nutrients by isolated epithelial cells of the rat colon. *Gastroenterology* **1982**, *83*, 424–429. [PubMed]

107. Vernia, P.; Marcheggiano, A.; Caprilli, R.; Frieri, G.; Corrao, G.; Valpiani, D.; Torsoli, A. Short-chain fatty acid topical treatment in distal ulcerative colitis. *Aliment. Pharmacol. Ther.* **1995**, *9*, 309–313. [CrossRef] [PubMed]

108. Kanauchi, O.; Suga, T.; Tochihara, M.; Hibi, T.; Naganuma, M.; Homma, T.; Andoh, A. Treatment of ulcerative colitis by feeding with germinated barley foodstuff: First report of a multicenter open control trial. *J. Gastroenterol.* **2002**, *37*, 67–72. [CrossRef] [PubMed]

109. Turner, D.; Steinhart, A.H.; Griffiths, A.M. Omega 3 fatty acids (fish oil) for maintenance of remission in ulcerative colitis. *Cochrane Database Syst. Rev.* **2007**. [CrossRef]

110. Shivananda, S.; Lennard-Jones, J.; Logan, R.; Fear, N.; Price, A.; Carpenter, L.; Van Blankenstein, M. Incidence of inflammatory bowel disease across Europe: Is there a difference between north and south? Results of the European Collaborative Study on Inflammatory Bowel Disease (EC-IBD). *Gut* **1996**, *39*, 690–697. [CrossRef] [PubMed]

111. Bach-Faig, A.; Berry, E.M.; Lairon, D.; Reguant, J.; Trichopoulou, A.; Dernini, S.; Serra-Majem, L. Mediterranean diet pyramid today. Science and cultural updates. *Public Health Nutr.* **2011**, *14*, 2274–2284. [CrossRef] [PubMed]

112. Gottschall, E. *Breaking the Viscous Cycle*; Kirkton Press: Baltimore, MD, USA, 1994.

113. Nieves, R.; Jackson, R.T. Specific carbohydrate diet in treatment of inflammatory bowel disease. *Tenn. Med.* **2004**, *97*, 407. [PubMed]

114. Cordain, L. The Paleo Diet. 2016. Available online: http://thepaleodiet.com/ (accessed on 30 September 2016).

115. Goel, A.; Kunnumakkara, A.B.; Aggarwal, B.B. Curcumin as "Curecumin": From kitchen to clinic. *Biochem. Pharmacol.* **2008**, *75*, 787–809. [CrossRef] [PubMed]

116. Losurdo, G.; Iannone, A.; Contaldo, A.; Ierardi, E.; Di Leo, A.; Principi, M. Escherichia coli Nissle 1917 in Ulcerative Colitis Treatment: Systematic Review and Meta-analysis. *J. Gastrointest. Liver Dis.* **2015**, *24*, 499–505.

117. Fujiya, M.; Ueno, N. Kohgo, Probiotics for maintenance of remission in inflammatory bowel diseases: A meta-anlysis of randomized controlled trials. *Clin. J.Gastroenterol.* **2014**, *1*, 1–13. [CrossRef]

118. Shen, J.; Ran, H.Z.; Yin, M.H.; Zhou, T.X.; Xiao, D.S. Meta-analysis: The effect and adverse events of Lactobacilli versus placebo in maintenance therapy for Crohn disease. *Intern. Med. J.* **2009**, *39*, 103–109. [CrossRef] [PubMed]

119. Naidoo, K.; Gordon, M.; Fagbemi, A.O.; Thomas, A.G.; Akobeng, A.K. Probiotics for maintenance of remission in ulcerative colitis. *Cochrane Database Syst. Rev.* **2011**. [CrossRef]

120. Shen, J.; Zuo, Z.X.; Mao, A.P. Effect of probiotics on inducing remission and maintaining therapy in ulcerative colitis, Crohn's disease, and pouchitis: Meta-analysis of randomized controlled trials. *Inflamm. Bowel Dis.* **2014**, *20*, 21–35. [CrossRef]

121. Mouli, V.P.; Ananthakrishnan, A.N. Review article: Vitamin D and inflammatory bowel diseases. *Aliment. Pharmacol. Ther.* **2014**, *39*, 125–136. [CrossRef] [PubMed]

122. Kabbani, T.A.; Koutroubakis, I.E.; Schoen, R.E.; Ramos-Rivers, C.; Shah, N.; Swoger, J.; Baidoo, L. Association of Vitamin D Level With Clinical Status in Inflammatory Bowel Disease: A 5-Year Longitudinal Study. *Am. J. Gastroenterol.* **2016**, *111*, 712–719. [CrossRef]

123. Ananthakrishnan, A.N.; Cheng, S.-C.; Cai, T.; Cagan, A.; Gainer, V.S.; Szolovits, P.; Kohane, I. Association between reduced plasma 25-hydroxy vitamin D and increased risk of cancer in patients with inflammatory bowel diseases. *Clin. Gastroenterol. Hepatol.* **2014**, *12*, 821–827. [CrossRef] [PubMed]

124. Gubatan, J.; Mitsuhashi, S.; Zenlea, T.; Rosenberg, L.; Robson, S.; Moss, A.C. Low Serum Vitamin D During Remission Increases Risk of Clinical Relapse in Patients With Ulcerative Colitis. *Clin. Gastroenterol Hepatol.* **2017**, *15*, 240–246. [CrossRef] [PubMed]

125. Hlavaty, T.; Krajcovicova, A.; Payer, J. Vitamin D therapy in inflammatory bowel diseases: Who, in what form, and how much? *J. Crohns Colitis* **2015**, *9*, 198–209. [CrossRef] [PubMed]

126. Jorgensen, S.P.; Agnholt, J.; Glerup, H.; Lyhne, S.; Villadsen, G.E.; Hvas, C.L.; Dahlerup, J.F. Clinical trial: Vitamin D3 treatment in Crohn's disease—A randomized double-blind placebo-controlled study. *Aliment. Pharmacol. Ther.* **2010**, *32*, 377–383. [CrossRef] [PubMed]

127. Zeevi, D.; Korem, T.; Zmora, N.; Israeli, D.; Rothschild, D.; Weinberger, A.; Suez, J. Personalized Nutrition by Prediction of Glycemic Responses. *Cell* **2015**, *163*, 1079–1095. [CrossRef] [PubMed]

128. Dolan, K.T.; Chang, E.B. Diet, gut microbes, and the pathogenesis of inflammatory bowel diseases. *Mol. Nutr. Food Res.* **2016**. [CrossRef] [PubMed]

Potential Impact of Diet on Treatment Effect from Anti-TNF Drugs in Inflammatory Bowel Disease

Vibeke Andersen [1,2,*], Axel Kornerup Hansen [3] and Berit Lilienthal Heitmann [4,5,6]

[1] Focused Research Unit for Molecular Diagnostic and Clinical Research, IRS-Centre Sonderjylland, Hospital of Southern Jutland, Åbenrå 6200, Denmark

[2] Institute of Molecular Medicine, University of Southern Denmark, Odense 5000, Denmark

[3] Department of Veterinary and Animal Sciences, University of Copenhagen, Frederiksberg 1871, Denmark; akh@sund.ku.dk

[4] Research Unit for Dietary Studies, Parker Institute, Frederiksberg 2000, Denmark; berit.lilienthal.heitmann@regionh.dk

[5] Section for General Medicine, Department of Public Health, University of Copenhagen, Copenhagen 1353, Denmark

[6] National Institute of Public Health, University of Southern Denmark, Odense 5000, Denmark

[*] Correspondence: vandersen@health.sdu.dk

Abstract: We wanted to investigate the current knowledge on the impact of diet on anti-TNF response in inflammatory bowel diseases (IBD), to identify dietary factors that warrant further investigations in relation to anti-TNF treatment response, and, finally, to discuss potential strategies for such investigations. PubMed was searched using specified search terms. One small prospective study on diet and anti-TNF treatment in 56 patients with CD found similar remission rates after 56 weeks among 32 patients with good compliance that received concomitant enteral nutrition and 24 with poor compliance that had no dietary restrictions (78% versus 67%, $p = 0.51$). A meta-analysis of 295 patients found higher odds of achieving clinical remission and remaining in clinical remission among patients on combination therapy with specialised enteral nutrition and Infliximab (IFX) compared with IFX monotherapy (OR 2.73; 95% CI: 1.73–4.31, $p < 0.01$, OR 2.93; 95% CI: 1.66–5.17, $p < 0.01$, respectively). In conclusion, evidence-based knowledge on impact of diet on anti-TNF treatment response for clinical use is scarce. Here we propose a mechanism by which Western style diet high in meat and low in fibre may promote colonic inflammation and potentially impact treatment response to anti-TNF drugs. Further studies using hypothesis-driven and data-driven strategies in prospective observational, animal and interventional studies are warranted.

Keywords: lifestyle factors; chronic inflammatory diseases; treatment result; treatment response; diet; meat intake; dietary pattern; food; mucosa associated bacteria; epithelium-associated bacteria; microbiome; fibre intake; personalized medicine; mucus; sulphate-reducing bacteria; mucin-degrading bacteria; Western style diet; anti-TNF

---

1. Introduction

Inflammatory bowel diseases (IBD), including Crohn's Disease (CD) and ulcerative colitis (UC), are chronic lifelong illnesses of early onset that substantially affect the life quality of the patients and their families [1–3]. Up to 1% of the population in the Western world is affected [4]. The disease burden is continuously rising in the Western world and in newly industrialised countries in Asia, South America, and the Middle East [5]. Thus, more patients will need medical treatment.

The management of IBD has changed significantly during the last two decades [6,7]. The inadequate response to conventional therapy in a large portion of patients and the advances in understanding the role of the inflammatory pathways in IBD [8], has led to the development of bioengineered therapeutic agents targeting key pro-inflammatory molecules. Anti-TNF acts through targeting and neutralising the effect of tumour necrosis factor (TNF-α), thereby diminishing the downstream effects of TNF-α activation. However, the pharmacodynamics of anti-TNF drugs seem to depend on other factors than simply the TNF-binding capacities [8]. Hence, their precise mechanism of action remains unclear. Anti-TNF drugs have proven highly effective for many patients, yet, a significant proportion of the patients do not respond to the treatment (i.e., "primary failures") or lose the effect over time (i.e., "secondary failures") [6–8]. Despite the introduction of biological treatment of IBD, surgery is still required in 30%–40% of patients with CD and in 25%–30% of patients with UC at some point during their lifetime [9,10]. Sub-therapeutic drug levels and the formation of anti-drug antibodies may decrease their efficacy [11]. Genetics have also been found to define the response to anti-TNF [12,13].

Many patients ask their health care professionals about recommendations for dietary intake, and for now we are not able to provide evidence-based answers. Dietary recommendations that can help to improve the outcome of anti-TNF drugs are thus highly warranted by patients. Furthermore, knowledge on diet that supports good treatment response is important for the health care system in order to improve the utilization of the health care resources, as the resources spent for the care of IBD patients are expected to increase exponentially in the coming years [5].

Given the important role of environment on the development of IBD, we hypothesised that lifestyle may impact the effect of anti-TNF drugs. We therefore set out to investigate the current knowledge on the impact of diet on anti-TNF response. Furthermore, we wanted to identify dietary factors that warrant further investigations in relation to anti-TNF treatment response, based on knowledge of their effects on gut inflammation. Finally, we discuss potential strategies for such investigations. For review of diet and risk of IBD please refer to recent papers by Lee et al. and Andersen et al. [14,15].

2. Materials and Methods

PubMed was searched using the search terms shown in Table 1. In general, the Boolean terms "OR" was used within the groups and "AND" between the groups. The "Similar articles", "Cited by" function in PubMed and references for key studies were used for finding more articles. Retrieved articles were evaluated for relevance by VA.

Table 1. Various combinations of these search terms were used. Both AND (between the groups) and OR (within the groups) were used. The "Similar articles", "Cited by" functions in PubMed and references for key studies were used for finding more articles.

Group 1	Group 2	Group 3	Group 4	Group 5	Group 6
intestinal bowel disease, Crohn's disease, ulcerative colitis, inflammatory bowel diseases, chronic inflammatory diseases	lifestyle factor, life style factors, diet, dietary, nutrients, dairy, dietary pattern, food, meat intake, fibre intake, vitamins, high salt diet	tumour necrosis factor, TNF, anti-TNF, treatment response, treatment outcome, treatment result, treatment efficacy, drug, infliximab, IFX, personalised medicine, personalized medicine	sulphate-reducing bacteria, mucolytic bacteria, mucosa-associated bacteria, epithelium-associated bacteria	metabolomics	prospective
IFX, Infliximab					

3. Results

3.1. Environmental Factors in IBD

When assessing the effect of lifestyle factors on disease risk, prospective studies are preferred over case-control or cross sectional studies in order to avoid recall bias and bias introduced by lifestyle changes due to the disease itself. Diet seems important [14,15] although strong clinical evidence is scarce [14,15]. In the recent years, prospective studies on diet have emerged. Findings from the European Investigation into Cancer and Nutrition (EPIC) Study and the Nurses' Health Study (NHS) are particularly noteworthy because of their large well-characterized cohorts [16–28]. These studies have investigated the involvement of dietary factors such as dietary patterns, vitamin D, dietary fibre, zinc, dairy products, *n*-3 and *n*-6 polyunsaturated fatty acids (PUFA), and protein, particularly animal protein, in IBD development [16–28]. The increases in IBD seen in developing countries as they adopt a Western lifestyle [5], and the high incidence among immigrants coming from low to high incidence areas, strongly suggest the involvement of other environmental factors such as lifestyle factors in disease aetiology [29]. Non-diet risk factors include family predisposition, birth by caesarean section, smoking, appendectomy, and antibiotics [30]. Smoking is the single most important environmental factor found to be involved in disease development [31]. Smoking increases the risk of CD and aggravates the disease course [31,32], whereas smoking cessation increases the risk of UC, and the risk of flares and the need for drugs in UC [31–33].

3.2. Intestinal Barrier Function and Effects of Anti-TNF

An essential function of the intestinal mucosa is to act as a barrier between luminal contents and the underlying immune system, at the same time allowing absorption of nutrients. The luminal surface of the intestinal mucosa is lined by a mucus layer, a hydrated gel, composed of mucins secreted by goblet cells. In the small intestine, where a large part of nutrient absorption takes place, the mucus layer is discontinuous. In the colon, where most of the gut microbes are present, there is a continuous mucus coat with two layers, an upper "sloppy" layer and a lower adherent layer [34]. In healthy individuals, the mucus prevents large particles and intact microbes from coming into direct contact with the underlying epithelium; thus, the lower adherent layer is generally free from microbes.

In case of defects in the mucus layer, microbes may get into contact with the epithelium. Molecular structures in bacteria known as microbial-associated molecular patterns (MAMPs) stimulate pattern-recognition receptors in the host, most importantly the Toll-like receptors (TLRs), thereby inducing inflammation [35]. Different types of MAMPs stimulate different TLRs dispersed on a variety of different cell types including the enterocytes, and MAMPs are also dispersed and shared between members of the microbiota [36]. Activation of TLRs, including TLR1, TLR2, TLR4, and TLR10 on the intestinal epithelial cells and local innate leukocytes, lead to the activation of the innate immune system via activation of the nuclear factor-κB (NF-κB) signaling pathway [35]. Next, the induction of pro-inflammatory cytokines, such as interleukin (IL)-1, IL-6, tumour necrosis factor-α (TNFα), and interferon-γ (IFNγ), and anti-inflammatory cytokines, such as IL-10, regulates cells of the adaptive immune system (T_H1, T_H17, T_H2, and regulatory T-cells) [35]. Treatment with antibodies targeting TNF neutralizes downstream TNF-α-mediated pro-inflammatory cell signalling and inhibit expression of pro-inflammatory genes (Figure 1).

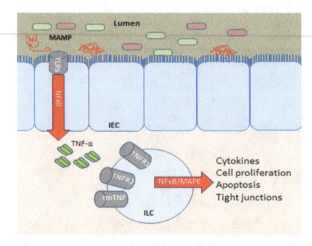

Figure 1. Tumour necrosis factor (TNF-α) is a pro-inflammatory cytokine produced by host cells such as intestinal epithelial cells, macrophages, and lymphocytes, and the principle of anti-TNF-α treatment

is the blocking of this [37]. One of the key enteric effector mechanisms of TNF-α production is caused through NF-κB, when microbial associated molecular patterns (MAMPs) contained in certain bacteria stimulate the toll-like receptors (TLRs) on a variety of host cells including the enterocytes (intestinal epithelia cells, IEC). The main biological activity of TNF-α is mediated by its binding to TNF receptor type 1 (TNFR1), type 2 (TNFR2), and transmembrane TNF receptors (tmTNFR) [37]. After binding to the receptors, e.g., on innate lymphocytic cells (ILC), TNF-α initiates pro-inflammatory signalling by activation of the MAPKs and NF-κB pathways, leading to the secretion of cytokines (pro-inflammatory TNF-α, IL-1β, IL-6, IFNγ, and anti-inflammatory IL-10), induction of cell proliferation (e.g., via effects on the pluripotent intestinal epithelial stem cells [38]), caspase-8 activation, apoptosis of intestinal cells, and induction of changes in the epithelial expression of tight junction proteins among patients with CD [8]. Anti-TNF treatment neutralizes downstream TNF-α-mediated pro-inflammatory cell signalling and inhibit expression of pro-inflammatory genes. Moreover, TNF inhibitors have been shown to induce apoptosis of TNF-α–producing immune cells, reducing the production of a variety of downstream pro-inflammatory cytokines from these and other cells, and may also induce regulatory macrophages [37,39]. Interestingly, activation of the membrane-bound form of TNF has been suggested to be involved in the downregulation of epithelial apoptosis [40].

3.3. Impact of Diet on Treatment Results from Anti-TNF Treatment

Exclusive enteral nutrition has been shown to induce remission in some patients with CD, in particular children, whereas, in UC, enteral nutrition had no effect (recently reviewed by Richman [41]). Specialised nutrition-based therapy for direct treatment of CD was first proposed in the 1970s. In patients with mild CD, enteral nutrition monotherapy may be sufficient to induce and maintain clinical remission [42]. A Cochrane meta-analysis on the use of sole enteral nutrition to induce remission in CD, concluded that "the effectiveness of enteral nutrition for the induction of remission in CD is evident from the remission rates" (up to 84%) [41,43].

Nutrition therapy has been established in the medical treatment of CD in Japan [44] in addition to conventional drug therapy. Elemental diet therapy (ED) is high-calorie liquid diets containing primarily amino acids that are absorbed by the small intestine without digestion, and was originally developed as food for astronauts who worked for the National Aeronautics and Space Administration in the 1960s [45].

One prospective study on diet and anti-TNF treatment in IBD was identified. The authors compared Infliximab (INF) and ED versus INF and no dietary restrictions in 56 patients with CD that had achieved clinical remission with INF induction therapy [46]. In total, 32 with good compliance were assigned to receive concomitant enteral nutrition, and 24 with poor compliance were assigned to a non-ED group. The 32 patients in the EN group received additional EN therapy with ED (1200–1500 mL) infusion during night-time and a low fat (20–30 g/day) diet during daytime. On an intention-to-treat basis, 25 patients in the EN group (78%) and 16 patients in the non-EN group (67%) remained in clinical remission during the 56-week observation ($p = 0.51$).

In a retrospective study of primary response in 110 CD patients that received either one single infusion (luminal disease) or three infusions (fistulising disease) with the anti-TNFα drug Infliximab (IFX), 51 patients concomitantly received ED [45]. CD activity index (CDAI) was assessed and CDAI < 150 was defined as clinical remission. The authors reported that 26 out of the 38 patients with inflammatory disease who responded to anti-TNF therapy at week 16, as opposed to 12 out of the 37 of the non-responders, had received concomitant ED treatment ($p = 0.0026$).

Likewise, Kamata et al. retrospectively studied loss of response in 125 patients with luminal CD treated with scheduled IFX maintenance therapy with a regular dosage [47]. Patients were classified into two groups based on the amount of daily ED intake. The ED group included patients who tolerated 900 kcal/day ED or more, and the non-ED group included those that tolerated less than 900 kcal/day ED at the start of IFX. Furthermore, more patients from the non-ED (32/65) than from the ED (4/24) group were smokers. Twenty-eight patients were categorized as the ED group and

97 patients as the non-ED group. In total, 21 patients developed loss of response in the observational period (mean follow up 799 ± 398 and 771 ± 497 days in the ED and non-ED group). The authors concluded that the ED group was significantly superior to the non-ED group ($p = 0.049$) in sustaining scheduled IFX maintenance therapy.

A recent meta-analysis by Nguyen et al. on the use of IFX monotherapy versus specialised enteral nutrition therapy combination with IFX reviewed 1 prospective study (56 patients) and 3 retrospective studies (in total 295 patients, including the study by Tanaka [45], but not the later study by Kamata [47]) [42]. The daily amount of enteral nutrition ranged from 600 kcal to 1500 kcal/day. Efficacy was measured by clinical response indices. Specialised enteral nutrition therapy with IFX resulted in 109 of 157 (69.4%) patients reaching clinical remission compared with 84 of 185 (45.4%) with IFX monotherapy. In the meta-analysis, there appeared to be more than a two-fold increase in the odds of achieving clinical remission among patients on combination therapy with specialised enteral nutrition and IFX compared with IFX monotherapy (odds ratio (OR) = 2.73; 95% confidence interval (95% CI): 1.73–4.31, $p < 0.01$). Similar results were achieved assessing the numbers that remained in clinical remission after one year (79 of 106 in combination therapy compared to 62 of 126 in monotherapy corresponding to an OR = 2.93; 95% CI: 1.66–5.17, $p < 0.01$). The authors were not able to conclude from the meta-analysis whether or not the type of enteral formula (elemental versus polymeric) made a difference in achieving clinical remission in patients on IFX. The authors stress that the included studies did not fully document the patients' compliance with the prescribed enteral nutrition formulation, and they concluded that, "Given the limitation of the existing studies, further randomized placebo controlled studies are needed".

These studies are subject to potential bias due to changes in diet as the consequence of the diseases and their symptoms. These studies need to be replicated in larger prospective, randomised studies before a final conclusion can be reached.

3.4. Impact of Diet on Disease Course and Treatment Results

No other studies on diet and treatment response in IBD patients on anti-TNF are available according to the authors' knowledge. There is, however, some evidence for the impact of diet on disease course and treatment results from other studies [14,33,41].

One study of 191 UC patients, with prospective sampling of diet information using a food frequency questionnaire (FFQ), reported 52 patients had a relapse according to the simple clinical colitis activity index (SCCAI) within one year [48]. A high intake of meat and meat products (particularly red and processed meats), eggs, protein, alcohol, energy, fat, sulphur, and sulphate was associated with an increased likelihood of relapse. Thus, the authors found a strong relationship between a high intake of meat, particularly of red meat and processed meat, and an increased risk of relapse (meat: OR = 3.2; 95% CI: 1.3–7.8, red and processed meat: OR = 5.19; 95% CI: 2.1–12.9). Meat contains essential n-6 PUFAs such as linoleic acid. Linoleic acid has been associated with high risk of UC [49].

A similar study of 1619 IBD patients from the Crohn's and Colitis Foundation of America Partners Internet cohort has been performed [50]. Data on diet was sampled by FFQ at entry, and participants were followed for 6 mo. Participants with longer duration of disease, past history of surgery, and past IBD hospitalization ate less fibre. Compared with those in the lowest quartile of fibre consumption, participants with Crohn's disease in the highest quartile were less likely to have a flare (adjusted OR = 0.58; 95% CI: 0.37–0.90). There was no association between fibre intake and flares in patients with ulcerative colitis (adjusted OR = 1.82; 95% CI: 0.92–3.60) [50].

A randomized controlled trial of 738 patients found no effect of n-3 fatty acid supplementation during 1 year in prevention of CD relapse [51], whereas other studies have found n-3 fatty acid (fish oil) supplementation to be associated with absence of relapse in CD [52]. In UC, no effect of n-3 fatty acid supplementation has been found in a meta-analysis or in a systematic review [41]. The authors of the negative studies have been criticised for use of unsatisfactory omega-3 preparations with variable bioactivity that may have attenuated the observed results of the studies [41,53].

A registry study of 3217 patients from a multi-institution cohort with established IBD reported that low plasma Vitamin D status was associated with an increased risk of surgery in CD patients but not in UC patients. Furthermore, CD patients who normalised their vitamin D status had a lower risk of subsequent surgery than those who remained deficient. The authors identified IBD patients with at least one measured plasma 25-hydroxy vitamin D (25(OH)D). Multivariable analysis in CD found that deficient vitamin D status (25(OH)D < 20 ng/mL) was associated with an increased risk of surgery (OR = 1.76; 95% CI: 1.24–2.51) compared with those with normal vitamin D status (25(OH)D > 30 ng/mL). The median lowest plasma 25(OH)D was 26 ng/mL (interquartile range, 17–35 ng/mL). In a subgroup of patients with CD, those who had an initial deficient level of 25(OH)D, but subsequently normalised their values, had a significantly lower likelihood of requiring surgery (OR = 0.56; 95% CI: 0.32–0.98) compared with those who remained deficient.

These studies, apart from the randomised study, are subject to potential bias, due to changes in diet and serum vitamin D levels as a consequence of the diseases and their symptoms.

3.5. Animal Studies of Potential Relevance for the Impact of Diet on Anti-TNF Treatment Results

Many experimental data suggest the association of dietary factors with gut inflammation in animal models [14,54,55].

3.5.1. A Diet High in Saturated Milk Fat Seems to Promote Colitis

Devkota et al. investigated the effects of three different diets on the enteric microbiota of IL-10-deficient and wild type mice [54]. The diets were low fat diet (LF), polyunsaturated (safflower oil) fat (PUFA) and saturated (milk-derived) fat (MF) diet. MF did not affect the onset and incidence of colitis in wild type mice, but increased onset and incidence in IL-10-deficient mice, driving it from a spontaneous rate of 25%–30% (on LF) to over 60% in a 6-month period. In contrast, the incidence of colitis in IL-10-deficient mice fed PUFA was no different than those fed LF. The colitis seen in mice fed MF was also more severe and extensive. The effects were mediated by MF-promoted taurine-conjugation of hepatic bile acids, which increased the availability of organic sulphur used by sulphate-reducing bacteria like *Bilophila wadsworthia*. When mice were fed a LF diet supplemented with taurocholic acid, but not with glycocholic acid, development of colitis were observed in IL-10-deficient mice. Taurocholic acid in contrast to glycocholic acid can be metabolised to hydrogen sulphide (H_2S). The data showed that dietary fats, by promoting changes in host bile acid composition, can dramatically alter conditions for gut microbial assemblage, resulting in dysbiosis that can perturb immune homeostasis.

Interestingly, another mouse study indicated that microbially produced hydrogen sulphide may open the protective mucus barrier and expose the epithelium to potential cytotoxic components, whereas antibiotics (by eliminating sulphate-reducing and mucin-degrading bacteria (e.g., Akkermansia)) blocked microbial sulphide production and thereby maintained the mucus barrier [56]. It was indicated that hydrogen sulphide reduced disulphide bonds in the mucus to trisulphides.

Conflicting results have been found in studies evaluating the effects of *n*-3 and *n*-6 PUFAs in mouse models [57]. However, some studies reported that feeding fish oil to mice decreased production of TNF-α, IL-1β and IL-6 by endotoxin-stimulated macrophages [58].

3.5.2. Vitamin D Deficiency Promotes Diarrhoea

The effect of vitamin D was evaluated in an IL-10-deficient mouse model of IBD [59]. Mice were made vitamin D-deficient, vitamin D-sufficient, or supplemented with active vitamin D (1,25-dihydroxycholecalciferol). Vitamin D–deficient IL-10-deficient mice developed diarrhoea and a wasting disease. In contrast, vitamin D–sufficient IL-10-deficient mice did not develop symptoms. Supplementation with vitamin D (cholecalciferol or 1,25-dihydroxycholecalciferol) significantly ameliorated symptoms, and vitamin D treatment for two weeks blocked the progression and ameliorated symptoms in IL-10-deficient mice with already established IBD. The small intestines from the vitamin D-deficient IL-10-deficient mice were enlarged compared to the vitamin D-sufficient IL-10-deficient mice [59]. Interestingly, administration of 1,25(OH)2D3 was found to suppress the TNF-α pathway [60].

3.5.3. Diet Low in Fibre Confers Susceptibility for Colitis

A recent study, using a simplified model of the human gut microbiome in gnotobiotic mice, found that low dietary intake of fibre increased the susceptibility of colitis by reducing the mucus layer [61]. Mice colonised with the simplified model of the human gut microbiome were fed a fibre-rich or fibre-free diet. Mice fed the fibre-free diet developed increased abundance of host mucosal polypeptide (mucin) degrading bacteria such as *Akkermansia muciniphila* at the cost of bacteria capable of degrading fibre [61]. In addition, gene transcripts from caecal samples showed increased amount of bacterial transcripts encoding enzymes for the metabolism of host polysaccharides such as mucosal O-glucans, at the cost of transcripts encoding for the metabolism of dietary fibre.

Another study found that oral intake of a specific multi-fibre mix (MFibre), designed to match the fibre content of a healthy diet, counteracted IBD-like intestinal inflammation and weight loss in dextran sodium sulphate (DSS)-treated mice [62]. The authors suggested that the reduction in inflammation might be brought about, at least in part, by the MFibre-induced decrease in inflammatory cytokines, including TNF-α, increase in IL-10, and relative increase in T-regulatory cells in the mesenteric lymph nodes.

3.5.4. High Salt Diet May Promote Colitis

Mice that received high salt diet (4%) developed a more severe colitis than controls when exposed to trinitrobenzene-sulfonic acid (TNBS) or DSS [63]. Sodium chloride was found to induce T_H17 cells characterized by up-regulation of TNF-α [64,65].

3.6. What is Already Known on Impact of Diet on Gut Inflammatory Mechanisms

Diet is considered to affect gut inflammatory pathways in various ways (Table 2).

Table 2. Previously suggested mechanisms whereby various diets may affect gut inflammation and potentially anti-TNF treatment response

Food Source	Nutrient	Potential Mechanisms	Reference	
Meat	Protein fermentation	NH_3 and H_2S > Mucosal toxicity	Yao, 2016	[66]
	N-6 PUFA	AA pathway > Pro- and anti-inflammatory prostaglandins and leukotrienes		[67]
Fish	Marine n-3 PUFA	EPA and DHA > Altered cell membrane phospholipid fatty acid composition Disruption of lipid rafts Inhibition of pro-inflammatory NFkB Activation of anti-inflammatory PPARγ Binding to GPR120	Calder, 2015	[58]
Vitamin D	1,25 D vitamin	signalling > Regulation of innate and adaptive immune response Decrease TNF-α secretion in animal models Regulation of antimicrobial peptides	Kamen, 2010	[68]
Vegetables, fruit, cereals, legumes	Fibre	Microbial degradation > SCFA > Fuel for enterocytes Regulation of GPRs and MAPKs Epigenetic regulation of gene transcription by inhibition of HDACs Decrease TNF-α secretion in animal models	Vinolo, 2011	[69]

SCFA; short chain fatty acids, GPRs; G protein-coupled receptors, MAPKs; mitogen-activated protein kinases, HDACs; histone deacetylases, AA; arachidonic acid, PUFA; polyunsaturated fatty acids, EPA; eicosapentaenoic acid, DHA; docosahexaenoic acid, NF-κB; nuclear factor-kappa B, PPARγ; peroxisome proliferator activated receptor γ

For example, dietary fat from meat, such as *n*-6 PUFA, may give rise to arachidonic acid, that may be incorporated in the cell membrane and metabolised to pro- and anti-inflammatory eicosanoids (prostaglandins and leukotrienes) [67]. Dietary protein, in particular from meat, may give rise to the release of marked quantities of branched chain fatty acids and compounds such as ammonia, phenols, and nitric oxide, in addition to sulphide compounds that may have toxic effects on the mucosal epithelium [66]. Dietary fibres from grains, fruit, and vegetables is usually metabolised by the gut microbiome to short chain fatty acids including butyrate, propionate, and acetate. These represent important fuel for the intestinal mucosa and are associated with various anti-inflammatory effects, including e.g. the regulation of G protein-coupled receptors (GPCRs) and mitogen-activated protein kinases (MAPKs) that are of importance for inflammatory processes, and epigenetic regulation of gene transcription by inhibition of histone deacetylases (HDACs) [69]. Vitamin D has impact on the innate and adaptive immune response, as well as the secretion of antimicrobial peptides in the small intestine [68]. Some of these mechanisms may also work in treatment response mechanisms, although the evidence for an involvement in anti-TNF treatment response is scarce.

3.7. New Understanding of Impact of Diet on Gut Inflammation

Low levels of fibre may change the gut microbial metabolism from primarily using microbial derived short chain fatty acids to using mucinous carbohydrates as the main energy source (Figure 2) [61].

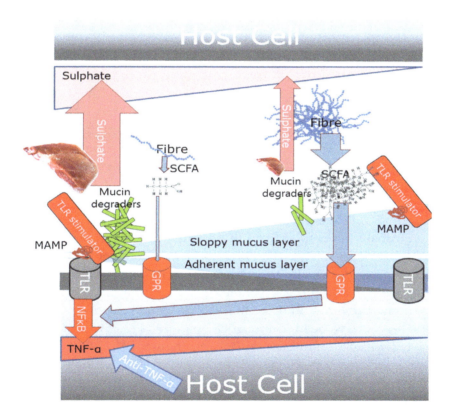

Figure 2. Potential mechanism whereby Western diet high in meat and low in fibre may impact gut inflammation and potentially anti-TNF treatment response. If the enteric mucus layer is thick and intact, the TLR-stimulating MAMP-containing bacteria will be contained in the sloppy mucus layer. If it is thin or disrupted, these bacteria will enter the adherent mucus layer and elicit their TLR stimulation. Dietary sulphate, from e.g. meat, weakens them. Apart from degrading the mucus layer and thereby increasing the potential for MAMP-TLR stimulation, mucus-degrading bacteria release sulphate during the degradation process. A high level of dietary fibres leads to a high level of short chain fatty acids (SCFAs), which stimulates the G protein-coupled receptors (GPRs), thereby counteracting the induction of TNF-α production. Supplementation of a plant fibre diet, as part of the theory, stimulates the mucus layer [41,70].

Mucolytic bacteria (*Ruminococcus gnavus*, *Ruminococcus torques*, *Akkermansia muciniphila*, and bacteria in the *Bifidobacterium* genus) are defined as mucus-degrading bacteria that are able to grow on mucin as its sole carbon substrate [71]. In IBD, an increased abundance of *Ruminococcus gnavus* and *Ruminococcus torques* and a reduced abundance of *Akkermansia muciniphila* compared to controls have been reported [71]. Degradation of mucus releases free sulphate, which would then become available for utilisation by sulphate-reducing bacteria (like *Bilophila wadsworthia*) for microbially produced hydrogen sulphide [72].

High intake of food containing organic sulphur and sulphate additives, such as meat, processed meat, milk, and wine, may increase the amount of sulphate for microbially produced hydrogen sulphide [66,73]. In fact, high amounts of sulphate-reducing bacteria (including *Bilophila wadsworthia*) [72,74] have been found in UC patients.

The resultant hydrogen sulphide from either low intake of fibre, high intake of meat and other sulphur, or both may reduce the disulphide bonds in the mucus network, rendering the mucus layer penetrable to bacteria [72,75]. Then, microbes may reach the epithelium and next activate the TLRs, inducing gut inflammation [35].

Additionally, diet may affect the systemic immune response. Intake of low-glycemic index diet was found to lower secretion of TNF-α and IL-6 from stimulated peripheral blood mononuclear cells from obese humans [76].

4. Discussion

Diet may impact the treatment response to anti-TNF drugs. We found that evidence-based knowledge on impact of diet on anti-TNF treatment response for clinical use is scarce. One small prospective study on diet and anti-TNF treatment in 56 patients with CD found similar remission rates after 56 weeks among 32 patients with good compliance that received concomitant enteral nutrition and 24 with poor compliance that had no dietary restrictions (78% versus 67%, $p = 0.51$). A meta-analysis of 295 patients found higher odds of achieving clinical remission and remaining in clinical remission among patients on combination therapy with specialised enteral nutrition and Infliximab (IFX) compared with IFX monotherapy (OR 2.73; 95% CI: 1.73–4.31, $p < 0.01$, OR 2.93; 95% CI: 1.66–5.17, $p < 0.01$, respectively). The animal studies provide understanding related to effects of high animal fat and fish oil diets on rates of colitis and cytokine expression. However, caution has to be taken when translating results from therapeutic studies in animals to humans with IBD. Here we hypothesised that Western style diet, high in meat (a rich source of fat, dietary sulphur, and protein) and low in fibre, may seriously impact treatment response in IBD. Such a diet could affect gut microbiome metabolism in a way that promotes gut inflammation and negatively affects medical treatment. There are some previous findings that support such processes in IBD, in particular UC. In fact, high sulphide levels have been found in UC patients [72,75]. Moreover, a defective mucus layer has been associated with UC in humans and colitis in mice [34,77,78]. Additionally, an increased number of epithelium-associated bacteria have been found in IBD, although more consistently in CD than UC [79,80]. Finally, our pharmacogenetics studies of gene-environment interactions in relation to development of colorectal cancer, suggest that intake of red and processed meat interacts with genes encoding TLRs and NF-κB [81], which may offer a potential link to anti-TNF treatment response.

The role of the microbiome in IBD is far from clear. The mucin-degrading bacteria have been suggested to control the abundance of mucosa-associated bacteria by providing substrate for non-mucus degrading bacteria [71]. In addition to their mucin-degrading properties, the mucin-degrading bacteria may have other and diverging abilities. For example, *Akkermansia muciniphila* have been associated with various anti-inflammatory actions [82]. Hence, in obese mice, an increase in number of *Akkermansia muciniphila* has been correlated with increased numbers of goblet cells [83]. Furthermore, *Irgm1* was found to regulate the levels of *Akkermansia muciniphila* in a metabolic mouse model [84]. *IRGM* has been associated with IBD susceptibility and with anti-TNF response in IBD in a pilot study [85] (Hubenthal et al., unpublished). Finally, a mouse study demonstrated that the effect of host genotype on the consumption of mucus glucans was dependent on diet [86]. First, the authors demonstrated impact of a genotype-dependent mucus phenotype (the presence or absence of host fucose) on the gut microbial composition. Next, upon switching to a diet low in polysaccharide, the observed differences seen on a standard diet were lost [86]. The impact of the gut microbiome on the gut immune system thus depends on both the diet and host genetics.

Pharmacogenetic studies may be used for identifying biological mechanisms underlying treatment effects. Our explorative genetic studies of 758 anti-TNF-treated IBD patients suggested that the driving mechanism underlying the inflammation may be individual, and hence, treatment may have to be targeted [12,13]. Our results suggest that IBD patients with genetic variants associated with high TNF inflammatory response were more likely to respond to anti-TNF treatment, whereas IBD patients with genetic variants associated with high IL-1β, IL-6 or INFγ were more likely to be non-responders [13]. Moreover, our ImmunoChip study of 592 anti-TNF-treated IBD patients suggested that *IRGM* and *HNF4G* are involved in defining treatment response. Thus, these results support the involvement of microbes in defining treatment response, as *IRGM* and *HNF4G* encodes proteins involved in autophagy, whereby microbes in the gut are degraded [87,88]. Hence, our exploratory pharmacogenetic studies indicate that the genetic make-up of the host may define the response to anti-TNF treatment and may involve gut-microbe interactions.

Different mechanisms likely define the treatment response in the small intestine and in colon. In the small intestine, a more intimate contact between various dietary components (e.g., gluten) is taking place. In colon, metabolites resulting from microbial degradation of the luminal content may drive the inflammation. Similarly, different mechanisms driving inflammation in CD versus UC may add to the complexity. In accordance, a recent study of genotype-phenotype associations in IBD found that disease location is an intrinsic aspect of disease. The authors demonstrated that IBD is better characterised as three groups (ileal Crohn's disease, colonic Crohn's disease, and ulcerative colitis) instead of CD and UC [89].

It has been suggested that plant fibre may be important for restoring the mucus layer [34,79]. Supplementation with complex oligosaccharides such as those present in soluble edible plant fibres was able to inhibit the adherence of pathogen bacteria to epithelial cells in a hen model [70]. Thus, diet modification may represent directions for future treatment and preventative strategies.

5. Conclusions

Diet and other lifestyle factors may potentially impact the treatment response to anti-TNF drugs. However, evidence-based knowledge for clinical use is generally scarce, although vitamin D supplementation to vitamin D-deficient IBD patients seems rational. Our results suggest complex interactions between diet, microbiome, and genetics in defining immune response and treatment response in IBD. Here we propose a mechanism by which a Western style diet high in meat and low in fibre may promote colonic inflammation and potentially affect treatment response to anti-TNF drugs. Further studies of the biological mechanisms of various food items, such as red meat and fibre rich foods, using hypothesis-driven and data-driven explorative strategies in observational studies, animal studies, and interventional studies, may help in understanding how diet may affect treatment results.

Acknowledgments: This work was supported by "Knud og Edith Erichsens Mindefond" (VA). Thank you to the Library at Regional Hospital Viborg and Hospital of Southern Jutland for help to retrieve articles. Also, thank you to the Focused research unit for Molecular Diagnostic and Clinical Research, IRS-Centre Sonderjylland, Hospital of Southern Jutland for the cost to publish in open access.

Author Contributions: V.A. collected the articles and wrote the first draft, A.K.H. performed Figure 2, V.A. Figure 1, and all authors critically reviewed for important intellectual content and approved the version to be submitted.

Conflicts of Interest: BLH has received funding from MatPrat, the Norwegian information office for egg and meat. VA reports to have received compensation from Merck (MSD) and Jansen for consultancy and as an advisory board member. AKH has received funding from NOVO Nordisk A/S. The founding sponsors had no role in the design of the study; in the collection, analyses, or interpretation of data; in the writing of the manuscript, and in the decision to publish the results.

References

1. Baumgart, D.C.; Carding, S.R. Inflammatory bowel disease: Cause and immunobiology. *Lancet* **2007**, *369*, 1627–1640. [CrossRef]

2. Baumgart, D.C.; Sandborn, W.J. Inflammatory bowel disease: Clinical aspects and established and evolving therapies. *Lancet* **2007**, *369*, 1641–1657. [CrossRef]

3. Strober, W.; Fuss, I.; Mannon, P. The fundamental basis of inflammatory bowel disease. *J. Clin. Investig.* **2007**, *117*, 514–521. [CrossRef] [PubMed]

4. Molodecky, N.A.; Soon, I.S.; Rabi, D.M.; Ghali, W.A.; Ferris, M.; Chernoff, G.; Benchimol, E.I.; Panaccione, R.; Ghosh, S.; Barkema, H.W.; et al. Increasing incidence and prevalence of the inflammatory bowel diseases with time, based on systematic review. *Gastroenterology* **2012**, *142*, 46–54. [CrossRef] [PubMed]

5. Kaplan, G.G. The global burden of IBD: From 2015 to 2025. *Nat. Rev. Gastroenterol. Hepatol.* **2015**, *12*, 720–727. [CrossRef] [PubMed]

6. Dignass, A.; van Assche, G.; Lindsay, J.O.; Lemann, M.; Soderholm, J.; Colombel, J.F.; Danese, S.; D'Hoore, A.; Gassull, M.; Gomollon, F.; et al. The second European evidence-based Consensus on the diagnosis and management of Crohn's disease: Current management. *J. Crohns Colitis* **2010**, *4*, 28–62. [CrossRef] [PubMed]

7. Dignass, A.; Lindsay, J.O.; Sturm, A.; Windsor, A.; Colombel, J.F.; Allez, M.; D'Haens, G.; D'Hoore, A.; Mantzaris, G.; Novacek, G.; et al. Second European evidence-based consensus on the diagnosis and management of ulcerative colitis part 2: Current management. *J. Crohns Colitis* **2012**, *6*, 991–1030. [CrossRef] [PubMed]

8. Pedersen, J.; Coskun, M.; Soendergaard, C.; Salem, M.; Nielsen, O.H. Inflammatory pathways of importance for management of inflammatory bowel disease. *World J. Gastroenterol.* **2014**, *20*, 64–77. [CrossRef] [PubMed]

9. Bouguen, G.; Peyrin-Biroulet, L. Surgery for adult Crohn's disease: What is the actual risk? *Gut* **2011**, *60*, 1178–1181. [CrossRef] [PubMed]

10. Hancock, L.; Mortensen, N.J. How often do IBD patients require resection of their intestine? *Inflamm. Bowel Dis.* **2008**, *14* (Suppl. 2), S68–S69. [CrossRef] [PubMed]

11. Khanna, R.; Sattin, B.D.; Afif, W.; Benchimol, E.I.; Bernard, E.J.; Bitton, A.; Bressler, B.; Fedorak, R.N.; Ghosh, S.; Greenberg, G.R.; et al. Review article: A clinician's guide for therapeutic drug monitoring of infliximab in inflammatory bowel disease. *Aliment. Pharmacol. Ther.* **2013**, *38*, 447–459. [CrossRef] [PubMed]

12. Bek, S.; Nielsen, J.V.; Bojesen, A.B.; Franke, A.; Bank, S.; Vogel, U.; Andersen, V. Systematic review: Genetic biomarkers associated with anti-TNF treatment response in inflammatory bowel diseases. *Aliment. Pharmacol. Therap.* **2016**, *44*, 554–567. [CrossRef] [PubMed]

13. Bank, S.; Andersen, P.S.; Burisch, J.; Pedersen, N.; Roug, S.; Galsgaard, J.; Turino, S.Y.; Brodersen, J.B.; Rashid, S.; Rasmussen, B.K.; et al. Associations between functional polymorphisms in the NF kappa B signaling pathway and response to anti-TNF treatment in Danish patients with inflammatory bowel disease. *Pharmacogenom. J.* **2014**, *14*, 526–534. [CrossRef] [PubMed]

14. Lee, D.; Albenberg, L.; Compher, C.; Baldassano, R.; Piccoli, D.; Lewis, J.D.; Wu, G.D. Diet in the pathogenesis and treatment of inflammatory bowel diseases. *Gastroenterology* **2015**, *148*, 1087–1106. [CrossRef] [PubMed]

15. Andersen, V.; Olsen, A.; Carbonnel, F.; Tjonneland, A.; Vogel, U. Diet and risk of inflammatory bowel disease. *Dig. Liver Dis.* **2012**, *44*, 185–194. [CrossRef] [PubMed]

16. Ananthakrishnan, A.N.; Khalili, H.; Higuchi, L.M.; Bao, Y.; Korzenik, J.R.; Giovannucci, E.L.; Richter, J.M.; Fuchs, C.S.; Chan, A.T. Higher predicted vitamin D status is associated with reduced risk of Crohn's disease. *Gastroenterology* **2012**, *142*, 482–489. [CrossRef] [PubMed]

17. Ananthakrishnan, A.N.; Khalili, H.; Konijeti, G.G.; Higuchi, L.M.; de Silva, P.; Fuchs, C.S.; Willett, W.C.; Richter, J.M.; Chan, A.T. Long-term intake of dietary fat and risk of ulcerative colitis and Crohn's disease. *Gut* **2014**, *63*, 776–784. [CrossRef] [PubMed]

18. Ananthakrishnan, A.N.; Khalili, H.; Konijeti, G.G.; Higuchi, L.M.; de Silva, P.; Korzenik, J.R.; Fuchs, C.S.; Willett, W.C.; Richter, J.M.; Chan, A.T. A prospective study of long-term intake of dietary fiber and risk of Crohn's disease and ulcerative colitis. *Gastroenterology* **2013**, *145*, 970–977. [CrossRef] [PubMed]

19. Ananthakrishnan, A.N.; Khalili, H.; Song, M.; Higuchi, L.M.; Richter, J.M.; Chan, A.T. Zinc intake and risk of Crohn's disease and ulcerative colitis: A prospective cohort study. *Int. J. Epidemiol.* **2015**, *44*, 1995–2005. [CrossRef] [PubMed]

20. Ananthakrishnan, A.N.; Khalili, H.; Song, M.; Higuchi, L.M.; Richter, J.M.; Nimptsch, K.; Wu, K.; Chan, A.T. High School Diet and Risk of Crohn's Disease and Ulcerative Colitis. *Inflamm. Bowel Dis.* **2015**, *21*, 2311–2319. [PubMed]

21. Chan, S.S.; Luben, R.; Olsen, A.; Tjonneland, A.; Kaaks, R.; Lindgren, S.; Grip, O.; Bergmann, M.M.; Boeing, H.; Hallmans, G.; et al. Association between high dietary intake of the *n*-3 polyunsaturated fatty acid docosahexaenoic acid and reduced risk of Crohn's disease. *Aliment. Pharmacol. Therap.* **2014**, *39*, 834–842. [CrossRef] [PubMed]

22. Chan, S.S.; Luben, R.; Olsen, A.; Tjonneland, A.; Kaaks, R.; Teucher, B.; et al. Body Mass Index and the Risk for Crohn's Disease and Ulcerative Colitis: Data From a European Prospective Cohort Study (The IBD in EPIC Study). *Am. J. Gastroenterol.* **2013**, *108*, 575–582. [CrossRef] [PubMed]

23. Chan, S.S.; Luben, R.; van Schaik, F.; Oldenburg, B.; Bueno-de-Mesquita, H.B.; Hallmans, G.; Karling, P.; Lindgren, S.; Grip, O.; Key, T.; et al. Carbohydrate intake in the etiology of Crohn's disease and ulcerative colitis. *Inflamm. Bowel Dis.* **2014**, *20*, 2013–2021. [CrossRef] [PubMed]

24. John, S.; Luben, R.; Shrestha, S.S.; Welch, A.; Khaw, K.T.; Hart, A.R. Dietary *n*-3 polyunsaturated fatty acids and the aetiology of ulcerative colitis: A UK prospective cohort study. *Eur. J. Gastroenterol. Hepatol.* **2010**, *22*, 602–606. [CrossRef] [PubMed]

25. De Silva, P.S.; Luben, R.; Shrestha, S.S.; Khaw, K.T.; Hart, A.R. Dietary arachidonic and oleic acid intake in ulcerative colitis etiology: A prospective cohort study using 7-day food diaries. *Eur. J. Gastroenterol. Hepatol.* **2014**, *26*, 11–18. [CrossRef] [PubMed]

26. De Silva, P.S.; Olsen, A.; Christensen, J.; Schmidt, E.B.; Overvaad, K.; Tjonneland, A.; Hart, A.R. An association between dietary arachidonic acid, measured in adipose tissue, and ulcerative colitis. *Gastroenterology* **2010**, *139*, 1912–1917. [CrossRef] [PubMed]

27. Hart, A.R.; Luben, R.; Olsen, A.; Tjonneland, A.; Linseisen, J.; Nagel, G.; Berglund, G.; Lindgren, S.; Grip, O.; Key, T.; et al. Diet in the aetiology of ulcerative colitis: A European prospective cohort study. *Digestion* **2008**, *77*, 57–64. [CrossRef] [PubMed]

28. Opstelten, J.; Leenders, M.; Dik, V.; Chan, S.; van Schaik, F.; Siersema, P.; Bueno-de-Mesquita, B.; Hart, A.; Oldenburg, B. Dairy products, dietary calcium and the risk of inflammatory bowel disease: Results from a European prospective cohort investigation. *J. Crohns Colitis* **2016**, *10*, S462. [CrossRef] [PubMed]

29. Benchimol, E.I.; Mack, D.R.; Guttmann, A.; Nguyen, G.C.; To, T.; Mojaverian, N.; Quach, P.; Manuel, D.G. Inflammatory bowel disease in immigrants to Canada and their children: A population-based cohort study. *Am. J. Gastroenterol.* **2015**, *110*, 553–563. [CrossRef] [PubMed]

30. Andersen, V.; Erichsen, R.; Froslev, T.; Sorensen, H.T.; Ehrenstein, V. Differential risk of ulcerative colitis and Crohn's disease among boys and girls after cesarean delivery. *Inflamm. Bowel Dis.* **2013**, *19*, E8–E10. [CrossRef] [PubMed]

31. Higuchi, L.M.; Khalili, H.; Chan, A.T.; Richter, J.M.; Bousvaros, A.; Fuchs, C.S. A prospective study of cigarette smoking and the risk of inflammatory bowel disease in women. *Am. J. Gastroenterol.* **2012**, *107*, 1399–1406. [CrossRef] [PubMed]

32. Parkes, G.C.; Whelan, K.; Lindsay, J.O. Smoking in inflammatory bowel disease: Impact on disease course and insights into the aetiology of its effect. *J. Crohns Colitis* **2014**, *8*, 717–725. [CrossRef] [PubMed]

33. Cosnes, J. Smoking and Diet: Impact on Disease Course? *Dig. Dis.* **2016**, *34*, 72–77. [CrossRef] [PubMed]

34. Merga, Y.; Campbell, B.J.; Rhodes, J.M. Mucosal barrier, bacteria and inflammatory bowel disease: Possibilities for therapy. *Dig. Dis.* **2014**, *32*, 475–483. [CrossRef] [PubMed]

35. Maloy, K.J.; Powrie, F. Intestinal homeostasis and its breakdown in inflammatory bowel disease. *Nature* **2011**, *474*, 298–306. [CrossRef] [PubMed]

36. Hansen, A.K.; Hansen, C.H.; Krych, L.; Nielsen, D.S. Impact of the gut microbiota on rodent models of human disease. *World J. Gastroenterol.* **2014**, *20*, 17727–17736. [PubMed]

37. Nielsen, O.H.; Ainsworth, M.A. Tumor necrosis factor inhibitors for inflammatory bowel disease. *N. Engl. J. Med.* **2013**, *369*, 754–762. [PubMed]

38. Peterson, L.W.; Artis, D. Intestinal epithelial cells: Regulators of barrier function and immune homeostasis. *Nat. Rev. Immunol.* **2014**, *14*, 141–153. [CrossRef] [PubMed]

39. Cader, M.Z.; Kaser, A. Recent advances in inflammatory bowel disease: Mucosal immune cells in intestinal inflammation. *Gut* **2013**, *62*, 1653–1664. [CrossRef] [PubMed]

40. Billmeier, U.; Dieterich, W.; Neurath, M.F.; Atreya, R. Molecular mechanism of action of anti-tumor necrosis factor antibodies in inflammatory bowel diseases. *World J. Gastroenterol.* **2016**, *22*, 9300–9313. [CrossRef] [PubMed]

41. Richman, E.; Rhodes, J.M. Review article: Evidence-based dietary advice for patients with inflammatory bowel disease. *Aliment. Pharmacol. Ther.* **2013**, *38*, 1156–1171. [CrossRef] [PubMed]

42. Nguyen, D.L.; Palmer, L.B.; Nguyen, E.T.; McClave, S.A.; Martindale, R.G.; Bechtold, M.L. Specialized enteral nutrition therapy in Crohn's disease patients on maintenance infliximab therapy: A meta-analysis. *Ther. Adv. Gastroenterol.* **2015**, *8*, 168–175. [CrossRef] [PubMed]

43. Zachos, M.; Tondeur, M.; Griffiths, A.M. Enteral nutritional therapy for induction of remission in Crohn's disease. *Cochrane Database Syst. Rev.* **2007**. [CrossRef]

44. Matsueda, K.; Shoda, R.; Takazoe, M.; Hiwatashi, N.; Bamba, T.; Kobayashi, K.; Saito, T.; Terano, A.; Yao, T. Therapeutic efficacy of cyclic home elemental enteral alimentation in Crohn's disease: Japanese cooperative Crohn's disease study. *J. Gastroenterol.* **1995**, *30* (Suppl. 8), 91–94. [PubMed]

45. Tanaka, T.; Takahama, K.; Kimura, T.; Mizuno, T.; Nagasaka, M.; Iwata, K.; Nakano, H.; Muramatsu, M.; Takazoe, M. Effect of concurrent elemental diet on infliximab treatment for Crohn's disease. *J. Gastroenterol. Hepatol.* **2006**, *21*, 1143–1149. [CrossRef] [PubMed]

46. Yamamoto, T.; Nakahigashi, M.; Umegae, S.; Matsumoto, K. Prospective clinical trial: Enteral nutrition during maintenance infliximab in Crohn's disease. *J. Gastroenterol.* **2010**, *45*, 24–29. [CrossRef] [PubMed]

47. Kamata, N.; Oshitani, N.; Watanabe, K.; Watanabe, K.; Hosomi, S.; Noguchi, A.; Yukawa, T.; Yamagami, H.; Shiba, M.; Tanigawa, T.; et al. Efficacy of concomitant elemental diet therapy in scheduled infliximab therapy in patients with Crohn's disease to prevent loss of response. *Dig. Dis. Sci.* **2015**, *60*, 1382–1388. [CrossRef] [PubMed]

48. Jowett, S.L.; Seal, C.J.; Pearce, M.S.; Phillips, E.; Gregory, W.; Barton, J.R.; Welfare, M.R. Influence of dietary factors on the clinical course of ulcerative colitis: A prospective cohort study. *Gut* **2004**, *53*, 1479–1484. [CrossRef] [PubMed]

49. Tjonneland, A.; Overvad, K.; Bergmann, M.M.; Nagel, G.; Linseisen, J.; Hallmans, G.; Palmqvist, R.; Sjodin, H.; Hagglund, G.; Berglund, G.; et al. Linoleic acid, a dietary *n*-6 polyunsaturated fatty acid, and the aetiology of ulcerative colitis: A nested case-control study within a European prospective cohort study. *Gut* **2009**, *58*, 1606–1611. [PubMed]

50. Brotherton, C.S.; Martin, C.A.; Long, M.D.; Kappelman, M.D.; Sandler, R.S. Avoidance of Fiber Is Associated With Greater Risk of Crohn's Disease Flare in a 6-Month Period. *Clin. Gastroenterol. Hepatol.* **2016**, *14*, 1130–1136. [CrossRef] [PubMed]

51. Feagan, B.G.; Sandborn, W.J.; Mittmann, U.; Bar-Meir, S.; D'Haens, G.; Bradette, M.; Cohen, A.; Dallaire, C.; Ponich, T.P.; McDonald, J.W.; et al. Omega-3 free fatty acids for the maintenance of remission in Crohn disease: The EPIC Randomized Controlled Trials. *J. Am. Med. Assoc.* **2008**, *299*, 1690–1697. [CrossRef] [PubMed]

52. Turner, D.; Zlotkin, S.H.; Shah, P.S.; Griffiths, A.M. Omega 3 fatty acids (fish oil) for maintenance of remission in Crohn's disease. *Cochrane Database Syst. Rev.* **2009**. [CrossRef]

53. Ferguson, L.R.; Smith, B.G.; James, B.J. Combining nutrition, food science and engineering in developing solutions to Inflammatory bowel diseases—Omega-3 polyunsaturated fatty acids as an example. *Food Funct.* **2010**, *1*, 60–72. [CrossRef] [PubMed]

54. Devkota, S.; Wang, Y.; Musch, M.W.; Leone, V.; Fehlner-Peach, H.; Nadimpalli, A.; Antonopoulos, D.A.; Jabri, B.; Chang, E.B. Dietary-fat-induced taurocholic acid promotes pathobiont expansion and colitis in Il10-/- mice. *Nature* **2012**, *487*, 104–108. [CrossRef] [PubMed]

55. Ejsing-Duun, M.; Josephsen, J.; Aasted, B.; Buschard, K.; Hansen, A.K. Dietary gluten reduces the number of intestinal regulatory T cells in mice. *Scand. J. Immunol.* **2008**, *67*, 553–559. [CrossRef] [PubMed]

56. Ijssennagger, N.; Belzer, C.; Hooiveld, G.J.; Dekker, J.; van Mil, S.W.; Muller, M.; Kleerebezem, M.; van der Meer, R. Gut microbiota facilitates dietary heme-induced epithelial hyperproliferation by opening the mucus barrier in colon. *Proc. Natl. Acad. Sci. USA* **2015**, *112*, 10038–10043. [CrossRef] [PubMed]

57. Nanau, R.M.; Neuman, M.G. Nutritional and probiotic supplementation in colitis models. *Dig. Dis. Sci.* **2012**, *57*, 2786–2810. [CrossRef] [PubMed]

58. Calder, P.C. Marine omega-3 fatty acids and inflammatory processes: Effects, mechanisms and clinical relevance. *Biochim. Biophys. Acta* **2015**, *1851*, 469–484. [CrossRef] [PubMed]

59. Cantorna, M.T.; Munsick, C.; Bemiss, C.; Mahon, B.D. 1,25-Dihydroxycholecalciferol prevents and ameliorates symptoms of experimental murine inflammatory bowel disease. *J. Nutr.* **2000**, *130*, 2648–2652. [PubMed]
60. Zhu, Y.; Mahon, B.D.; Froicu, M.; Cantorna, M.T. Calcium and 1 alpha,25-dihydroxyvitamin D3 target the TNF-alpha pathway to suppress experimental inflammatory bowel disease. *Eur. J. Immunol.* **2005**, *35*, 217–224. [CrossRef] [PubMed]
61. Desai, M.S.; Seekatz, A.M.; Koropatkin, N.M.; Kamada, N.; Hickey, C.A.; Wolter, M.; Pudlo, N.A.; Kitamoto, S.; Terrapon, N.; Muller, A.; et al. A Dietary Fiber-Deprived Gut Microbiota Degrades the Colonic Mucus Barrier and Enhances Pathogen Susceptibility. *Cell* **2016**, *167*, 1339–1353. [CrossRef] [PubMed]
62. Hartog, A.; Belle, F.N.; Bastiaans, J.; de Graaff, P.; Garssen, J.; Harthoorn, L.F.; Vos, A.P. A potential role for regulatory T-cells in the amelioration of DSS induced colitis by dietary non-digestible polysaccharides. *J. Nutr. Biochem.* **2015**, *26*, 227–233. [CrossRef] [PubMed]
63. Monteleone, I.; Marafini, I.; Dinallo, V.; Di Fusco, D.; Troncone, E.; Zorzi, F.; Laudisi, F.; Monteleone, G. Sodium chloride-enriched Diet Enhanced Inflammatory Cytokine Production and Exacerbated Experimental Colitis in Mice. *J. Crohns Colitis* **2017**, *11*, 237–245. [CrossRef] [PubMed]
64. Kleinewietfeld, M.; Manzel, A.; Titze, J.; Kvakan, H.; Yosef, N.; Linker, R.A.; Muller, D.N.; Hafler, D.A. Sodium chloride drives autoimmune disease by the induction of pathogenic TH17 cells. *Nature* **2013**, *496*, 518–522. [CrossRef] [PubMed]
65. Wu, C.; Yosef, N.; Thalhamer, T.; Zhu, C.; Xiao, S.; Kishi, Y.; Regev, A.; Kuchroo, V.K. Induction of pathogenic TH17 cells by inducible salt-sensing kinase SGK1. *Nature* **2013**, *496*, 513–517. [CrossRef] [PubMed]
66. Yao, C.K.; Muir, J.G.; Gibson, P.R. Review article: Insights into colonic protein fermentation, its modulation and potential health implications. *Aliment. Pharmacol. Ther.* **2016**, *43*, 181–196. [CrossRef] [PubMed]
67. Wang, D.; Dubois, R.N. Eicosanoids and cancer. *Nat. Rev. Cancer* **2010**, *10*, 181–193. [CrossRef] [PubMed]
68. Kamen, D.L.; Tangpricha, V. Vitamin D and molecular actions on the immune system: Modulation of innate and autoimmunity. *J. Mol. Med. (Berl. Ger.)* **2010**, *88*, 441–450. [CrossRef] [PubMed]
69. Vinolo, M.A.; Rodrigues, H.G.; Nachbar, R.T.; Curi, R. Regulation of inflammation by short chain fatty acids. *Nutrients* **2011**, *3*, 858–876. [CrossRef] [PubMed]
70. Parsons, B.N.; Wigley, P.; Simpson, H.L.; Williams, J.M.; Humphrey, S.; Salisbury, A.M.; Watson, A.J.; Fry, S.C.; O'Brien, D.; Roberts, C.L.; et al. Dietary supplementation with soluble plantain non-starch polysaccharides inhibits intestinal invasion of Salmonella Typhimurium in the chicken. *PLoS ONE* **2014**, *9*, e87658. [CrossRef] [PubMed]
71. Png, C.W.; Linden, S.K.; Gilshenan, K.S.; Zoetendal, E.G.; McSweeney, C.S.; Sly, L.I.; McGuckin, M.A.; Florin, T.H. Mucolytic bacteria with increased prevalence in IBD mucosa augment in vitro utilization of mucin by other bacteria. *Am. J. Gastroenterol.* **2010**, *105*, 2420–2428. [CrossRef] [PubMed]
72. Gibson, G.R.; Macfarlane, G.T.; Cummings, J.H. Sulphate reducing bacteria and hydrogen metabolism in the human large intestine. *Gut* **1993**, *34*, 437–439. [CrossRef] [PubMed]
73. Windey, K.; de Preter, V.; Louat, T.; Schuit, F.; Herman, J.; Vansant, G.; Verbeke, K. Modulation of protein fermentation does not affect fecal water toxicity: A randomized cross-over study in healthy subjects. *PLoS ONE* **2012**, *7*, e52387. [CrossRef] [PubMed]
74. Jia, W.; Whitehead, R.N.; Griffiths, L.; Dawson, C.; Bai, H.; Waring, R.H.; Ramsden, D.B.; Hunter, J.O.; Cauchi, M.; Bessant, C.; et al. Diversity and distribution of sulphate-reducing bacteria in human faeces from healthy subjects and patients with inflammatory bowel disease. *FEMS Immunol. Med. Microbiol.* **2012**, *65*, 55–68. [CrossRef] [PubMed]
75. Ijssennagger, N.; van der Meer, R.; van Mil, S.W. Sulfide as a Mucus Barrier-Breaker in Inflammatory Bowel Disease? *Trends Mol. Med.* **2016**, *22*, 190–199. [CrossRef] [PubMed]
76. Kelly, K.R.; Haus, J.M.; Solomon, T.P.; Patrick-Melin, A.J.; Cook, M.; Rocco, M.; Barkoukis, H.; Kirwan, J.P. A low-glycemic index diet and exercise intervention reduces TNF(alpha) in isolated mononuclear cells of older, obese adults. *J. Nutr.* **2011**, *141*, 1089–1094. [CrossRef] [PubMed]
77. Sheng, Y.H.; Hasnain, S.Z.; Florin, T.H.; McGuckin, M.A. Mucins in inflammatory bowel diseases and colorectal cancer. *J. Gastroenterol. Hepatol.* **2012**, *27*, 28–38. [CrossRef] [PubMed]
78. Chen, S.J.; Liu, X.W.; Liu, J.P.; Yang, X.Y.; Lu, F.G. Ulcerative colitis as a polymicrobial infection characterized by sustained broken mucus barrier. *World J. Gastroenterol. WJG* **2014**, *20*, 9468–9475. [PubMed]
79. Flanagan, P.; Campbell, B.J.; Rhodes, J.M. Bacteria in the pathogenesis of inflammatory bowel disease. *Biochem. Soc. Trans.* **2011**, *39*, 1067–1072. [CrossRef] [PubMed]

80. Strober, W. Impact of the gut microbiome on mucosal inflammation. *Trends Immunol.* **2013**, *34*, 423–430. [CrossRef] [PubMed]

81. Kopp, T.I.; Andersen, V.; Tjonneland, A.; Vogel, U. Polymorphisms in NFκB1 and TLR4 and interaction with dietary and life style factors in relation to colorectal cancer in a Danish prospective case-cohort study. *PLoS ONE* **2015**, *10*, e0116394. [CrossRef] [PubMed]

82. Shin, N.R.; Lee, J.C.; Lee, H.Y.; Kim, M.S.; Whon, T.W.; Lee, M.S.; Bae, J.W. An increase in the Akkermansia spp. population induced by metformin treatment improves glucose homeostasis in diet-induced obese mice. *Gut* **2014**, *63*, 727–735. [CrossRef] [PubMed]

83. Li, J.; Lin, S.; Vanhoutte, P.M.; Woo, C.W.; Xu, A. Akkermansia Muciniphila Protects Against Atherosclerosis by Preventing Metabolic Endotoxemia-Induced Inflammation in Apoe-/- Mice. *Circulation* **2016**, *133*, 2434–2446. [CrossRef] [PubMed]

84. Greer, R.L.; Dong, X.; Moraes, A.C.; Zielke, R.A.; Fernandes, G.R.; Peremyslova, E.; Vasquez-Perez, S.; Schoenborn, A.A.; Gomes, E.P.; Pereira, A.C.; et al. Akkermansia muciniphila mediates negative effects of IFN gamma on glucose metabolism. *Nat. Commun.* **2016**, *7*, 13329. [CrossRef] [PubMed]

85. Jostins, L.; Ripke, S.; Weersma, R.K.; Duerr, R.H.; McGovern, D.P.; Hui, K.Y.; Lee, J.C.; Schumm, L.P.; Sharma, Y.; Anderson, C.A.; et al. Host-microbe interactions have shaped the genetic architecture of inflammatory bowel disease. *Nature* **2012**, *491*, 119–124. [CrossRef] [PubMed]

86. Kashyap, P.C.; Marcobal, A.; Ursell, L.K.; Smits, S.A.; Sonnenburg, E.D.; Costello, E.K.; Higginbottom, S.K.; Domino, S.E.; Holmes, S.P.; Relman, D.A.; et al. Genetically dictated change in host mucus carbohydrate landscape exerts a diet-dependent effect on the gut microbiota. *Proc. Natl. Acad. Sci. USA* **2013**, *110*, 17059–17064. [CrossRef] [PubMed]

87. Delgado, M.; Singh, S.; De Haro, S.; Master, S.; Ponpuak, M.; Dinkins, C.; Ornatowski, W.; Vergne, I.; Deretic, V. Autophagy and pattern recognition receptors in innate immunity. *Immunol. Rev.* **2009**, *227*, 189–202. [CrossRef] [PubMed]

88. Randall-Demllo, S.; Chieppa, M.; Eri, R. Intestinal epithelium and autophagy: Partners in gut homeostasis. *Front. Immunol.* **2013**, *4*, 301. [CrossRef] [PubMed]

89. Cleynen, I.; Boucher, G.; Jostins, L.; Schumm, L.P.; Zeissig, S.; Ahmad, T.; Andersen, V.; Andrews, J.M.; Annese, V.; Brand, S.; et al. Inherited determinants of Crohn's disease and ulcerative colitis phenotypes: A genetic association study. *Lancet* **2016**, *387*, 156–167. [CrossRef]

4

Intestinal Anti-Inflammatory Effect of a Peptide Derived from Gastrointestinal Digestion of Buffalo (*Bubalus bubalis*) Mozzarella Cheese

Gian Carlo Tenore [1,†], Ester Pagano [1,†], Stefania Lama [2], Daniela Vanacore [2], Salvatore Di Maro, Maria Maisto, Raffaele Capasso [4], Francesco Merlino [1], Francesca Borrelli [1,*], Paola Stiuso [2,*] and Ettore Novellino [1]

[1] Department of Pharmacy, School of Medicine and Surgery, University of Naples Federico II, Via D. Montesano 49, 80131 Naples, Italy; giancarlo.tenore@unina.it (G.C.T.); ester.pagano@unina.it (E.P.); maria.maisto@unina.it (M.M.); francesco.merlino@unina.it (F.M.); ettore.novellino@unina.it (E.N.)

[2] Department of Precision Medicine, University of Campania "Luigi Vanvitelli", Via De Crecchio 7, 80138 Naples, Italy; stefania.lama@unicampania.it (S.L.); daniela.vanacore@unicampania.it (D.V.)

[3] DiSTABiF, Università degli Studi della Campania "Luigi Vanvitelli", via Vivaldi 43, 81100 Caserta, Italy; salvatore.dimaro@unicampania.it

[4] Department of Agricultural Sciences, University of Naples Federico II, 80055 Portici, Italy; raffaele.capasso@unina.it

* Correspondence: franborr@unina.it (F.B.); paola.stiuso@unicampania.it (P.S.)

† These two authors equally contributed to this work.

Abstract: Under physiological conditions, the small intestine represents a barrier against harmful antigens and pathogens. Maintaining of the intestinal barrier depends largely on cell–cell interactions (adherent-junctions) and cell–matrix interactions (tight-junctions). Inflammatory bowel disease is characterized by chronic inflammation, which induces a destructuring of the architecture junctional epithelial proteins with consequent rupture of the intestinal barrier. Recently, a peptide identified by *Bubalus bubalis* milk-derived products (MBCP) has been able to reduce oxidative stress in intestinal epithelial cells and erythrocytes. Our aim was to evaluate the therapeutic potential of MBCP in inflammatory bowel disease (IBD). We studied the effect of MBCP on (i) inflamed human intestinal Caco2 cells and (ii) dinitrobenzene sulfonic acid (DNBS) mice model of colitis. We have shown that MBCP, at non-cytotoxic concentrations, both *in vitro* and *in vivo* induced the adherent epithelial junctions organization, modulated the nuclear factor (NF)-κB pathway and reduced the intestinal permeability. Furthermore, the MBCP reverted the atropine and tubocurarine injury effects on adherent-junctions. The data obtained showed that MBCP possesses anti-inflammatory effects both *in vitro* and *in vivo*. These results could have an important impact on the therapeutic potential of MBCP in helping to restore the intestinal epithelium integrity damaged by inflammation.

Keywords: intestinal inflammation; inflammatory bowel disease; epithelial adherens junctions; bioactive peptides

---

1. Introduction

Inflammatory bowel disease (IBD) is a term used to describe conditions that are characterized by chronic inflammation of the gastrointestinal tract. Crohn's disease and ulcerative colitis are the principal types of inflammatory bowel disease. Worldwide, the prevalence and incidence of IBD is increasing mainly in newly industrialized countries whose societies have become more Westernized [1]. Although the etiology of IBD is still unknown, it arises as a result of the interaction of environmental or genetic factors and the immune responses [2]. IBD treatment involves the use of anti-inflammatory drugs (such as 5-aminosalicylic acid), corticosteroids, monoclonal antibodies [anti-tumor necrosis factor (TNF)-α antibodies] and vascular adhesion molecules [2,3] (anti-integrin antibodies). However, these drugs are not curative therapies and are mainly used as induction and maintenance therapy. Moreover, for most of these drugs, a high inter-individual variability in a positive response has been reported [3]. Therefore, it is essential to find clinical efficacious alternatives for the treatment of inflammatory bowel disease (IBD). Recently, intestinal permeability has been recognized as a new target for IBD prevention and therapy [4,5]. In physiological conditions, the intestinal epithelium selectively absorbs nutrients and represents an efficient barrier to noxious antigens and pathogens. Disruption of the intestinal barrier has been considered a major factor in several inflammatory intestinal diseases [6]. The architecture and function of the intestinal epithelium requires close coordination between enterocyte proliferation and apoptosis, both highly dependent on cell–cell and cell–matrix interactions. Enterocytes are joined to each other by tight junctions and adherens junctions. The main molecular component of the adherens junctions is E-cadherin, a transmembrane protein with five extracellular domains that interdigitate with those of an adjacent cell in a calcium-dependent homophilic manner to form a continuous linear "zipper" structure [7,8]. E-cadherin exerts functional adhesion activity when it is connected to the actin cytoskeleton by the cytoplasmic complex α-, β-, or γ-catenin in a mutually exclusive manner [7,8]. It is well established that, in IBD patients, these junctional complexes undergo a disruption leading to a breaking of the intestinal barrier [9]. Moreover, mucosal biopsies from patients with IBD have increased levels of cytokines, able to regulate intercellular permeability, such as interferon-gamma (IFN-γ) and tumor necrosis factor (TNF-α), have been observed [10].

Buffalo (*Bubalus bubalis*) milk is a source of many bioactive peptides that have been demonstrated to play a relevant role in preventing various disorders [11–14]. These bioactive peptides are mainly released during gastrointestinal digestion of milk and milk-products. Recently, novel peptides have been identified from buffalo milk-derived products (MBCP) that are able to reduce H_2O_2-induced oxidative stress in intestinal epithelial cells and in erythrocytes [15,16]. Among these, MBCP, a peptide isolated from the buffalo milk after *in vitro* digestion of *Mozzarella di Bufala Campana DOP*, has demonstrated possession of a good stability to brush border exopeptidases and a high bioavailability [16]. In this paper, we evaluated the therapeutic potential of MBCP in IBD. For this purpose, we investigated the effect of MBCP on (i) adjacent junctions conformation and permeability under inflammatory conditions in an intestinal epithelial cell line, Caco-2 cells and (ii) intestinal inflammation and the associated changes in motility in mice.

2. Material and Methods

2.1. Peptide Synthesis

MBCP was synthetised using the solid-phase method and purified via HPLC after deprotection, as previously described [16]. MBCP was dissolved in water for *in vitro* and *in vivo* experiments.

2.2. Drugs and Reagents

2,4,6-dinitrobenzenesulfonic acid (DNBS), croton oil, fluorescein isothiocyanate (FITC)-conjugated dextran (molecular mass 3–5 kDa), betamethasone, atropine, tubocurarine and neutral red (NR) solution were purchased from Sigma (Milan, Italy). TNF-α was obtained from R&D Systems, Space Import-Export SRL (Milano, Italy). All reagents for cell cultures were obtained from Sigma, Bio-Rad Laboratories (Milan, Italy) and Microtech Srl (Naples, Italy). All chemicals and reagents employed in this study were of analytical grade.

2.3. Cell Culture

Caco-2 cells (American Type Culture Collection, Rockville, MD, USA), a human colorectal adenocarcinoma epithelial cell line, were grown at 37 °C in a 5% CO_2 atmosphere in h-glucose Minimum essential medium MEM containing 1% non-essential amino acids and supplemented with 10% de-complemented fetal bovine serum (FBS), 100 U·mL^{-1} penicillin, 100 mg·mL^{-1} streptomycin, 1% L-glutamine and 1% sodium pyruvate. The growth of the cells was measured by counting the cells with a Coulter counter (Nexcelom, Lawrence, MA, USA, Cellometer Auto1000). All experiments were performed in triplicate.

2.4. Animals

Male adult ICR mice, weighing 20–25 g for upper gastrointestinal transit experiments and 25–30 g for colitis experiments, were purchased from Charles River Laboratories (Calco, Lecco, Italy) and housed in polycarbonate cages under controlled temperature (23 ± 2 °C), constant humidity (60%) and a 12 h light/dark cycle. The animals were acclimatized to their environment at least 1 week under the above reported standard conditions with free access to tap water. Mice were fed *ad libitum* with a standard rodent diet, except for the 24 h immediately before the intracolonic administration of DNBS or the oral administration of the charcoal meal and for 2-h before the oral gavage of croton oil or MBCP. Mice were randomly allocated to different experimental groups and outcome assessments were performed in single-blind. All experiments were approved by the Institutional Animal Ethics Committee for the use of experimental animals and conformed to guidelines for the safe use and care of experimental animals in accordance with the Italian D.L. no. 116 of 27 January 1992 and associated guidelines in the European Communities Council (86/609/ECC and 2010/63/UE).

2.5. Cytotoxicity Studies

We evaluated the effect of MBCP on Caco-2 cell viability by using a microplate colorimetric assay that measures the ability of viable cells to incorporate and bind the neutral red (NR), a weak cationic dye, in lysosomes. Cells were plated at the appropriate density to obtain a model of undifferentiated and differentiated cells; then, 5×10^3 and 20×10^3 cells per well in 96-well plates for undifferentiated and differentiated cells, respectively. After 24 hours, cells were exposed to various concentrations of MBCP (9–375 µM) for 48-h. Then, cells were incubated with NR dye solution (50 µg/mL) for 3-h at 37 °C, and finally washed with phosphate buffered saline (PBS) and lysed with 1% acetic acid. The absorbance was read at 540 nm (iMarkTM microplate reader, Bio-Rad, Milano, Italy).

2.6. Alkaline Phosphatase (ALP) Activity

ALP activity was used as marker of the degree of differentiation of human Caco-2 cells. Attached and floating cells were washed and lysed with 0.25% sodium deoxycholate. ALP activity was determined using Sigma Diagnostics ALP reagent (no. 245). Total cellular protein content of the samples was determined in a microassay procedure using the Coomassie protein assay reagent kit (Pierce). ALP activity was calculated as nmol/min/mg of protein.

2.7. Western Blotting

For cell extract preparation, the cells were washed twice with ice-cold PBS/bovine serum albumin (BSA), scraped and centrifuged for 30 min at 4 °C in 1 mL of lysis buffer (1% Triton, 0.5% sodium deoxycholate, 0.1 M NaCl, 1mM Ethylenediamine tetra-acetic acid (EDTA), pH 7.5, 10 mM Na_2HPO_4, pH 7.4, 10 mM Phenylmethyl sulfonyl fluoride, 25 mM benzamidin, 1 mM leupeptin, 0.025 units/mL aprotinin). Colon tissue were lysed in a specific buffer (1% NP-40, 0.1% SDS, 100 mM sodium ortovanadate, 0.5% sodium deoxycholate in RIPA buffer) in the presence of protease inhibitors (4 mg/mL of leupeptin, aprotinin, pepstatin A, chymostatin, PMSF and 5 mg/mL of chymotrypsin-like proteases (TPCK)). The homogenates were sonicated twice by three strokes (20 Hz for 20 s each); after centrifugation for 30 min at $10,000 \times g$, the supernatants were stored at 80 °C. Equal amounts of cell and tissues proteins were separated by SDS-PAGE, electrotransferred to nitrocellulose and reacted with the different antibodies. Blots were then developed using enhanced chemoluminescence detection reagents (SuperSignal West Pico, Pierce) and exposed to X-ray film. All films were scanned by using Quantity One software (BioRad laboratories, Hercules, CA, USA).

2.8. Immunostaining and Confocal Microscopy

After 24-h and 48-h of incubation with TNF-α (10 μM), TNF-α plus MBCP (18 μM) or TNF-α plus betamethasone (10 μM), Caco-2 cells were fixed for 20 min with a 3% (*w/v*) paraformaldehyde solution and permeabilized for 10 min with 0.1% (*w/v*) Triton X-100 in PBS at room temperature. To prevent nonspecific interactions of antibodies, cells were treated for 2 h in 5% BSA in PBS. In another set of experiments, Caco-2 cells were treated with the acetylcholine receptor antagonists atropine (10 μM) and tubocurarine (10 μM) for 6-h. Immunostaining was carried out by incubation with anti-E-cadherin, anti-actin and anti-β-catenin antibodies (1:500, Alexa Fluor®, BD Pharmingen™). The slides were mounted on microscope slides by Mowiol. The analyses were performed with a Zeiss LSM 510 microscope equipped with a plan-apochromat objective X 63 (NA 1.4) in oil immersion. The nuclei were stained with 4′,6-diamidino-2-phenylindole (DAPI).

2.9. Permeability Assay on Caco-2 Cells

To evaluate cell permeability, Caco-2 cells were seeded into a transwell filters with a pore diameter of 8 μm in 24-well plates at a density of 2.0×10^5 cells/insert. Further cultivation in the same medium as above allowed the cells to spontaneously differentiate and polarize into the epithelial monolayer within 21 days. The basolateral compartment contained 1.5 mL of culture medium while apical compartment contained 0.2 mL. After seeding, the cells were treated with 0.07 μM of MBCP. The culture medium was replaced 3 times/wk. After 21 days, the filters containing the cell monolayers (with or without MBCP) were treated for 2 h with TNF-α (10 μM) and then with a mannitol-lactulose solution (0.05 mmol/L, 0.25 mol/L, 0.2 mL). After 3 hours, the basolateral solution was collected and both mannitol and lactulose concentration were measured by liquid chromatography-mass spectrometry (LC-MS).

2.10. Induction of Experimental Colitis

Colitis was induced in the anesthetized mice by the intracolonic administration of 2,4,6-dinitrobenzene sulfonic acid (DNBS) as previously described [17]. Briefly, DNBS (150 mg/kg), dissolved in 50% ethanol (150 μL/mouse), was administrated into the distal colon using a polyethylene catheter (1 mm in diameter) via the rectum (4.5 cm from the anus). Three days after the DNBS administration, all mice were euthanized by asphyxiation with CO_2, the mice abdomen was opened by a midline incision and the colon removed, isolated from surrounding tissues, length measured, opened along the antimesenteric border, rinsed and weighed and then fixed in 10% formaldehyde for histopathological analysis. MBCP was administrated by oral gavage (10–100 mg/kg) once a day for 3 consecutive days starting 24 h after DNBS administration. Animals were euthanized 2 hours after the last administration of MBCP.

2.11. Haematoxylin-Eosin Staining

Paraffin-embedded colon tissues were cut into 5-mm sections. The sections were dewaxed in xylene for 10 min and dehydrated in gradient alcohol. The sections were then stained with haematoxylin for 8 min and eosin for 5 min. After dehydration, the sections were sealed and examined under a light microscope (Leica DM 2500). Photographs were taken using the Leica DFC320 R2 digital camera [18].

2.12. Immuno-Fluorescence Microscopy

The fixed slides of colon tissue, were dewaxed, rehydrated and processed. Briefly, antigen retrieval was performed by pressure-cooking slides for 3 min in 0.01 M citrate buffer (pH 6.0). To prevent nonspecific interactions of antibodies, the slides were treated for 2 h in 5% BSA in PBS. Immunostaining was carried out by incubation, overnight at 4 °C, with anti-E-cadherin and anti-β-Catenin antibodies (1:100, Alexa Fluor®, BD Pharmingen™). The slides were mounted on microscope slides by Mowiol + DAPI for nuclear staining, and then observed under the optical microscope (Leica DM 5000 B + CTR 5000).

2.13. Intestinal Permeability Measurement

The effect of MBCP, at a dose of 100 mg/kg, was also tested on intestinal permeability, using the FITC-Dextran method.Briefly, 2 days after the induction of colitis, mice were gavaged with 600 mg/kg of FITC–conjugated dextran (molecular mass 3–5 kDa). After 24 h, blood was collected by cardiac puncture, and the FITC-derived fluorescence was immediately analyzed in the serum by a microplate reader (GloMax Explorer System, Promega; excitation wavelengths 485 ± 14 nm, emission wavelengths 520 ± 25 nm). Serial-diluted FITC dextran was used to generate a standard curve. Intestinal permeability was expressed as the concentrations of FITC (μM) detected in the serum.

2.14. Induction of Intestinal Hypermotility and Upper Gastrointestinal Transit in Mice

Upper gastrointestinal transit was measured in both physiological and pathological conditions. The hypermotility was induced by the inflammatory agent croton oil (CO) as previously described [19]. Briefly, two doses of CO (20 μL/mouse) were given for two consecutive days by oral gavage and the upper gastrointestinal transit was measured 4 days after the first administration of CO [20] (i.e., when the maximal inflammatory response associated to the intestinal hypermotility was reported). Mice were deprived of food overnight and then the upper gastrointestinal transit was evaluated by identifying the leading front of an intragastrically administered charcoal meal marker (10% charcoal suspension in 5% gum Arabic, 10 mL/kg) in the small intestine as previously described [19]. Twenty minutes after charcoal administration, mice were euthanized and the small intestine was isolated by cutting at the pyloric and ileocaecal junctions. The distance traveled by the marker was measured and expressed as a percentage of the total length of the small intestine from pylorus to caecum. MBCP was administrated by oral gavage (5–50 mg/kg) 30 min prior to charcoal administration.

2.15. Statistical Analysis

Data are expressed as the mean $\pm$ S.E.M. or S.D. of n experiments. Statistical significance was assessed using the Student's t-test for comparing a single treatment mean with a control mean, and a one-way ANOVA followed by a Tukey multiple comparisons test for the analysis of multiple treatment means. Values of $p < 0.05$ were considered significant. The IC_{50} (concentration that produced 50% inhibition of cell viability) values were calculated using sigmoidal dose response curve-fitting models (Graphpad Prism Software, version 5.03, Inc. Avendia de la Playa La Jolla, CA, USA).

3. Results

3.1. In Vitro Study

3.1.1. MBCP Induces Cytotoxic Effects in Caco-2 Cells at Very High Concentrations

In order to characterize a safety profile of MBCP, we evaluated its effect on the cell viability of pre- (undifferentiated exponentially growing) and post-confluent (differentiated) Caco-2 cells. MBCP (9–375 μM), induced in undifferentiated and differentiated Caco-2 cells, a concentration-dependent cell viability inhibition at 48 h with an IC_{50} of 65 μM (Figure 1). Therefore, to characterize the anti-inflammatory effects of MBCP on Caco-2 cells, subsequent experiments were performed using a

MBCP concentration that did not induce significant cytotoxic effect in both pre and post-confluent cells (i.e., 18 μM).

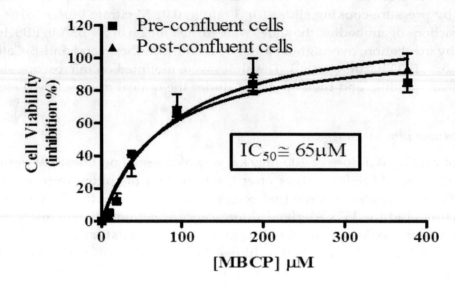

Figure 1. MBCP reduces cell viability in Caco-2 cells. Cell viability was evaluated by the Neutral Red assay in pre and post-confluent Caco-2 cells. Cells were incubated with increasing concentration of MBCP (9–375 μM) for 48 h. Each point represents the mean ± SD of three independent experiments.

3.1.2. MBCP Stimulates Differentiation in Growing Caco-2 Cells

The effect of MBCP on cell differentiation was evaluated by measuring the activity of alkaline phosphatase, with the enzyme frequently used as a marker of colon cells differentiation [21]. A treatment of undifferentiated Caco-2 cells with MBCP (18 μM for 48 h) induced a significantly increase ($p < 0.05$) of alkaline phosphatase activity (APA) of about 14% compared to the untreated Caco-2 cells (control). The APA value was in the Caco-2 cells of 8.6 ± 0.4 (nmol/min/mg protein), while, in MBCP treated Caco-2 cells, it was 10 ± 0.7 (mean ± SD, $n = 3$, * $p < 0.05$)

3.1.3. MBCP Modulates Adherent Junctions Formation in Control and TNF-α-Stimulated Caco-2 Cells

In order to investigate the role of MBCP on adherent junctions (AJs) formation, we studied the cellular organization of E-cadherin and actin in pre-confluent Caco-2 cells by confocal miscroscopy. Caco-2 cells, after 24 h from seeding, showed a strong cytoplasmic localization of both E-cadherin and actin proteins (Figure 2A–C) that was ameliorated by MBCP treatment (Figure 2D–F). At 48 h, the E-cadherin-actin complex presented a not homogeneous membranous localization in untreated Caco-2 cells (Figure 2G–I). MBCP treatment induced a strong cell–cell contact membranous localization of E-cadherin-Actin complex (Figure 2M–O).

To assess whether MBCP could counteract the AJ-destructuration induced by the pro-inflammatory mediator TNF-α, we examined the β-catenin organization in TNF-α-stimulated cells. Caco-2 cells treated with TNF-α (10 μM, for 48-h) showed a cytoplasmic compartment β-catenin localization (Figure 3D–F) compared to untreated cells (CTR) (Figure 3A–C). A treatment of Caco-2 cell with MBCP (18 μM) induced an enhancement of both E-cadherin and β-catenin localization at AJs (Figure 2G–I) compared to TNF-α alone. Since corticosteroids are the effective first-line treatment in cytokine-induced inflammation, we treated the Caco-2 cells (stimulated with TNF-α) with betamethasone. Betamethasone (10 μM) treatment induced a membranous E-cadherin and β-catenin organization, although a β-catenin cytoplasmic immunoreactivity persisted (Figure 3L–N). In our experimental conditions (Caco-2 cells treated or not with TNF-α), MBCP accelerated and induced an organization of adjacent junctions in the cells, without changes the E-cadherin, actin and β-catenin protein expression evaluated by Western blot analysis (data not shown).

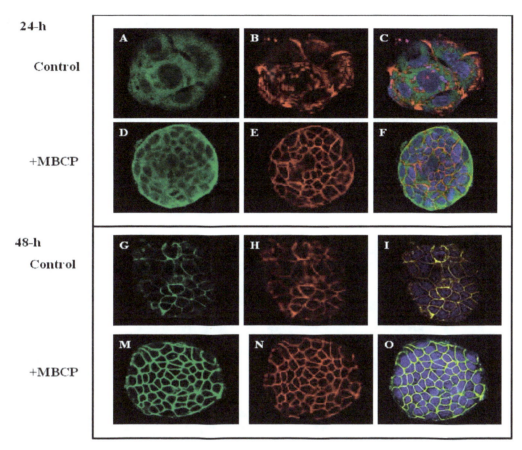

Figure 2. MBCP accelerates the formation of adherens junctions. Confocal microscopy images of Caco-2 cells (**A–C,G–I**) and MBCP treated Caco-2 cells (panel (**D–F,M–O**). Cells were treated for 24-h and 48-h with MBCP at 18 μM concentration. The merged image is on the right (green, actin; red, E-cadherin; blue, dapi).

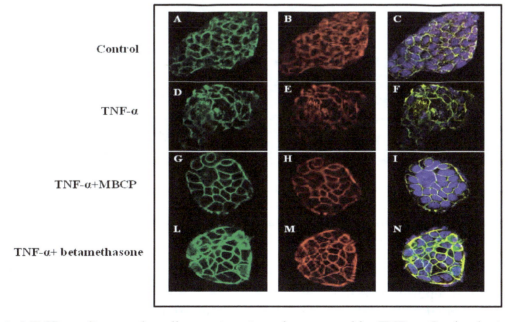

Figure 3. MBCP ameliorates the adherens junctions destructured by TNF-α. Confocal microscopy images of untreated Caco-2 cells (panel (**A–C**), Caco-2 cells treated for 48 h with TNF-α (10 μM, (**D–F**)), TNFα 10μM plus MBCP (18 μM, (**G–I**)) or with TNF-α (10 μM) plus betamethasone (**L–N**). On the right, merged image (green, β-catenin; red, E-cadherin; blue, dapi).

3.1.4. MBCP Counteracts the TNF-α Inflammatory Effect by Modulating the NF-κB Pathway

It is well known that TNF-α causes the activation of transcription factors, including NF-κB. NF-κB regulates host inflammatory, immune responses and also stimulates the expression of inducible cyclooxygenase enzymes (COX-2) that contribute to the pathogenesis of the inflammatory process. Therefore, we evaluated, by Western blot analysis, the effects of MBCP on NF-κB, pNF-κB, COX-2 and 5-Lipoxygenases (LOX) expression in TNF-α treated Caco-2 cells. A treatment with TNF-α induced an increase of 5-LOX, p-NF-κB and COX-2 expression. MBCP (18 μM) was able to reduce the expression of p-NF-κB, 5-LOX and COX-2 expression increased by TNF-α (Figure 4). Moreover, MBCP (18 μM) reduced the basal expression of NF-κB in untreated Caco-2 cells. Betamethasone (10 μM), used as a positive control, significantly reduced 5-LOX expression, but not the NF-κB, p-NF-κB and COX-2 expression, increased by TNF-α.

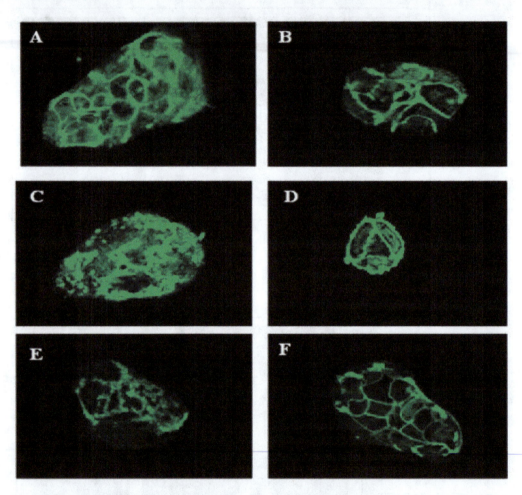

Figure 4. MBCP ameliorates the adherens junctions destructured by atropine and tubocurarine. Confocal microscopy images of untreated Caco-2 cells (**A**) or Caco-2 cells treated for six hours with MBCP (18 μM, (**B**)), tubocurarine (10 μM, (**C**)), Tubocurarine plus MBCP (**D**), atropine (10 μM, (**E**)) and atropine plus MBCP (**F**). The color green represents β-catenin.

3.1.5. MBCP Reduces Atropine and Tubocurarine-Induced Adherens Junctions Disorganization

Several studies reported that the stimulation of the acetylcholine receptors (AChR) enhances epithelial barrier formation [22,23] and ameliorates TNF-α induced barrier dysfunction in intestinal epithelial cells [24]. According to literature, treatment of Caco-2 cells with the AChR antagonists atropine (10 μM) or tubocurarine (10 μM) induced an disorganization of adherents junctions (Figure 5). MBCP (18 μM) attenuated both atropine and tubocurarine AChR antagonist effects on Caco-2 cells adherens junctions, indicating that MBCP treatment could affect the AChR pathway (Figure 5).

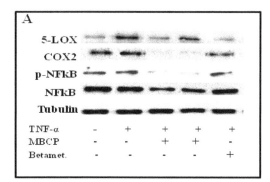 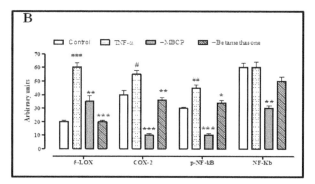

Figure 5. MBCP reduces the expression of 5-LOX, COX-2, p-NF-κB and NF-κB. (**A**) Western blot analysis of Caco-2 cells alone or treated with MBCP or betamethasone. Bands associated with the expression of 5-LOX, COX-2, p-NF-κB, NF-κB, and house-keeping γ-tubulin, after 48 h of treatment with MBCP (18 μM) and betamethasone (10 μM). The expression of the house-keeping protein γ-tubulin was used as loading control. (**B**) The expression levels of the above proteins are reported as a percentage with respect to the level of the protein in untreated cells, used as control. Bars show the mean ± SD of three different determinations. # $p < 0.05$, ## $p < 0.01$ and ### $p < 0.001$ vs. control; * $p < 0.05$, ** $p < 0.01$ and *** $p < 0.001$ vs. TNF-α alone.

3.1.6. MBCP Inhibits the TNF-α-Increased Caco-2 Permeability

The intestinal epithelial cell line Caco-2 has been used extensively as a model of the human epithelium, as it can be grown in the Transwell system as a differentiated cell monolayer that has selective paracellular permeability to ions and solutes. We used both mannitol and lactulose, intestinal permeability probes, to evaluate the permeability changes in Caco-2 stimulated with TNF-α. Treatment of the Caco-2 cell (see Section 2.9) with TNF-α (10 μM) increased the concentration of mannitol in the basolateral solution by about twofold compared to the control cells (cells without TNF-α treatment). [Control of mannitol concentration (mmol/L): 0.01 ± 0.004; TNF-α 0.023 ± 0.005 *; mean ± SD; * $p < 0.05$]. The mannitol concentration in the basolateral side of the Caco-2 cells pretreated with MBCP and then incubated with TNF-α (0.009 ± 0.003 mmol/L, mean ± SD; n = 3, * $p < 0.05$) was decreased twofold compared to the TNF-α treated Caco-2 cells. The MBCP induced any change of the lactulose permeability in the same inflammatory cell condition.

3.2. In Vivo Study

3.2.1. MBCP Reduces the Inflammation in the DNBS Model of Colitis

The DNBS murine model of colitis was used to assess the in vivo intestinal anti-inflammatory effects of MBCP. DNBS administration (150 mg/kg) caused inflammatory damage, as indicated by the approximately twofold increase in colon weight/colon length *ratio* (mg/cm), a simple and reliable marker of inflammation and damage (Figure 6A). MBCP (10–100 mg/kg, by oral gavage), administered for three consecutive days after the inflammatory insult, significantly and in a dose-dependent manner, reduced the effect of DNBS on colon weight/colon length *ratio*. The effect was significant starting from 30 mg/kg dose (Figure 6A). The anti-inflammatory effect MBCP was further confirmed by histological analysis. As shown in Figure 6B, DNBS caused a severe inflammatory cellular infiltration and complete destruction of the colon epithelium, compared to control mice (Figure 6B). Our data showed that oral MBCP (100 mg/kg) reduced the colonic damage induced by DNBS (Figure 6B).

Considering that the peptide inhibited the phosphorylation of NF-κB in vitro, we investigated if this pathway was involved in the in vivo anti-inflammatory effect of MBCP. As shown in Figure 6C, the phosphorylation of IκBα and active NF-κB expression were increased in the colons of mice treated with DNBS. MBCP (100 mg/kg) was able to significantly reduce these changes induced by DNBS. These results demonstrated that MBCP suppressed NF-κB activation both in the experimental model of colitis and in TNFα-stimulated Caco-2 cells.

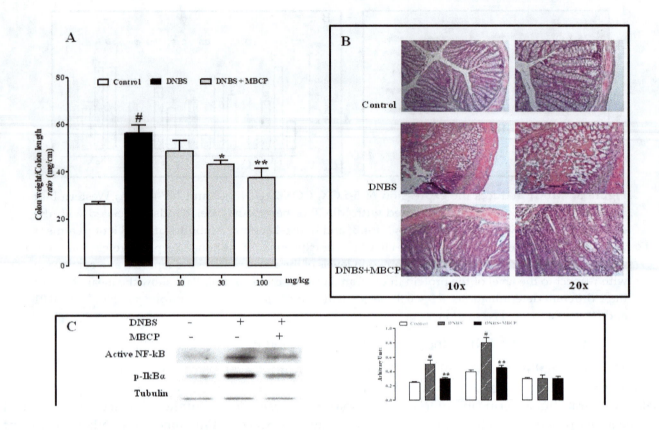

Figure 6. MBCP reduces colon weight/colon length *ratio* in DNBS-induced colitis in mice. (**A**) MBCP (10–100 mg/kg, by oral gavage) was administered once a day starting 24 h after the induction of colitis by DNBS (150 mg/kg). Colons were collected three days after DNBS. (**B**) representative hematoxylin & eosin stained colon cross-sections of mice treated with vehicle (control), DNBS and DNBS plus MBCP (100 mg/kg by oral gavage). Colons were collected three days after the induction of colitis by DNBS. Original magnification 10× and 20× (A). (**C**) Western blot analysis of p-NF-κB, NF-κB, and house-keeping γ-tubulin expression in normal mice colon and after the induction of colitis by DNBS. All data are represented as mean ± SEM of seven mice for each experimental group. Statistical significance was calculated using one-way ANOVA test. # $p < 0.001$ vs. control, * $p < 0.05$ and ** $p < 0.01$ vs. DNBS alone.

3.2.2. MBCP Reduces the Intestinal Permeability in Vivo

The intestinal permeability was increased of the intracolonic administration of DNBS, as revealed by the high concentration of FITC-conjugated dextran in the serum (see Supplementary Files Figure S1). While MBCP (100 mg/kg), given by oral gavage for three consecutive days, synergistically ($p < 0.01$) partially counteracted the DNBS-induced increase in intestinal permeability (see Supplementary Files Figure S1). Moreover, immunofluorescence analysis showed that DNBS administration caused a destructuration of the colonic AJs associated with an increase of the citoplasmatic expression of E-cadherin and β-catenin. MBCP (100 mg/kg) counteracted the effect of DNBS on AJs, (Figure 7), thus confirming the *in vitro* results on TNF-α-stimulated Caco-2 cells.

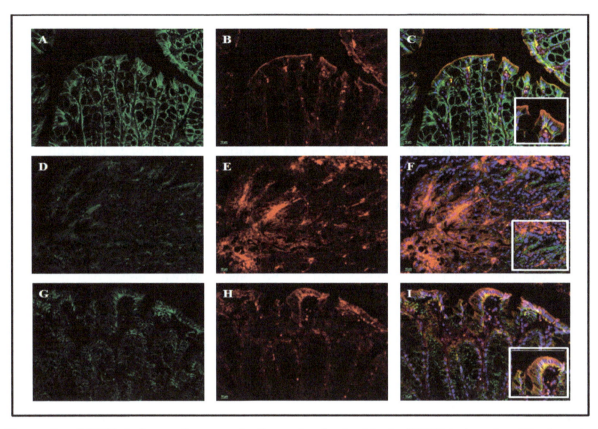

Figure 7. MBCP induces the organization of colonic AJs in DNBS-induced colitis in mice. Immunofluorescence analysis showing the expression of E-cadherin (red) and β-catenin (green) in control (**A–C**), DNBS (**D–F**) and DNBS plus MBCP (**G–I**) (100 mg/kg) mice. Original magnification 20×. A magnified portion of the immunofluorescence was shown at higher magnification in the inset of panel (**C,F,I**). The DNBS-induced colitis in mice was treated for three consecutive days after the inflammatory insults with MBCP (100 mg/kg, by oral gavage).

3.2.3. MBCP Counteracts the Accelerated Upper Gastrointestinal Transit Induced by Croton Oil

The administration of the flogogen agent croton oil (CO) induced an accelerated upper gastrointestinal transit (GT) 4 days after its first administration. The physiological GT percentage in the mice (control) was of 49.8 ± 1.4; whereas GT significantly increased up to values of 65.50 ± 6.26* (mean ± SEM; * $p < 0.05$) in CO treated mice. MBCP (5–50 mg/kg), given by oral gavage 30 min before the administration of the charcoal, in a dose dependent manner restored the intestinal motility to physiological conditions (% of GT MBCP 5 mg/kg: 59.43 ± 2.75; MBCP 10 mg/kg: 56.14 ± 3.63; MBCP 50 mg/kg: 39.87 ± 6.38 **; ** $p < 0.01$). MBCP, at the high dose (50 mg/kg), did not modify the upper gastrointestinal transit in control mice (% of GT: control 55 ± 3.53; MBCP 48.60 ± 4.38 (mean ± SEM)).

4. Discussion

In mammals, the enterocytes are renewed continuously every 4–8 days through an organized series of events involving proliferation, differentiation and programmed cell death. The proliferation to differentiation transition (PDT) is a critical step in the continual renewal of a normal intestinal epithelium [25]. A useful *in vitro* model to study the effects of food ingredients on the gut epithelial layer is based on the use of Caco-2 cells for their functional similarity to colonic enterocytes [26]. Indeed, Caco-2 cells express tight junctions, microvilli, enzymes and transporters functionally similar to colonic enterocyte [26]. Moreover, this cell line has the ability to elicit a pro-inflammatory reaction in response to stimulants like TNF-α, a known mediator of gastrointestinal mucosal barrier injury [5,27]. In this study, we have shown that a peptide (MBCP) obtained from gastrointestinal digestion of *Mozzarella of Bufala Campana DOP* is able to modulate the differentiation and permeability in Caco-2 cells stimulated with TNF-α and to attenuate inflammation and hypermotility in murine models of intestinal inflammation.

4.1. MBPC Modulates the Differentiation and Permeability in Caco-2 Cells

Proliferating Caco-2 cells spontaneously initiate the differentiation process when they have reached confluence. The differentiation program starts when specific biochemical events induce the cell–cell contact, through the E-Cadherin/actin/β-Catenin complex [28]. Here, we have found that MBCP, at a non-cytotoxic concentration (i.e., 18 μM), induced an increase of intestinal alkaline phosphatase activity in undifferentiated Caco2 cells. Intestinal alkaline phosphatase is a well-known cell differentiation marker and its activity has been inversely correlated with an increased risk of intestinal inflammation development [29]. Moreover, we also found that MBCP treatment, already after 24 h, induced the differentiation program accelerating the E-cadherin-actin membranous organization, thus suggesting a beneficial effect on the AJ. This result is further supported by the experiments with TNF-α. According to previous studies [30], we have shown that Caco-2 treatment with TNF-α induced molecular alterations of the E-cadherin organization and consequently a passage of mannitol through the Caco-2 monolayer. MBCP treatment was able to restore the cell–cell junctions, counteracting the breakdown of E-cadherin-β-catenin complex and reducing the increase of mannitol permeability inducted by TNF-α.

According to previous studies, we found that un-stimulated Caco-2 cells over-expressed COX-2 and NF-κB and TNF-α-stimulated Caco-2 cells increased 5-LOX expression. NF-κB transcription factor is a master regulator of the inflammatory response and it is essential for the homeostasis of the immune system. NF-κB regulates the transcription of genes, such as LOX and COX-2, which control inflammation [31]. Our results demonstrated that MBCP reduced the phosphorylation of NF-κB as well as COX-2 and 5-LOX expression in TNF-α stimulated cells.

Many mechanisms are responsible for the regulation and stability of adherens junction proteins, one of these possibilities could be the AChR activation. Furthermore, previous studies indicate that cholinergic agonists interfere with NF-κB pathways preventing IkBα breakdown and p65 nuclear translocation [24,32]. Moreover, cholinergic agonists could prevent gut barrier failure after severe burn injury maintaining intestinal barrier integrity. McGilligan has showed that nicotine decrease Caco-2 permeability by regulating the expression of TJ proteins [33]. Therefore, we measured changes in localization of β-catenin to determine whether modulation of this protein correlates with the adherens junctions disorganization induced by cholinergic antagonists like atropine and tubocurarine. Confocal microscopy analysis confirmed that both atropine and tubocurarine treatment induced a cytoplasmic accumulation of β-catenin in Caco-2 cells. These detrimental effects induced by cholinergic antagonists were counteracted by MBCP treatment.

4.2. MBPC Ameliorates Murine Colitis

The ability of MBCP to restore cell–cell contacts as well as to exert an anti-inflammatory actions was subsequently evaluated *in vivo* by using the mice model of DNBS-induced colitis. According to previous studies [34,35] intracolonic administration of DNBS induced intestinal inflammation associated to an increase of epithelial permeability. Oral MBCP administration was able to reduce intestinal inflammation as demonstrated by the reduction of colon weight colon length *ratio* (a simple and reliable marker of inflammation and damage), histological alterations, IkBα phosphorylation and of NF-κB activation associated with DNBS administration.

Intestinal permeability plays a crucial role in the development of IBD as well as in the IBD ongoing bowel symptoms [5,36]. Moreover, inflammation reduces barrier integrity and affects the normal intestinal permeability [4]. Studies on Caco-2 cells have shown that MBCP restored tight junctions altered by TNF-α. Tight junctions are multi-protein complexes that maintain the intestinal barrier while regulating permeability [9]. Therefore, we investigated the effect of MBPC on intestinal permeability in vivo. We adopted an immunofluorescent method through which an orally-administered marker (i.e., FITC-conjugated dextran) can be detected in the blood if permeability is impaired. As expected, intestinal permeability increased after DNBS administration and, more importantly, MBCP restored the impaired permeability.

4.3. MBPC Normalizes Inflammation-Induced Murine Intestinal Hypermotility

It is clinically well established that inflammation in the gut causes debilitating symptoms due to motility disturbances [37]. To investigate the effect of MBCP on intestinal motility, we administered mice croton oil, which is a flogogen agent able to induce hypermotility as a consequence of intestinal inflammation. By using this experimental model, we have shown that MBCP did not affect motility in healthy mice, but normalized the exaggerated intestinal transit caused by the inflammatory insult. The lack of effect of MBPC in control mice is clinically relevant in the light of the observation that constipation is a very common side effect associated with drugs clinically used to reduce intestinal motility [38,39].

5. Conclusions

In conclusion, the data obtained in our study shown that MBCP, a peptide isolated from the buffalo milk after *in vitro* digestion of *Mozzarella di Bufala Campana DOP*, exerts anti-inflammatory effects both *in vitro* and *in vivo*. This anti-inflammatory effect could be related to its beneficial effects on adherens junctions mainly during an inflammatory process. These results could have an important impact on the therapeutic potential of MBCP in helping to restore the intestinal epithelium integrity damaged by inflammation, thereby reducing the risk of colorectal cancer.

Author Contributions: G.C.T.; P.S.; and E.N.: conceived and designed the experiments; S.L.; E.P.; D.V.; M.M.; R.C.; F.M. and S.D.M.: performed the experiments and analyzed the data; P.S. and F.B.: wrote the paper. G.C.T.; P.S.; E.N.; and F.B.: discussed and confirmed the final manuscript.

References

1. Ng, S.C.; Shi, H.Y.; Hamidi, N.; Underwood, F.E.; Tang, W.; Benchimol, E.I.; Panaccione, R.; Ghosh, S.; Wu, J.C.Y.; Chan, F.K.L.; et al. Worldwide incidence and prevalence of inflammatory bowel disease in the 21st century: A systematic review of population-based studies. *Lancet* **2018**, *390*, 2769–2778. [CrossRef]
2. Sairenji, T.; Collins, K.L.; Evans, D.V. An Update on Inflammatory Bowel Disease. *Prim Care* **2017**, *44*, 673–692. [CrossRef]
3. Lucafò, M.; Franca, R.; Selvestrel, D.; Curci, D.; Pugnetti, L.; Decorti, G.; Stocco, G. Pharmacogenetics of treatments for inflammatory bowel disease. *Expert Opin. Drug Metab. Toxicol.* **2018**, *14*, 1209–1223. [CrossRef] [PubMed]
4. Bischoff, S.C.; Barbara, G.; Buurman, W.; Ockhuizen, T.; Schulzke, J.D.; Serino, M.; Tilg, H.; Watson, A.; Wells, J.M. Intestinal permeability—A new target for disease prevention and therapy. *BMC Gastroenterol.* **2014**, *14*, 189. [CrossRef] [PubMed]
5. Michielan, A.; D'Incà, R. Intestinal Permeability in Inflammatory Bowel Disease: Pathogenesis, Clinical Evaluation, and Therapy of Leaky Gut. *Mediat. Inflamm.* **2015**, *2015*, 628157. [CrossRef]
6. Fasano, A.; Shea-Donohue, T. Mechanisms of disease: The role of intestinal barrier function in the pathogenesis of gastrointestinal autoimmune diseases. *Nat. Clin. Pract. Gastroenterol. Hepatol.* **2005**, *2*, 416–422. [CrossRef] [PubMed]
7. Coopman, P.; Djiane, A. Adherens Junction and E-Cadherin complex regulation by epithelial polarity. *Cell. Mol. Life Sci.* **2016**, *73*, 3535–3553. [CrossRef]
8. Brüser, L.; Bogdan, S. Adherens Junctions on the Move-Membrane Trafficking of E-Cadherin. *Cold Spring Harb. Perspect. Biol.* **2017**, *9*, a029140. [CrossRef] [PubMed]
9. Edelblum, K.L.; Turner, J.R. The tight junction in inflammatory disease: Communication breakdown. *Curr. Opin. Pharmacol.* **2009**, *9*, 715–720. [CrossRef]
10. Utech, M.; Brüwer, M.; Nusrat, A. Tight junctions and cell-cell interactions. *Methods Mol. Biol.* **2006**, *341*, 185–195.

11. De Simone, C.; Picariello, G.; Mamone, G.; Stiuso, P.; Dicitore, A.; Vanacore, D.; Chianese, L.; Addeo, F.; Ferranti, P. Characterisation and cytomodulatory properties of peptides from Mozzarella di Bufala Campana cheese whey. *J. Pept. Sci.* **2009**, *15*, 251–258. [CrossRef] [PubMed]

12. De Simone, C.; Ferranti, P.; Picariello, G.; Scognamiglio, I.; Dicitore, A.; Addeo, F.; Chianese, L.; Stiuso, P. Peptides from water buffalo cheese whey induced senescence cell death via ceramide secretion in human colon adenocarcinoma cell line. *Mol. Nutr. Food Res.* **2011**, *55*, 229–238. [CrossRef] [PubMed]

13. Mohanty, D.P.; Mohapatra, S.; Misra, S.; Sahu, P.S. Milk derived bioactive peptides and their impact on human health—A review. *Saudi J. Biol. Sci.* **2016**, *23*, 577–583. [CrossRef] [PubMed]

14. Chanu, K.V.; Thakuria, D.; Kumar, S. Antimicrobial peptides of buffalo and their role in host defenses. *Vet. World* **2018**, *11*, 192–200. [CrossRef] [PubMed]

15. Basilicata, M.G.; Pepe, G.; Adesso, S.; Ostacolo, C.; Sala, M.; Sommella, E.; Scala, M.C.; Messore, A.; Autore, G.; Marzocco, S.; et al. Antioxidant Properties of Buffalo-Milk Dairy Products: A β-Lg Peptide Released after Gastrointestinal Digestion of Buffalo Ricotta Cheese Reduces Oxidative Stress in Intestinal Epithelial Cells. *Int. J. Mol. Sci.* **2018**, *19*, 1955. [CrossRef] [PubMed]

16. Tenore, G.C.; Ritieni, A.; Campiglia, P.; Stiuso, P.; Di Maro, S.; Sommella, E.; Pepe, G.; D'Urso, E.; Novellino, E. Antioxidant peptides from "Mozzarella di Bufala Campana DOP" after simulated gastrointestinal digestion: In vitro intestinal protection, bioavailability, and anti-haemolytic capacity. *J. Funct. Foods* **2015**, *15*, 365–375.

17. Pagano, E.; Capasso, R.; Piscitelli, F.; Romano, B.; Parisi, O.A.; Finizio, S.; Lauritano, A.; Marzo, V.D.; Izzo, A.A.; Borrelli, F. An Orally Active Cannabis Extract with High Content in Cannabidiol attenuates Chemically-induced Intestinal Inflammation and Hypermotility in the Mouse. *Front. Pharmacol.* **2016**, *7*, 341. [CrossRef]

18. Venditti, M.; Fasano, C.; Santillo, A.; Aniello, F.; Minucci, S. First evidence of DAAM1 localization in mouse seminal vesicles and its possible involvement during regulated exocytosis. *C. R. Biol.* **2018**, *341*, 228–234. [CrossRef] [PubMed]

19. Capasso, R.; Orlando, P.; Pagano, E.; Aveta, T.; Buono, L.; Borrelli, F.; Di Marzo, V.; Izzo, A.A. Palmitoylethanolamide normalizes intestinal motility in a model of post-inflammatory accelerated transit: Involvement of CB_1 receptors and TRPV1 channels. *Br. J. Pharmacol.* **2014**, *171*, 4026–4037. [CrossRef] [PubMed]

20. Pol, O.; Puig, M.M. Reversal of tolerance to the antitransit effects of morphine during acute intestinal inflammation in mice. *Br. J. Pharmacol.* **1997**, *122*, 1216–1222. [CrossRef] [PubMed]

21. Matsumoto, H.; Erickson, R.H.; Gum, J.R.; Yoshioka, M.; Gum, E.; Kim, Y.S. Biosynthesis of alkaline phosphatase during differentiation of the human colon cancer cell line Caco-2. *Gastroenterology* **1990**, *98*, 1199–1207. [CrossRef]

22. Pelissier-Rota, M.; Lainé, M.; Ducarouge, B.; Bonaz, B.; Jacquier-Sarlin, M. Role of cholinergic receptors in colorectal cancer: Potential therapeutic implications of vagus nerve stimulation? *J. Cancer Ther.* **2013**, *4*, 1116–1131. [CrossRef]

23. Lesko, S.; Wessler, I.; Gäbel, G.; Petto, C.; Pfannkuche, H. Cholinergic modulation of epithelial integrity in the proximal colon of pigs. *Cells Tissues Organs* **2013**, *197*, 411–420. [CrossRef] [PubMed]

24. Khan, M.R.; Uwada, J.; Yazawa, T.; Islam, M.T.; Krug, S.M.; Fromm, M.; Karaki, S.; Suzuki, Y.; Kuwahara, A.; Yoshiki, H.; et al. Activation of muscarinic cholinoceptor ameliorates tumor necrosis factor-α-induced barrier dysfunction in intestinal epithelial cells. *FEBS Lett.* **2015**, *589*, 3640–3647. [CrossRef] [PubMed]

25. Yang, B.; Cao, L.; Liu, B.; McCaig, C.D.; Pu, J. The transition from proliferation to differentiation in colorectal cancer is regulated by the calcium activated chloride channel A1. *PLoS ONE* **2013**, *8*, e60861. [CrossRef]

26. Tanoue, T.; Nishitani, Y.; Kanazawa, K.; Hashimoto, T.; Mizuno, M. In vitro model to estimate gut inflammation using co-cultured Caco-2 and RAW264.7 cells. *Biochem. Biophys. Res. Commun.* **2008**, *374*, 565–569. [CrossRef]

27. Tatiya-Aphiradee, N.; Chatuphonprasert, W.; Jarukamjorn, K. Immune response and inflammatory pathway of ulcerative colitis. *J. Basic Clin. Physiol. Pharmacol.* **2018**, *30*, 1–10. [CrossRef]

28. Buhrke, T.; Lengler, I.; Lampen, A. Analysis of proteomic changes induced upon cellular differentiation of the human intestinal cell line Caco-2. *Dev. Growth Differ.* **2011** *53*, 411–426. [CrossRef]

29. Bilski, J.; Mazur-Bialy, A.; Wojcik, D.; Zahradnik-Bilska, J.; Brzozowski, B.; Magierowski, M.; Mach, T.; Magierowska, K.; Brzozowski, T. The Role of Intestinal Alkaline Phosphatase in Inflammatory Disorders of Gastrointestinal Tract. *Mediat. Inflamm.* **2017**, *2017*, 9074601. [CrossRef]

30. Yi, J.Y.; Jung, Y.J.; Choi, S.S.; Chung, E. TNF-alpha Downregulates E-cadherin and Sensitizes Response to γ-irradiation in Caco-2 Cells. *Cancer Res. Treat.* **2009**, *41*, 164–170. [CrossRef]

31. Christian, F.; Smith, E.L.; Carmody, R.J. The Regulation of NF-κB Subunits by Phosphorylation. *Cells* **2016**, *5*, 12. [CrossRef]

32. Rioux, N.; Castonguay, A. The induction of cyclooxygenase-1 by a tobacco carcinogen in U937 human macrophages is correlated to the activation of NF-kappaB. *Carcinogenesis* **2000**, *21*, 1745–1751. [CrossRef] [PubMed]

33. McGilligan, V.E.; Wallace, J.M.; Heavey, P.M.; Ridley, D.L.; Rowland, I.R. The effect of nicotine in vitro on the integrity of tight junctions in Caco-2 cell monolayers. *Food. Chem. Toxicol.* **2007**, *45*, 1593–1598. [CrossRef] [PubMed]

34. Borrelli, F.; Fasolino, I.; Romano, B.; Capasso, R.; Maiello, F.; Coppola, D.; Orlando, P.; Battista, G.; Pagano, E.; Di Marzo, V.; et al. Beneficial effect of the non-psychotropic plant cannabinoid cannabigerol on experimental inflammatory bowel disease. *Biochem. Pharmacol.* **2013**, *85*, 1306–1316. [CrossRef] [PubMed]

35. Borrelli, F.; Romano, B.; Petrosino, S.; Pagano, E.; Capasso, R.; Coppola, D.; Battista, G.; Orlando, P.; Di Marzo, V.; Izzo, A.A. Palmitoylethanolamide, a naturally occurring lipid, is an orally effective intestinal anti-inflammatory agent. *Br. J. Pharmacol.* **2015**, *172*, 142–158. [CrossRef] [PubMed]

36. Chang, J.; Leong, R.W.; Wasinger, V.C.; Ip, M.; Yang, M.; Phan, T.G. Impaired Intestinal Permeability Contributes to Ongoing Bowel Symptoms in Patients with Inflammatory Bowel Disease and Mucosal Healing. *Gastroenterology* **2017**, *153*, 723–731. [CrossRef] [PubMed]

37. Brierley, S.M.; Linden, D.R. Neuroplasticity and dysfunction after gastrointestinal inflammation. *Nat. Rev. Gastroenterol. Hepatol.* **2014**, *11*, 611–627. [CrossRef]

38. Corsetti, M.; Tack, J. Naloxegol, a new drug for the treatment of opioid-induced constipation. *Expert Opin. Pharmacother.* **2015**, *16*, 399–406. [CrossRef]

39. Rao, S.S.; Rattanakovit, K.; Patcharatrakul, T. Diagnosis and management of chronic constipation in adults. *Nat. Rev. Gastroenterol. Hepatol.* **2016**, *13*, 295–305. [CrossRef]

The Role of Vitamin D in Inflammatory Bowel Disease: Mechanism to Management

Jane Fletcher [1,*], Sheldon C. Cooper [2], Subrata Ghosh [3,4] and Martin Hewison [5]

[1] Nutrition Nurses, University Hospitals Birmingham NHS Trust, Queen Elizabeth Hospital Birmingham, Mindelsohn Way, Edgbaston, Birmingham B15 2TH 1, UK

[2] Gastroenterology Department, University Hospitals Birmingham NHS Trust, Queen Elizabeth Hospital Birmingham, Mindelsohn Way, Edgbaston, Birmingham B15 2WB 2, UK; sheldon.cooper@uhb.nhs.uk

[3] NIHR Biomedical Research Centre, University Hospitals Birmingham NHS Foundation Trust, Queen Elizabeth Hospital Birmingham, Mindelsohn Way, Edgbaston, Birmingham B15 2TH, UK; s.ghosh@bham.ac.uk

[4] Institute of Translational Medicine, University of Birmingham, Birmingham B15 2TH, UK

[5] Institute of Metabolism and Systems Research, The University of Birmingham, Birmingham B15 2TT, UK; m.hewison@bham.ac.uk

[*] Correspondence: jane.fletcher@uhb.nhs.uk

Abstract: Vitamin D has been linked to human health benefits that extend far beyond its established actions on calcium homeostasis and bone metabolism. One of the most well studied facets of extra-skeletal vitamin D is its activity as an immuno-modulator, in particular its potent anti-inflammatory effects. As a consequence, vitamin D deficiency has been associated with inflammatory diseases including inflammatory bowel disease (IBD). Low serum levels of the major circulating form of vitamin D, 25-hydroxyvitamin D (25-OH-D) are significantly more prevalent in patients with IBD, particularly in the winter and spring months when UV-induced synthesis of vitamin D is lower. Dietary malabsorption of vitamin D may also contribute to low serum 25(OH)D in IBD. The benefits of supplementation with vitamin D for IBD patients are still unclear, and improved vitamin D status may help to prevent the onset of IBD as well as ameliorating disease severity. Beneficial effects of vitamin D in IBD are supported by pre-clinical studies, notably with mouse models, where the active form of vitamin D, 1,25-dihydroxyvitamin D (1,25-(OH)2D) has been shown to regulate gastrointestinal microbiota function, and promote anti-inflammatory, tolerogenic immune responses. The current narrative review aims to summarise the different strands of data linking vitamin D and IBD, whilst also outlining the possible beneficial effects of vitamin D supplementation in managing IBD in humans.

Keywords: vitamin D; IBD; Crohn's disease; ulcerative colitis; supplementation; deficiency

---

1. Introduction

Inflammatory bowel diseases (IBD) are chronic, disabling diseases precipitating inflammation and ulceration throughout the gastro-intestinal tract (GIT). IBD is characterised by diarrhea, nocturnal defecation, abdominal pain, weight loss, and fatigue. The two principal forms of IBD are Crohn's disease (CD) and ulcerative colitis (UC). Where UC usually only affects the colon, CD may affect the entire GIT from mouth to anus. IBD is common in developed, westernised countries with highest prevalence estimates of; UC 505 per 100,000 and CD 322 per 100,000 population in Europe and UC 249 per 100,000 and CD 319 per 100,000 population in North America [1]. The incidence of IBD is rapidly increasing in newly industrialised countries strongly implicating environmental factors [2]. The pathogenesis of IBD is not fully understood, but key influences are thought to include genetics, environmental factors, immune response, and gut microbiota [3]. The gut microbiota has emerged as an important feature in innate and adaptive immunity [4], with microbial colonisation of the gut being essential for the development of a mature immune system [5]. One explanation for the ongoing increase in IBD is the adverse effect of modern lifestyles on the composition and function of gut microbiota, including high saturated fat/high sugar diets and the use of antibiotics [6].

It is recognised that the availability of vitamin D is important in regulating gut mucosal immunity [3]; with studies suggesting that vitamin D may affect gut epithelial integrity, innate immune barrier function, and the development and function of T cells [7–9]. Although vitamin D deficiency is common in people with IBD it is not established if this is a cause or a consequence of the disease. However, there are suggestions that in genetically predisposed individuals, vitamin D deficiency may be a contributing factor in the development of IBD [7]. There is growing evidence that vitamin D status may affect disease activity. As such consideration should be given to screening and management of vitamin D deficiency in this patient group [10–12].

This narrative review explores the prevalence of vitamin D deficiency in people with IBD and the possible benefits to patients in treating this deficiency. Consideration is given to the management of vitamin D deficiency via exposure to sunlight, dietary sources and supplementation.

2. Vitamin D Deficiency in IBD

2.1. Defining Vitamin D Deficiency

Vitamin D-deficiency is a common health issue across the globe, but it is especially prevalent in Northern European countries. Despite this, defining vitamin D deficiency in human populations remains a contentious issue. In 2010 the Institute of Medicine (IOM) defined vitamin deficiency as serum concentrations of 25-OH-D less than 20 ng/mL (50 nmol/L) [13]. Subsequently the Endocrine Society issued slightly different guidelines, defining vitamin D insufficiency as being serum 25-OH-D levels below 30 ng/mL (75 nmol/L) [14]. In the UK, the Scientific Advisory Committee on Nutrition (SACN) have taken a different approach [15], recommending that a serum 25-hydroxyvitamin D (25-OH-D) level of <25 nmol/L is the threshold at which vitamin D deficiency, and associated complications such as poor musculoskeletal health, is likely to develop. However, other guidelines and studies suggest that levels of 25-OH-D below 25–50 nmol/L constitute deficiency with levels >75 nmol/L indicating sufficiency [14,16–19]. The threshold between 51–74 nmol/L 25-OH-D may then be termed insufficiency. Crucially, these varying recommendations for vitamin D sufficiency and insufficiency continue to be based on the classical skeletal actions of vitamin D, and there are no current recommendations for more recently reported extra-skeletal actions of vitamin D and additional effects are associated with pharmacologic doses of vitamin D.

Both the Endocrine Society [14] and the National Osteoporosis Society [20] recommend that screening for vitamin D deficiency should be carried out in those at risk of vitamin D deficiency; they include people with IBD/malabsorptive disorders in the at risk group. Treatment for deficiency is recommended at a cut off of <50 nmol/L [14,20]. Nonetheless, current UK National Institute for Health and Care Excellence (NICE) and American College of Gastroenterology (ACG) guidance on the management of patients with CD and UC [21–24] do not address vitamin D deficiency in these patients.

2.2. Prevalence of Deficiency in IBD

Vitamin D deficiency is a public health concern with the NICE recommending oral supplementation in specific population groups including infants and children under 4 years, pregnant or breastfeeding women, people over 65 years of age and those who have low or no exposure to the sun. For example, those who cover their skin for cultural reasons, are housebound or confined indoors [25]. The population prevalence of vitamin D deficiency (serum 25-OH-D <40 nmol/L) in some westernised countries is reported to be between 30% [26,27] and 47% [28] with the highest levels reported for those people with darkly pigmented skin. However, people with IBD are likely to be at increased risk of developing vitamin D deficiency for a number of reasons including: impaired absorption of nutrients and bile salt malabsorption, restricted dietary intake, and medical advice to avoid/protect against sunlight exposure while taking immuno-suppressive treatments such as thiopurines [29].

A number of studies have evaluated the prevalence of vitamin D deficiency and insufficiency in people with IBD [30] (Table 1). Prevalence of vitamin D deficiency is highest during winter and spring and lowest during summer and autumn [31]. Where available reported prevalence in Table 1 corresponds with winter/spring levels. These studies suggest that vitamin D deficiency is generally higher in patients with CD than UC and usually higher than that of the general population. However, previous work by the authors suggest it is not standard clinical practice to measure vitamin D in these groups [30]. It is also important to recognise that whilst serum 25-OH-D deficiency has been widely reported for CD and UC, this may not necessarily reflect the status of other vitamin D metabolites. Notably analysis of the active form of vitamin D, 1,25-dihydroxyvitamin D (1,25-(OH)2D) has shown higher serum levels of this metabolite in patients with CD relative to UC patients [32]. The suggestion from this and other studies is that the increased inflammation in CD is associated with enhanced extra-renal conversion of 25-OH-D to 1,25-(OH)2D to support gastrointestinal anti-inflammatory immune responses. Measurement of serum levels of 1,25-(OH)2D is generally rare, but it is interesting to note that serum levels of this metabolite correlated inversely with bone mineral density in CD patients [32]. The functional impact of vitamin D on skeletal homeostasis in IBD is still unclear, and it is possible that link between elevated serum 1,25-(OH)2D and bone loss simply reflects the greater severity of inflammatory disease. Inflammation itself can drive osteopenia through pro-inflammatory cytokines [33]. Impaired vitamin D status has been reported to be a risk factor for low bone mineral density (BMD) in IBD patients in some studies [34], but not in others [35], and single nucleotide polymorphism variants of the gene for the vitamin D receptor (*VDR*) have been shown to protect against low BMD in patients with IBD [36]. Supplementation with vitamin D and calcium has been shown to improve BMD in pediatric [37] and adult [38] IBD patients.

Table 1. Prevalence of vitamin D deficiency and insufficiency in inflammatory bowel disease (IBD) [30].

Study	n	Age Years Mean (SD)	Condition	25(OH)D <75nmol/L (%)	25(OH)D <50nmol/L (%)	25(OH)D <30nmol/L (%)
Bours et al [39]	185	50 (15)	UC		34	
	131	47 (15)	CD		44	
Caviezel et al [40]	57	41 (13)	UC		44	
	99	41 (14)	CD		58	
	25	48 (15)	IBS		28	
Frigstad et al [41]	178	39	UC		44	7
	230	40	CD		53	8
Gilman et al [42]	50	38 (10)	CD		44	6
Kabbani et al [43]	368	44 (10)	UC	29.9		
	597		CD	30		
Kuwabara et al [44]	41	39 (15)	UC		60	
	29	32 (7)	CD		100	
McCarthy et al [45]	32	37 (11)	CD		50	41
	32	37 (11)	HC		25	1
Pappa et al [46]	36	15 (3)	UC			25
	94	15 (4)	CD			38
Sentongo et al [47]	112	16 (4)	CD			16
Siffledeen et al [48]	242	40 (10)	CD		22	8
Suibhne et al [49]	81	36 (11)	CD	90	63	
	70	36 (9)	HC		51	
Ulitsky et al [50]	101	42	UC	67	46	
	403	43	CD	76	51	
Veit et al [51]	18	16 (2)	UC	83	50	28
	40	17 (2)	CD	73	40	15
	116	15 (2)	HC	75	27	10

UC = Ulcerative colitis; CD = Crohn's disease; IBS = irritable bowel syndrome; HC = healthy control.

2.3. Vitamin D Deficiency in IBD—Cause or Consequence

Though vitamin D deficiency in IBD is well documented it is unclear if this is a cause or a consequence of the disease. It is notable that the highest prevalence of the disease appears in more temperate climates with lower levels of sunlight [8]. Some studies have suggested a correlation between vitamin D deficiency and increased disease activity [41,43,52–54]. Low vitamin D levels associated with IBD may be due to dietary restriction or low UV light exposure, but it is also important to recognise that genetic factors also contribute to variations in circulating vitamin D [55]. Single nucleotide polymorphisms (SNP) for components of the vitamin D system have been shown to contribute to the variation of serum 25-OH-D levels in IBD patients [56]. However, the contribution of SNPs to serum levels of 25-OH-D in IBD patients is very small (3%) [56], and subsequent Mendelian randomisation analyses have not shown any link between genetic determinants of vitamin D status and risk of IBD [57]. It is still unclear whether these observations support a causative relationship between vitamin D status and the development of IBD. A prospective cohort study of 72,719 women (age, 40–73 years) enrolled in the Nurses' Health Study found that a higher predicted vitamin D status was associated with a reduced risk of developing CD [58]. However, it would seem that grounds for a causative relationship are most likely to be found in laboratory evidence of the functional effects of vitamin D, suggesting an effect of the active form of vitamin D on immune responses related to IBD [59].

3. Functional Effects of Vitamin D in IBD—Analysis of In Vitro and In Vivo Models

The mechanistic basis for a role for vitamin D in IBD stems firstly from studies of immuno-modulatory properties of 1,25-(OH)2D. These include antibacterial [60–62] and anti-inflammatory [63,64] actions on cell from the innate and adaptive immune system that modulate the pathology of gastrointestinal dysregulation and inflammation. Vitamin D also appears to play a pivotal role in the maintenance of gastrointestinal barrier integrity by regulating proteins associated with epithelial cell gap junctions [65–67]. The barrier function of vitamin D is also linked to its impact on the gastrointestinal microbiota, with serum 25-OH-D status in humans being correlated with changes in gastrointestinal bacterial genera associated with inflammatory immune responses [68,69]. In this way vitamin D has the potential to both prevent the onset of IBD via effects on barrier function and microbiota homeostasis, and also ameliorate disease progression through anti-inflammatory immune responses.

The beneficial effects of vitamin D on gastrointestinal barrier function and immune surveillance are strongly supported by studies of mouse models that have incorporated dietary vitamin D restriction and genetic manipulation of the vitamin D metabolic and signaling system. Mice lacking the gene for the vitamin D receptor (VDR) that binds 1,25-(OH)2D show increased severity of experimentally-induced colitis that mimics IBD [70]. Similar observations have also been made for mice lacking the gene for 1α-hydroxylase, the enzyme that converts 25-OH-D to 1,25-(OH)2D [71]. Thus, in mice, inability to synthesise or recognise 1,25-(OH)2D was associated with increased IBD severity. This is due, in part, to impaired anti-inflammatory adaptive immune function [70], but has also been linked to disruption of the normal gastrointestinal epithelial barrier [66]. Interestingly, in mice with dietary vitamin D restriction increased colitis severity was associated with elevated levels of normal commensal bacteria within the gastrointestinal sub-mucosal epithelium, further underlining the importance of vitamin D in maintaining barrier integrity and surveillance of the gut microbiota [72]. The bioavailability of vitamin D for barrier and immunomodulatory activity within the gastrointestinal tract may also be influenced by the serum vitamin D binding protein (DBP) that transports vitamin D metabolites in the circulation. Although 25-OH-D binds with high affinity to DBP, it has been reported that the unbound or 'free' fraction of serum 25-OH-D is the most biologically active for immune responses to vitamin D [73]. Thus, the interaction between DBP and 25-OH-D may play a key role in gastrointestinal responses to vitamin D. For example, mice raised on diets containing exclusively vitamin D2 showed much lower serum levels of 25-OH-D compared to mice raised on vitamin D3 only. However, because 25-OH-D2 binds with lower affinity to DBP than 25-OH-D3, the levels of free 25-OH-D were similar in the two groups of mice and both showed similar patterns of experimentally induced colitis [74]. These observations suggest that free 25-OH-D may be a more sensitive marker of the protective effects of vitamin D on IBD. In addition to observations from mouse models, evidence from studies of humans also supports a link between vitamin D and IBD. This includes reports that 1,25-(OH)2D is a potent stimulator of nucleotide-binding oligomerisation domain containing 2 (NOD2), an intracellular pathogen-recognition receptor [75]. Mutations in the gene for NOD2 (CARD15) are associated with the development of CD [76,77], and vitamin D status may therefore act as a key environmental trigger for those individuals who are genetically predisposed to CD. Figure 1 is a schematic representation of the expression of VDR and the CYP27B1 gene (responsible for the production of 1α-hydroxylase) in human colonic epithelial cells and antigen presenting cells.

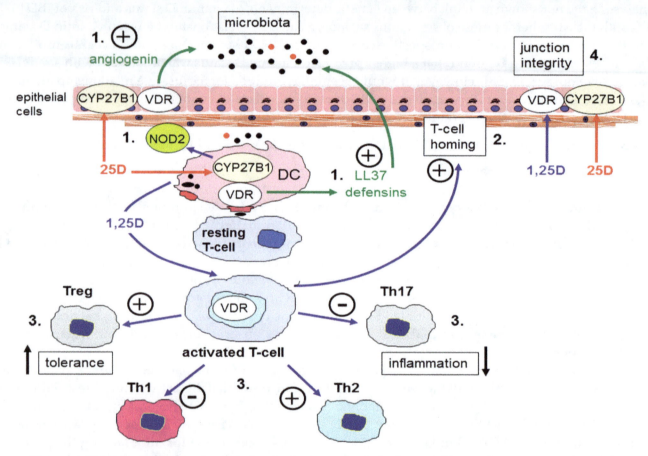

Figure 1. Vitamin D and barrier function in the gastrointestinal tract. Schematic representation of the expression of the vitamin D receptor (VDR) and vitamin D-activating enzyme (CYP27B1) in human colonic epithelial cells, antigen presenting cells such as dendritic cells (DC), and T cells. Immune responses to vitamin D occur either via systemic 1,25-dihydroxyvitamin D (1,25-(OH)2D) or local conversion of 25-hydroxyvitamin D (25-OH-D) to 1,25-(OH)2D. Possible target mechanisms include: 1) interface with microbiota (induction of antibacterials such as angiogenin, cathelcidin (LL37), defensins or intracellular pathogen recognition proteins such as nucleotide-binding oligomerisation domain containing 2 (NOD2)); 2) T cell homing to sites of inflammation; 3) suppression of inflammatory Th17 and Th1 cells and induction of tolerogenic Treg and Th2 cells; 4) enhanced expression of epithelial membrane junction proteins

4. Managing Vitamin D Deficiency in IBD—Sources of Vitamin D

4.1. Sunlight Exposure

The main source of vitamin D in humans is via synthesis in the body stimulated by sunlight exposure [78]. The vitamin D precursor 7-dehydrocholesterol is produced by the liver and is stored in the skin. On exposure of the skin to ultraviolet B-light, this is converted to pre-vitamin D3 and enters the circulation. In the liver pre-vitamin D3 is converted to the inactive form 25(OH)D3. Renal conversion of 25(OH)D3 produces active form 1,25-(OH)2D3 [78].

Lack of adequate exposure to sunlight is likely to lead to vitamin D deficiency with levels <25 nmol/L [15]. However, it is difficult to determine what adequate exposure is. The British Dermatology Association in their 2010 consensus statement on the use of sun-exposure to prevent vitamin D deficiency noted the results of Rhodes et al [79]; the time to produce vitamin D is generally short and certainly before skin begins to burn or redden. The study found that sunlight exposure for an equivalent of 13 minutes of UK summer midday sun (approximate latitude 53.4808° N, 2.2426° W), three times per week over a six-week period was sufficient to increase serum vitamin D levels above 50 nmol/L. The study was carried out in Caucasian participants with one third of their skin exposed to simulated sunlight and wearing no sunscreen [79]. Darker skin required a longer exposure to sunlight to produce vitamin D, so, it would not be possible to have a single recommendation for all skin types. In addition, Rhodes et al note that excessive cutaneous exposure to sunlight may in fact lead to degradation of vitamin D but they do not quantify what excessive exposure is [79]. A more recent global consensus statement on the treatment and prevention of rickets suggests that the use of sunlight exposure to prevent or treat vitamin D deficiency is not feasible [80]. The authors note that there is no safe threshold of ultra violet exposure that allows for sufficient vitamin D synthesis without increasing the risk of skin cancer [80]. This is of particular relevance to patients with IBD, where there is an increased risk of non-melanoma skin cancer in those who have received thiopurines to treat IBD [81].

4.2. Dietary Sources

The majority of naturally occurring vitamin D in food is found in animal products [82] and, as in humans, the quantity of vitamin D found in animal products will vary according to the vitamin D status of the animal. This will be influenced by the animal's diet, if they receive vitamin D supplementation in their feed and their exposure to sunlight [83]. In the USA the addition of vitamin D to livestock feed has been shown to improve the quality of the meat [84]. Despite the emphasis on animal sources of vitamin D, Black et al [85], stress the importance of further research in to edible plant-based foods in providing vitamin D in the diet.

SACN [15] confirmed that the recommended daily intake for vitamin D from all sources (food and oral supplementation) is 400 IU per day for those aged 4 years and above. SACN estimate that this is a sufficient amount to maintain vitamin D levels >25 nmol/L. However, this remains below the levels recommended by the Endocrine Society and National Osteoporosis Society [14,20]. Nonetheless, maintaining this moderate intake from food sources alone is difficult where there are few foods containing significant quantities of vitamin D.

NHS Choices [86] recommend the following sources of vitamin D:

- oily fish—such as herring, mackerel, salmon and sardines
- liver
- red meat
- egg yolks
- fortified foods—such as fat spreads and breakfast cereals

There are notable differences in the amount of vitamin D in each of these foods. Oily fish is a good source of vitamin D even though there are inter-source variations, such as differences between wild salmon and farmed salmon. However, oily fish may not be commonly consumed in some national diets. An analysis of UK Biobank dietary intake data showed that, of 164,573 sets of participant data, only 20% reported consuming two portions of oily fish per week [87]. The main dietary sources of vitamin D intake in UK adults aged 19–64 were; oily fish (11% of vitamin D intake), cereals (13%), eggs and egg dishes (13%), fortified fats (19%), and meat (providing 30% of total vitamin D intake) [15].

The UK National Diet and Nutrition Survey [88] reports that in adults aged 19–64 years, mean daily intake of vitamin D from dietary sources alone was 112 IU. When oral supplementation was included intakes increased to 356 IU in men and 136 IU in women, still below the modest recommended 400 IU/day.

Dietary Intake of Vitamin D in People with IBD

Studies have suggested that people with IBD may restrict their diet to help manage the symptoms of their disease. This has been shown particularly in people with CD and CD-related strictures [89] and even in remission diet may be sub-optimal. A cross sectional study was carried out with 67 CD patients in remission in Canada. Results showed that intake of vitamins C, D, niacin, thiamin, magnesium, phosphorus, potassium, and zinc were all significantly lower in CD patients compared to a control sample ($p < 0.05$) [90]. A recent UK cross sectional study of 67 patients with IBD (40 CD, 23 UC) found that 97% of patients reported food avoidance [91]. Commonly avoided foods were vegetables and wheat products. Mean vitamin D intake was 283 IU/day in the reported cohort. A further small cross-sectional [92] study of dietary intake in 31 patients with IBD in Iceland reported that patients avoided dairy (60%) and processed meat products (55%) to manage symptoms of their IBD. Some patients reported that fish had a positive effect on their symptoms (22%). A cross-sectional study carried out in the Netherlands [93] of 165 patients with IBD compared to healthy controls, demonstrated that patients with IBD consumed more meat and poultry with an average difference of 15.0g/day (95% CI 8.50–21.4); less dairy products at −36.3 g/day (95% CI −65.8––6.84); and slightly less fish at −1.42 g/day (95% CI −0.94––3.79). The findings of these studies would suggest that patients with IBD are unlikely to consume adequate amounts of vitamin D rich foods to achieve the moderate recommended intake.

4.3. Vitamin D Supplementation

Oral supplements containing vitamin D are widely available both over the counter and in the form of prescription only medicines. Some may be single or multi-nutrient preparations. Supplements usually contain either ergocalciferol (vitamin D2) or cholecalciferol (vitamin D3); both forms of vitamin D are metabolised by the liver to 25(OH)D. However, studies suggest that vitamin D2 appears to yield less 25-OH-D than an equal amount of vitamin D3, with vitamin D3 being more effective at raising blood levels of 25-OH-D in humans [94,95]. For this reason, vitamin D3 supplementation is often recommended [14,20].

The dose of vitamin D supplementation required to prevent deficiency is an issue for debate. The European Food Safety Authority [96] has set an upper tolerable limit for vitamin D supplementation of 4,000 IU daily in adults. In line with the SACN report [15], current NICE [25] recommendations are 400 IU vitamin D daily. The IOM [13] suggest an intake of 600 IU daily to maintain a 25-OH-D level of >50 nmol/L, with the Endocrine Society [14] recommending a daily intake for adults of 1500 IU–2000IU. However, these guidelines do not address the risks for people with inflammatory, malabsorptive diseases such as IBD. A recent review has suggested that in IBD doses of 1800 IU–10,000 IU daily may be required [97]. With such a wide dosing range it is difficult to determine the amount that is likely to be most effective.

5. Benefits of Treating Vitamin D Deficiency in IBD

It is widely accepted that vitamin D supplementation should be provided during corticosteroid treatment in IBD for prevention of deterioration of bone health, forming standard guidance. There is increasing interest in research investigating prescribing vitamin D supplementation for modulating inflammatory biochemical processed in IBD [97]. Oral supplementation of vitamin D has been shown to be safe with only minor side-effects which on the whole are generally tolerated among children, with no difference with dosage regimes such as 2000 IU/day versus 50,000 IU/week [98,99]. Adult studies show similar safety profiles [97], with meta-analysis confirming this with the most common side-effects including thirst, nausea, dry mouth, headaches, minor gastrointestinal upset, drowsiness, and fatigue [100,101].

Supplementation of 40,000IU of cholecalciferol weekly successfully significantly increased vitamin D levels in patients with active UC and among subjects with inactive UC and non-UC sufferers. Moreover, there was an associated significant reduction in inflammatory markers of colitis: both C-reactive protein (CRP) and fecal calprotectin [69]. This is not a finding in every study, however. A study from Korea whilst establishing a negative correlation between vitamin D levels and CRP in those with CD, supplementation had no impact upon CRP and disease indices; no association seen with vitamin D levels, CRP and disease indices in those with UC [102]. Whilst not meeting statistical significance ($p = 0.06$) relapse of CD was less common among subjects supplemented with 1200IU of vitamin D3, a group also showing an increase in serum vitamin D3 with supplementation [101].

With immuno-modulatory and biologic therapy increasing the incidence of infections, it is of interest that upper respiratory tract infections were less commonly observed in those supplemented, and indeed the greatest protective effect was observed among those with vitamin D deficiency provided with a modest 500 IU per day (versus placebo) [103].

Vitamin D also impacts upon hospitalisation and need for surgery. In an observational study of patients with both UC and CD, those with an insufficient serum vitamin D (25-OH-D) had an increased risk of requiring both hospitalisation and surgical intervention than those who were never deficient. This was independent of treatment strategies with immuno-modulators and anti-TNF alpha medication. This study measured vitamin D levels and different time points and identified those in whom the levels rose to normal, the majority of whom were taking supplements. This group significantly reduced their risk of requiring surgery with a drop in CRP also noted [12]. Whilst the study by Govani et al [104] did not examine vitamin D levels, they used the US National inpatient sample database, identifying patients with CD requiring surgery and established a UV exposure index based at 3-digit zip-code level. It was identified that those exposed to greater UV had a reduced risk of surgical intervention [104].

Vitamin D deficiency has been shown to be a risk for the development of colo-rectal cancer in people with IBD [105]. Whilst the study by Ananthakrishnan et al does not examine supplementation of vitamin D, their study of 2809 patients with vitamin D assay results (at least one) and development of cancer revealed that deficiency of vitamin D was associated with an increased risk of cancer: odds ratio 1.82 (95%CI 1.25–2.65), with an 8% reduction in risk for every 1 ng/mL increase in vitamin D level [105]. A recent randomised controlled trial on recurrence of adenoma in people without an inflammatory bowel disease showed less-promising results [106]. In the trial participants were randomised to receive either vitamin D, calcium, both agents, or placebo. No significant difference was found in any of the treatment regimens on the recurrence of adenoma. However, it is important to note that only participants with 25-OH-D levels >30 nmol/L <225 nmol/L were included [106]. Therefore, it can be argued that these results do not relate to a population who are vitamin D deficient such as those with IBD. Further research is warranted into the effects of treatment of vitamin D deficiency in IBD and the impact on the development of colo-rectal cancers in this group.

IBD and anemia are linked, with the action of hepcidin implicated. Observational data has confirmed vitamin D deficiency is associated with increased hepcidin concentration and anemia [107]. This observational data has been strengthened with an interventional study revealing that even a short period of two-weeks of vitamin D supplementation was sufficient to not only increase serum vitamin D, but reduce serum CRP and hepcidin levels [108].

Vitamin D effects have been postulated to have an immuno-modulatory effect; a vitamin D analogue was shown to act as a TNF-alpha inhibitor of peripheral blood mononuclear cells, especially when used in conjunction with Infliximab, a TNF-alpha inhibitor [109]. Observation among 173 subjects receiving anti-TNF alpha medication showed those with a normal vitamin D level had an increased odds ratio 2.64 (95% CI 1.31–5.32, $p = 0.0067$) of having achieved remission at 3-months compared with those with low levels [110]. This finding is echoed in another retrospective observational study revealing that patients with IBD with an insufficient vitamin D level at initiation of anti-TNF alpha treatment were more likely to stop treatment due to loss of response (HR 3.49; 95%CI 1.34–9.09), again suggesting a beneficial effect of vitamin D repletion [111].

Meta-analysis of randomised control trials have been clear in identifying that supplementation, whilst on the whole was well tolerated and did increase serum vitamin D levels, were too heterogeneous in nature with regards to dosing and follow up-periods to draw any significant findings with improvements in serum inflammatory markers of CRP and ESR. There was however recognition that there were significantly fewer relapses in those supplemented with vitamin D (OR 0.34; 95%CI 0.20–0.58) but analysis by dosing did not yield further significant findings [100].

6. Conclusions

Vitamin D plays a significant role in the maintenance of gastrointestinal barrier integrity, surveillance of the gut microbiota and inflammatory immune responses. These mechanisms are important in both preventing the development of IBD and ameliorating symptoms of the disease. Nonetheless, vitamin D deficiency is common in people with IBD with prevalence being higher than the general population and somewhat higher in CD than UC [30]. The reasons for this are multi-factorial but include lack of sun exposure due to immuno-suppressive treatments, dietary restrictions [90], and impaired absorption of nutrients.

Whilst vitamin D deficiency is more common among those with IBD, data has been unable to establish if the relationship is causative or as a result of inflammation. Many serum markers of nutrition are affected by inflammation, making it challenging to understand cause or effect. However, through understanding of the mechanisms of action there is emerging evidence that vitamin D deficiency may be implicated in disease severity, if not in part the etiology of IBD.

There is a wealth of evidence revealing that intervention with oral vitamin D supplementation is safe and well tolerated. It has been more challenging to identify the advantages of restoring vitamin D levels in clinical disease progression, but more studies are beginning to reveal benefits. Aside from the well recognised skeletal effects, there is growing evidence for IBD disease outcome benefits from the normalisation of 25-OH-D serum levels in people with IBD. Benefits include: reduced risk of surgery in those with CD [12], reduction in inflammatory markers [69], reduction in the development of anemia [112], improved response to anti-TNF alpha treatment [111], and a reduction in the risk of colo-rectal cancer [105]. One study revealed a reduction in upper respiratory tract infections [91]. These benefits warrant attention to the vitamin D status of people with IBD. Several key questions remain to be answered. Firstly, it is still unclear what is the optimal circulating level(s) of 25-OH-D for prevention and/or management of IBD. Current guidelines such as the Institute of Medicine in North America [13], and Science Advisory Council on Nutrition in the UK [15] have been developed based on the regulation of calcium homeostasis and bone metabolism. As yet there are no similar guidelines for extra-skeletal effects of vitamin D. This is further complicated by the recent report of a human subject with homozygous deletion of the vitamin D binding protein (DBP) gene [113]. The woman in question had almost undetectable circulating levels of 25-OH-D but was nevertheless normocalcemic and had only had mild changes in bone metabolism, but had severe ankylosing spondylitis. This case report suggests that total serum measurement of 25-OH-D may not be the most accurate determinant of vitamin D 'status', but rather unbound or free 25-OH-D (which was relatively normal in the woman with the DBP gene deletion) is the driving force behind many actions of vitamin D [114]. This is likely to be an important consideration in future studies of vitamin D supplementation and clinical impact.

Maintaining or improving vitamin D intake by diet or increased sun exposure is problematic for people with IBD. Improvement in vitamin D status can be achieved by oral supplementation. There is however a lack of consistent outcome data for significant improvement in IBD outcomes, with variation in duration and dosing of supplementation, and many studies being retrospective in nature. The data surrounding enhanced response to biologic therapies with normalised vitamin D levels suggest that, with more interventional, double-blind, placebo controlled randomised trials, that individualisation of

IBD management with supplementation of vitamin D in those who are deficient offers an important strategy in improving clinical outcomes.

Author Contributions: Conceptualisation, J.F., S.C.C. and M.H.; Writing—Original Draft Preparation, J.F., S.C.C., S.G. and M.H.; Writing—Review and Editing, J.F., S.C.C., S.G. and M.H.; Visualisation, J.F.; Supervision, S.C.C. and M.H.

References

1. Molodecky, N.A.; Soon, I.S.; Rabi, D.M.; Ghali, W.A.; Ferris, M.; Chernoff, G.; Benchimol, E.I.; Panaccione, R.; Ghosh, S.; Barkema, H.W.; et al. Increasing Incidence and Prevalence of the Inflammatory Bowel Diseases With Time, Based on Systematic Review. *Gastroenterology* **2012**, *142*, 46–54. [CrossRef]
2. Ng, S.C.; Shi, H.Y.; Hamidi, N.; Underwood, F.E.; Tang, W.; Benchimol, E.I.; Panaccione., R.; Ghosh, S.; Wu, J.C.Y.; et al. Worldwide incidence and prevalence of inflammatory bowel disease in the 21st century: A systematic review of population-based studies. *Lancet* **2018**, *390*, 2769–2778. [CrossRef]
3. De Souza, H.S.P.; Fiocchi, C. Immunopathogenesis of IBD: current state of the art. *Nat. Rev. Gastroenterol. Hepatol.* **2015**, *13*, 13–27. [CrossRef]
4. Alexander, K.L.; Targan, S.R.; Elson, C.O., III. Microbiota activation and regulation of innate and adaptive immunity. *Immunol. Rev.* **2014**, *260*, 206–220. [CrossRef] [PubMed]
5. Maynard, C.L.; Elson, C.O.; Hatton, R.D.; Weaver, C.T. Reciprocal Interactions of the Intestinal Microbiota and Immune System. *Nat. Cell Boil.* **2012**, *489*, 231–241. [CrossRef] [PubMed]
6. Bernstein, C.N.; Shanahan, F. Disorders of a modern lifestyle: reconciling the epidemiology of inflammatory bowel diseases. *Gut* **2008**, *57*, 1185–1191. [CrossRef]
7. Cantorna, M.T. Vitamin D and its role in immunology: Multiple sclerosis, and inflammatory bowel disease. *Prog. Biophys. Mol. Boil.* **2006**, *92*, 60–64. [CrossRef]
8. Raman, M.; Milestone, A.N.; Walters, J.R.; Hart, A.L.; Ghosh, S. Vitamin D and gastrointestinal diseases: Inflammatory bowel disease and colorectal cancer. *Therap. Adv. Gastroenterol.* **2011**, *4*, 49–62. [CrossRef]
9. Raftery, T.; Martineau, A.R.; Greiller, C.L.; Ghosh, S.; McNamara, D.; Bennett, K.; Meddings, J.; O'Sullivan, M. Effects of vitamin D supplementation on intestinal permeability, cathelicidin and disease markers in Crohn's disease: Results from a randomised double-blind placebo-controlled study. *United Eur. Gastroenterol. J.* **2015**, *3*, 294–302. [CrossRef] [PubMed]
10. Yang, L.; Weaver, V.; Smith, J.P.; Bingaman, S.; Hartman, T.J.; Cantorna, M.T. Therapeutic Effect of Vitamin D Supplementation in a Pilot Study of Crohn's Patients. *Clin. Transl. Gastroenterol.* **2013**, *4*, e33. [CrossRef]
11. Bancil, A.S.; Poullis, A.; Samman, S.; Darnton-Hill, I. The Role of Vitamin D in Inflammatory Bowel Disease. *Healthcare* **2015**, *3*, 338–350. [CrossRef] [PubMed]
12. Ananthakrishnan, A.N.; Cagan, A.; Gainer, V.S.; Cai, T.; Cheng, S.-C.; Savova, G.; Chen, P.; Szolovits, P.; Xia, Z.; De Jager, P.L.; et al. Normalization of Plasma 25-hydroxy Vitamin D is Associated with Reduced Risk of Surgery in Crohn's Disease. *Inflamm. Bowel Dis.* **2013**, *19*, 1921–1927. [CrossRef] [PubMed]
13. Ross, A.C.; Manson, J.E.; Abrams, S.A.; Aloia, J.F.; Brannon, P.M.; Clinton, S.K.; Durazo-Arvizu, R.A.; Gallagher, J.C.; Gallo, R.L.; Jones, G.; et al. The 2011 Report on Dietary Reference Intakes for Calcium and Vitamin D From the Institute of Medicine: What Clinicians Need to Know. *Obstet. Gynecol.* **2011**, *66*, 356–357.
14. Holick, M.F.; Binkley, N.C.; Bischoff-Ferrari, H.A.; Gordon, C.M.; Hanley, D.A.; Heaney, R.P.; Murad, M.H.; Weaver, C.M. Evaluation, Treatment, and Prevention of Vitamin D Deficiency: an Endocrine Society Clinical Practice Guideline. *J. Clin. Endocrinol. Metab.* **2011**, *96*, 1911–1930. [CrossRef]
15. Scientific Advisory Committee on Nutrition. *SACN Vitamin D and Health Report*; Scientific Advisory Committee on Nutrition: London, UK, 2016.
16. Institute of Medicine (US) Committee to Review Dietary Reference Intakes for Vitamin D and Calcium. *Dietary Reference Intakes for Calcium and Vitamin D*; Ross, A.C., Taylor, C.L., Yaktine, A.L., Del Valle, H.B., Eds.; National Academies Press (US): Washington, DC, USA, 2011.
17. Dawson-Hughes, B.; Mithal, A.; Bonjour, J.-P.; Boonen, S.; Burckhardt, P.; Fuleihan, G.E.-H.; Josse, R.G.; Lips, P.; Morales-Torres, J.; Yoshimura, N. IOF position statement: vitamin D recommendations for older adults. *Osteoporos. Int.* **2010**, *21*, 1151–1154. [CrossRef]

18. Hanley, D.A.; Cranney, A.; Jones, G.; Whiting, S.J.; Leslie, W.D.; Cole, D.E.; Atkinson, S.A.; Josse, R.G.; Feldman, S.; Kline, G.A.; et al. Vitamin D in adult health and disease: a review and guideline statement from Osteoporosis Canada. *Can. Med Assoc. J.* **2010**, *182*, E610–E618. [CrossRef]

19. Okazaki, R.; Ozono, K.; Fukumoto, S.; Inoue, D.; Yamauchi, M.; Minagawa, M.; Michigami, T.; Takeuchi, Y.; Matsumoto, T.; Sugimoto, T. Assessment criteria for vitamin D deficiency/insufficiency in Japan: Proposal by an expert panel supported by the Research Program of Intractable Diseases, Ministry of Health, Labour and Welfare, Japan, the Japanese Society for Bone and Mineral Research and the Japan Endocrine Society [Opinion]. *J. Bone Miner. Metab.* **2017**, *35*, 1–5. [PubMed]

20. Francis, R.; Aspray, T.; Bowring, C.; Fraser, W.; Gittoes, N.; Javaid, M.; Macdonald, H.; Patel, S.; Selby, P.; Tanna, N. National Osteoporosis Society practical clinical guideline on vitamin D and bone health. *Maturitas* **2015**, *80*, 119–121. [CrossRef]

21. National Institute for Health and Care Excellence. *CG 152 Crohn's disease: Management in adults, children and young people*; NICE: London, UK, 2012.

22. National Institute for Health and Care Excellence. *CG 166 Ulcerative Colitis: Management in Adults, Children and Young People*; NICE: London, UK, 2013.

23. Lichtenstein, G.R.; Loftus, E.V.; Isaacs, K.L.; Regueiro, M.D.; Gerson, L.B.; E Sands, B. ACG Clinical Guideline: Management of Crohn's Disease in Adults. *Am. J. Gastroenterol.* **2018**, *113*, 481–517. [CrossRef]

24. Rubin, D.T.; Ananthakrishnan, A.N.; Siegel, C.A.; Sauer, B.G.; Long, M.D. ACG Clinical Guideline: Ulcerative Colitis in Adults. *Am. J. Gastroenterol.* **2019**, *114*, 384–413. [CrossRef]

25. National Institute for Health and Care Excellence. *Vitamin D: Supplement Use in Specific Population Groups PH56*; NICE: London, UK, 2017.

26. Larose, T.L.; Chen, Y.; Camargo, C.A., Jr.; Langhammer, A.; Romundstad, P.; Mai, X.M. Factors associated with vitamin D deficiency in a Norwegian population: the HUNT Study. *J. Epidemiol. Community Health* **2014**, *68*, 165–170. [CrossRef]

27. Schwalfenberg, G.; Genuis, S.; Hiltz, M.; Schwalfenberg, G. Addressing vitamin D deficiency in Canada: A public health innovation whose time has come. *Public Health* **2010**, *124*, 350–359. [CrossRef]

28. Hypponen, E.; Power, C. Hypovitaminosis D in British adults at age 45 y: nationwide cohort study of dietary and lifestyle predictors. *Am. J. Clin. Nutr.* **2007**, *85*, 860–868. [CrossRef]

29. Fletcher, J. Vitamin D deficiency in patients with inflammatory bowel disease. *Br. J. Nurs.* **2016**, *25*, 846–851. [CrossRef] [PubMed]

30. Fletcher, J.; Swift, A. Vitamin D screening in patients with inflammatory bowel disease. *Gastrointest. Nurs.* **2017**, *15*, 16–23. [CrossRef]

31. Hossein-Nezhad, A.; Holick, M.F. Vitamin D for Health: A Global Perspective. *Mayo Proc.* **2013**, *88*, 720–755. [CrossRef] [PubMed]

32. Abreu, M.T.; Kantorovich, V.; A Vasiliauskas, E.; Gruntmanis, U.; Matuk, R.; Daigle, K.; Chen, S.; Zehnder, D.; Lin, Y.-C.; Yang, H.; et al. Measurement of vitamin D levels in inflammatory bowel disease patients reveals a subset of Crohn's disease patients with elevated 1,25-dihydroxyvitamin D and low bone mineral density. *Gut* **2004**, *53*, 1129–1136. [CrossRef]

33. Ghosh, S.; Cowen, S.; Hannan, W.; Ferguson, A. Low bone mineral density in Crohn's disease, but not in ulcerative colitis, at diagnosis. *Gastroenterology* **1994**, *107*, 1031–1039. [CrossRef]

34. Abraham, B.P.; Prasad, P.; Malaty, H.M. Vitamin D deficiency and corticosteroid use are risk factors for low bone mineral density in inflammatory bowel disease patients. *Am. J. Dig. Dis.* **2014**, *59*, 1878–1884. [CrossRef]

35. Maratova, K.; Hradsky, O.; Matyskova, J.; Copova, I.; Soucek, O.; Sumnik, Z.; Bronsky, J. Musculoskeletal system in children and adolescents with inflammatory bowel disease: normal muscle force, decreased trabecular bone mineral density and low prevalence of vertebral fractures. *Eur. J. Pediatr.* **2017**, *176*, 1355–1363. [CrossRef] [PubMed]

36. Szymczak-Tomczak, A.; Krela-Kaźmierczak, I.; Kaczmarek-Ryś, M.; Hryhorowicz, S.T.; Stawczyk-Eder, K.; Szalata, M.; Skrzypczak-Zielińska, M.; Łykowska-Szuber, L.; Eder, P.; Michalak, M.; et al. Vitamin D receptor (VDR) TaqI polymorphism, vitamin D and bone mineral density in patients with inflammatory bowel diseases. *Adv. Clin. Exp. Med.* **2019**, *28*. [CrossRef]

37. Maratova, K.; Matyskova, J.; Copova, I.; Zarubova, K.; Sumnik, Z.; Hradsky, O.; Soucek, O.; Bronsky, J. Supplementation with 2000 IU of Cholecalciferol Is Associated with Improvement of Trabecular Bone Mineral Density and Muscle Power in Pediatric Patients with IBD. *Inflamm. Bowel Dis.* **2017**, *23*, 514–523.

38. Bakker, S.F.; Dik, V.K.; Witte, B.I.; Lips, P.; Roos, J.C.; Van Bodegraven, A.A. Increase in bone mineral density in strictly treated Crohn's disease patients with concomitant calcium and vitamin D supplementation. *J. Crohn's Coliti* **2013**, *7*, 377–384. [CrossRef]

39. Bours, P.H.; Wielders, J.P.; Vermeijden, J.R.; van de Wiel, A. Seasonal variation of serum 25-hydroxyvitamin D levels in adult patients with inflammatory bowel disease. *Osteoporos Int.* **2011**, *22*, 2857–2867. [CrossRef] [PubMed]

40. Caviezel, D.; Maissen, S.; Niess, J.H.; Kiss, C.; Hruz, P. High Prevalence of Vitamin D Deficiency among Patients with Inflammatory Bowel Disease. *Inflamm. Intest. Dis.* **2017**, *2*, 200–210. [CrossRef] [PubMed]

41. Frigstad, S.O.; Høivik, M.; Jahnsen, J.; Dahl, S.R.; Cvancarova, M.; Grimstad, T.; Berset, I.; Huppertz-Hauss, G.; Hovde, Ø.; Torp, R. Vitamin D deficiency in inflammatory bowel disease: prevalence and predictors in a Norwegian outpatient population. *Scand. J. Gastroenterol.* **2017**, *52*, 100–106. [CrossRef]

42. Gilman, J.; Shanahan, F.; Cashman, K.D. Determinants of vitamin D status in adult Crohn's disease patients, with particular emphasis on supplemental vitamin D use. *Eur. J. Clin. Nutr.* **2006**, *60*, 889–896. [CrossRef]

43. A Kabbani, T.; E Koutroubakis, I.; E Schoen, R.; Ramos-Rivers, C.; Shah, N.; Swoger, J.; Regueiro, M.; Barrie, A.; Schwartz, M.; Hashash, J.G.; et al. Association of Vitamin D Level With Clinical Status in Inflammatory Bowel Disease: A 5-Year Longitudinal Study. *Am. J. Gastroenterol.* **2016**, *111*, 712–719. [CrossRef]

44. Kuwabara, A.; Tanaka, K.; Tsugawa, N.; Nakase, H.; Tsuji, H.; Shide, K.; Kamao, M.; Chiba, T.; Inagaki, N.; Okano, T.; et al. High prevalence of vitamin K and D deficiency and decreased BMD in inflammatory bowel disease. *Osteoporos Int.* **2009**, *20*, 935–942. [CrossRef]

45. McCarthy, D.; Duggan, P.; O'Brien, M.; Kiely, M.; McCarthy, J.; Shanahan, F.; Cashman, K.D. Seasonality of vitamin D status and bone turnover in patients with Crohn's disease. *Aliment. Pharmacol. Ther.* **2005**, *21*, 1073–1083. [CrossRef]

46. Pappa, H.M.; Gordon, C.M.; Saslowsky, T.M.; Zholudev, A.; Horr, B.; Shih, M.-C.; Grand, R.J. Vitamin D Status in Children and Young Adults With Inflammatory Bowel Disease. *PEDIATRICS* **2006**, *118*, 1950–1961. [CrossRef] [PubMed]

47. Sentongo, A.T.; Semaeo, E.J.; Stettler, N.; A Piccoli, D.; A Stallings, V.; Zemel, B.S. Vitamin D status in children, adolescents, and young adults with Crohn disease. *Am. J. Clin. Nutr.* **2002**, *76*, 1077–1081. [CrossRef]

48. Siffledeen, J.S.; Siminoski, K.; Steinhart, H.; Greenberg, G.; Fedorak, R.N. The Frequency of Vitamin D Deficiency in Adults with Crohn's Disease. *Can. J. Gastroenterol.* **2003**, *17*, 473–478. [CrossRef]

49. Suibhne, T.N.; Cox, G.; Healy, M.; O'Morain, C.; O'Sullivan, M. Vitamin D deficiency in Crohn's disease: Prevalence, risk factors and supplement use in an outpatient setting. *J. Crohns Colitis* **2012**, *6*, 182–188. [CrossRef]

50. Ulitsky, A.; Ananthakrishnan, A.N.; Naik, A.; Skaros, S.; Zadvornova, Y.; Binion, D.G.; Issa, M. Vitamin D deficiency in patients with inflammatory bowel disease: association with disease activity and quality of life. *JPEN* **2011**, *35*, 308–316. [CrossRef]

51. Veit, L.E.; Maranda, L.; Fong, J.; Nwosu, B.U. The Vitamin D Status in Inflammatory Bowel Disease. *PLoS ONE* **2014**, *9*, e101583. [CrossRef]

52. Hassan, V.; Hassan, S.; Seyed-Javad, P.; Ahmad, K.; Asieh, H.; Maryam, S.; Farid, F.; Siavash, A. Association between Serum 25 (OH) Vitamin D Concentrations and Inflammatory Bowel Diseases (IBDs) Activity. *Med J.* **2013**, *68*, 34–38.

53. Garg, M.; Rosella, O.; Lubel, J.S.; Gibson, P.R. Association of Circulating Vitamin D Concentrations with Intestinal but Not Systemic Inflammation in Inflammatory Bowel Disease. *Inflamm. Bowel Dis.* **2013**, *19*, 2634–2643. [CrossRef] [PubMed]

54. Jørgensen, S.P.; Hvas, C.L.; Agnholt, J.; Christensen, L.A.; Heickendorff, L.; Dahlerup, J.F. Active Crohn's disease is associated with low vitamin D levels. *J. Crohn's Colitis* **2013**, *7*, e407–e413.

55. Wang, T.J.; Zhang, F.; Richards, J.B.; Kestenbaum, B.; Van Meurs, J.B.; Berry, D.; Kiel, D.P.; Streeten, E.A.; Ohlsson, C.; Koller, D.L.; et al. Common genetic determinants of vitamin D insufficiency: a genome-wide association study. *Lancet* **2010**, *376*, 180–188. [CrossRef]

56. Ananthakrishnan, A.N.; Cagan, A.; Cai, T.; Gainer, V.S.; Shaw, S.Y.; Churchill, S.; Karlson, E.W.; Murphy, S.N.; Kohane, I.; Liao, K.P.; et al. Common genetic variants influence circulating vitamin D levels in inflammatory bowel diseases. *Inflamm. Bowel Dis.* **2015**, *21*, 2507–2514. [CrossRef]

57. Lund-Nielsen, J.; Vedel-Krogh, S.; Kobylecki, C.J.; Brynskov, J.; Afzal, S.; Nordestgaard, B.G. Vitamin D and Inflammatory Bowel Disease: Mendelian Randomization Analyses in the Copenhagen Studies and UK Biobank. *J. Clin. Endocrinol. Metab.* **2018**, *103*, 3267–3277. [CrossRef]

58. Ananthakrishnan, A.N.; Khalili, H.; Higuchi, L.M.; Bao, Y.; Korzenik, J.R.; Giovannucci, E.L.; Richter, J.M.; Fuchs, C.S.; Chan, A.T. Higher predicted vitamin D status is associated with reduced risk of Crohn's disease. *Gastroenterology* **2012**, *142*, 482–489. [CrossRef]

59. Ananthakrishnan, A.N. Editorial: Vitamin D and IBD: Can We Get Over the "Causation" Hump? *Am. J. Gastroenterol.* **2016**, *111*, 720–722. [CrossRef]

60. Liu, P.T.; Stenger, S.; Li, H.; Wenzel, L.; Tan, B.H.; Krutzik, S.R.; Ochoa, M.T.; Schauber, J.; Wu, K.; Meinken, C.; et al. Toll-Like Receptor Triggering of a Vitamin D-Mediated Human Antimicrobial Response. *Science* **2006**, *311*, 1770–1773. [CrossRef] [PubMed]

61. Bacchetta, J.; Zaritsky, J.J.; Sea, J.L.; Chun, R.F.; Lisse, T.S.; Zavala, K.; Nayak, A.; Wesseling-Perry, K.; Westerman, M.; Hollis, B.W.; et al. Suppression of iron-regulatory hepcidin by vitamin D. *J. Am. Soc. Nephrol.* **2014**, *25*, 564–572. [CrossRef]

62. Hewison, M. Antibacterial effects of vitamin D. *Nat. Rev. Endocrinol.* **2011**, *7*, 337–345. [CrossRef] [PubMed]

63. Cantorna, M.T. Vitamin D, multiple sclerosis and inflammatory bowel disease. *Arch. Biochem. Biophys.* **2012**, *523*, 103–106. [CrossRef] [PubMed]

64. Adams, J.S.; Hewison, M. Unexpected actions of vitamin D: new perspectives on the regulation of innate and adaptive immunity. *Nat. Clin. Pr. Endocrinol. Metab.* **2008**, *4*, 80–90. [CrossRef]

65. Zhang, Y.-G.; Wu, S.; Lu, R.; Zhou, D.; Zhou, J.; Carmeliet, G.; Petrof, E.; Claud, E.C.; Sun, J. Tight junction CLDN2 gene is a direct target of the vitamin D receptor. *Sci. Rep.* **2015**, *5*, 10642. [CrossRef]

66. Liu, W.; Chen, Y.; Golan, M.A.; Annunziata, M.L.; Du, J.; Dougherty, U.; Kong, J.; Musch, M.; Huang, Y.; Pekow, J.; et al. Intestinal epithelial vitamin D receptor signaling inhibits experimental colitis. *J. Clin. Investig.* **2013**, *123*, 3983–3996. [CrossRef]

67. Kong, J.; Zhang, Z.; Musch, M.W.; Ning, G.; Sun, J.; Hart, J.; Bissonnette, M.; Li, Y.C. Novel role of the vitamin D receptor in maintaining the integrity of the intestinal mucosal barrier. *Am. J. Physiol. Liver Physiol.* **2008**, *294*, 208–216. [CrossRef]

68. Luthold, R.V.; Fernandes, G.R.; Franco-De-Moraes, A.C.; Folchetti, L.G.; Ferreira, S.R.G. Gut microbiota interactions with the immunomodulatory role of vitamin D in normal individuals. *Metab. Clin. Exp.* **2017**, *69*, 76–86. [CrossRef]

69. Garg, M.; Hendy, P.; Ding, J.N.; Shaw, S.; Hold, G.; Hart, A. The Effect of Vitamin D on Intestinal Inflammation and Faecal Microbiota in Patients with Ulcerative Colitis. *J. Crohn?s Coliti* **2018**, *12*, 963–972. [CrossRef]

70. Froicu, M.; Weaver, V.; Wynn, T.A.; McDowell, M.A.; Welsh, J.E.; Cantorna, M.T. A Crucial Role for the Vitamin D Receptor in Experimental Inflammatory Bowel Diseases. *Mol. Endocrinol.* **2003**, *17*, 2386–2392. [CrossRef]

71. Liu, N.; Nguyen, L.; Chun, R.F.; Lagishetty, V.; Ren, S.; Wu, S.; Hollis, B.; DeLuca, H.F.; Adams, J.S.; Hewison, M. Altered Endocrine and Autocrine Metabolism of Vitamin D in a Mouse Model of Gastrointestinal Inflammation. *Endocrinology* **2008**, *149*, 4799–4808. [CrossRef] [PubMed]

72. Lagishetty, V.; Misharin, A.V.; Liu, N.Q.; Lisse, T.S.; Chun, R.F.; Ouyang, Y.; McLachlan, S.M.; Adams, J.S.; Hewison, M. Vitamin D deficiency in mice impairs colonic antibacterial activity and predisposes to colitis. *Endocrinology* **2010**, *151*, 2423–2432. [CrossRef]

73. Chun, R.F.; Lauridsen, A.L.; Suon, L.; Zella, L.A.; Pike, J.W.; Modlin, R.L.; Martineau, A.R.; Wilkinson, R.J.; Adams, J.; Hewison, M. Vitamin D-Binding Protein Directs Monocyte Responses to 25-Hydroxy- and 1,25-Dihydroxyvitamin D. *J. Clin. Endocrinol. Metab.* **2010**, *95*, 3368–3376. [CrossRef]

74. Larner, D.P.; Jenkinson, C.; Chun, R.F.; Westgate, C.S.J.; Adams, J.S.; Hewison, M. Free versus total serum 25-hydroxyvitamin D in a murine model of colitis. *J. Steroid Biochem. Mol. Biol.* **2019**, *189*, 204–209. [CrossRef] [PubMed]

75. Wang, T.T.; Dabbas, B.; Laperriere, D.; Bitton, A.J.; Soualhine, H.; Tavera-Mendoza, L.E.; Dionne, S.; Servant, M.J.; Bitton, A.; Seidman, E.G.; et al. Direct and indirect induction by 1,25-dihydroxyvitamin D3 of

the NOD2/CARD15-defensin beta2 innate immune pathway defective in Crohn disease. *J. Biol. Chem.* **2010**, *285*, 2227–2231. [CrossRef] [PubMed]

76. Ogura, Y.; Bonen, D.K.; Inohara, N.; Nicolae, D.L.; Chen, F.F.; Ramos, R.; Britton, H.; Moran, T.; Karaliuskas, R.; Kirschner, B.S.; et al. A frameshift mutation in NOD2 associated with susceptibility to Crohn's disease. *Nature* **2001**, *411*, 603–606. [CrossRef] [PubMed]

77. Hugot, J.P.; Chamaillard, M.; Zouali, H.; Lesage, S.; Cézard, J.P.; Belaiche, J.; Almer, S.; Tysk, C.; O'Morain, C.A.; Gassull, M.; et al. Association of NOD2 leucine-rich repeat variants with susceptibility to Crohn's disease. *Nature* **2001**, *411*, 599–603. [CrossRef]

78. Reich, K.M.; Fedorak, R.N.; Madsen, K.; I Kroeker, K. Vitamin D improves inflammatory bowel disease outcomes: Basic science and clinical review. *World J. Gastroenterol.* **2014**, *20*, 4934–4947. [CrossRef] [PubMed]

79. Rhodes, L.E.; Webb, A.R.; Fraser, H.I.; Kift, R.; Durkin, M.T.; Allan, D.; O'Brien, S.J.; Vail, A.; Berry, J.L. Recommended Summer Sunlight Exposure Levels Can Produce Sufficient but Not the Proposed Optimal 25(OH)D Levels at UK Latitudes. *J. Invest. Dermatol.* **2010**, *130*, 1411–1418. [CrossRef] [PubMed]

80. Munns, C.F.; Shaw, N.; Kiely, M.; Specker, B.L.; Thacher, T.D.; Ozono, K.; Michigami, T.; Tiosano, D.; Mughal, M.Z.; Mäkitie, O.; et al. Global Consensus Recommendations on Prevention and Management of Nutritional Rickets. *J. Clin. Endocrinol. Metab.* **2016**, *101*, 394–415. [CrossRef] [PubMed]

81. Magro, F.; Peyrin-Biroulet, L.; Sokol, H.; Aldeger, X.; Costa, A.; Higgins, P.D.; Joyce, J.C.; Katsanos, K.H.; Lopez, A.; De Xaxars, T.M.; et al. Extra-intestinal malignancies in inflammatory bowel disease: Results of the 3rd ECCO Pathogenesis Scientific Workshop (III). *J. Crohn's Colitis* **2014**, *8*, 31–44. [CrossRef] [PubMed]

82. Schmid, A.; Walther, B. Natural Vitamin D Content in Animal Products1. *Adv. Nutr. Int. J.* **2013**, *4*, 453–462. [CrossRef]

83. Roseland, J.; Phillips, K.M.; Patterson, K.Y.; Pehrsson, P.R.; Taylor, C.L. Chapter 60: Vitamin D in foods: An evolution of knowledge. In *Vitamin D*; Feldman, D., Ed.; Elsevier: New York, NY, USA, 2018; pp. 41–77.

84. Carnagey, K.M.; Huff-Lonergan, E.; Trenkle, A.; Wertz-Lutz, A.E.; Horst, R.L.; Beitz, D.C. Use of 25-hydroxyvitamin D3 and vitamin E to improve tenderness of beef from the longissimus dorsi of heifers1,2. *J. Sci.* **2008**, *86*, 1649–1657. [CrossRef]

85. Black, L.J.; Lucas, R.M.; Sherriff, J.L.; Björn, L.O.; Bornman, J.F. In Pursuit of Vitamin D in Plants. *Nutrients* **2017**, *9*, 136. [CrossRef]

86. NHS. Vitamins and Minerals: Vitamin D. Available online: https://www.nhs.uk/conditions/vitamins-and-minerals/vitamin-d/ (accessed on 15 April 2019).

87. Shafique, M.; Russell, S.; Murdoch, S.; Bell, J.D.; Guess, N. Dietary intake in people consuming a low-carbohydrate diet in the UK Biobank. *J. Hum. Nutr. Diet.* **2018**, *31*, 228–238. [CrossRef]

88. Public Health England. *National Diet and Nutrition Survey: Results from Years 1, 2, 3 and 4*; Crown Copyright: London, UK, 2017.

89. Bergeron, F.; Bouin, M.; LeMoyne, M.; Presse, N.; D'Aoust, L.; D'Aoust, L. Food avoidance in patients with inflammatory bowel disease: What, when and who? *Clin. Nutr.* **2018**, *37*, 884–889. [CrossRef] [PubMed]

90. Taylor, L.; Almutairdi, A.; Shommu, N.; Fedorak, R.; Ghosh, S.; Reimer, R.A.; Panaccione, R.; Raman, M. Cross-Sectional Analysis of Overall Dietary Intake and Mediterranean Dietary Pattern in Patients with Crohn's Disease. *Nutrients* **2018**, *10*, 1761. [CrossRef] [PubMed]

91. Krishnamoorthy, R.; Jeanes, Y. PWE-115 Dietary patterns in inflammatory bowel disease-intolerances, quality of life and calcium/vitamin D intake. *Gut* **2018**, *67*, A175–A176.

92. Vidarsdottir, J.B.; Johannsdottir, S.E.; Thorsdottir, I.; Björnsson, E.; Ramel, A. A cross-sectional study on nutrient intake and -status in inflammatory bowel disease patients. *Nutr. J.* **2016**, *15*, 219. [CrossRef] [PubMed]

93. Opstelten, J.L.; De Vries, J.H.; Wools, A.; Siersema, P.D.; Oldenburg, B.; Witteman, B.J. Dietary intake of patients with inflammatory bowel disease: A comparison with individuals from a general population and associations with relapse. *Clin. Nutr.* **2018**, (in press). [CrossRef]

94. Tripkovic, L.; Lambert, H.; Hart, K.; Smith, C.P.; Bucca, G.; Penson, S.; Chope, G.; Hyppönen, E.; Berry, J.; Vieth, R.; et al. Comparison of vitamin D2 and vitamin D3 supplementation in raising serum 25-hydroxyvitamin D status: a systematic review and meta-analysis123. *Am. J. Clin. Nutr.* **2012**, *95*, 1357–1364. [CrossRef]

95. Glendenning, P.; Chew, G.T.; Inderjeeth, C.A.; Taranto, M.; Fraser, W.D. Calculated free and bioavailable vitamin D metabolite concentrations in vitamin D-deficient hip fracture patients after supplementation with cholecalciferol and ergocalciferol. *Bone* **2013**, *56*, 271–275. [CrossRef]

96. EFSA Panel on Dietetic Products, Nutrition and Allergies (NDA). Scientific Opinion on the Tolerable Upper Intake Level of vitamin D. *EFSA J.* **2012**, *10*, 2813.

97. Hlavaty, T.; Krajcovicova, A.; Payer, J. Vitamin D therapy in inflammatory bowel diseases: Who, in what form, and how much? *J Crohns Colitis* **2015**, *9*, 198–209. [CrossRef] [PubMed]

98. Pappa, H.M.; Mitchell, P.D.; Jiang, H.; Kassiff, S.; Filip-Dhima, R.; DiFabio, D.; Quinn, N.; Lawton, R.C.; Bronzwaer, M.E.S.; Koenen, M.; et al. Maintenance of Optimal Vitamin D Status in Children and Adolescents With Inflammatory Bowel Disease: A Randomized Clinical Trial Comparing Two Regimens. *J. Clin. Endocrinol. Metab.* **2014**, *99*, 3408–3417. [CrossRef] [PubMed]

99. Pappa, H.M.; Mitchell, P.D.; Jiang, H.; Kassiff, S.; Filip-Dhima, R.; DiFabio, D.; Quinn, N.; Lawton, R.C.; Varvaris, M.; Van Straaten, S.; et al. Treatment of Vitamin D Insufficiency in Children and Adolescents with Inflammatory Bowel Disease: A Randomized Clinical Trial Comparing Three Regimens. *J. Clin. Endocrinol. Metab.* **2012**, *97*, 2134–2142. [CrossRef]

100. Li, J.; Chen, N.; Wang, D.; Zhang, J.; Gong, X. Efficacy of vitamin D in treatment of inflammatory bowel disease: A meta-analysis. *Medicine* **2018**, *97*, e12662. [CrossRef]

101. Jørgensen, S.P.; Agnholt, J.; Glerup, H.; Lyhne, S.; Villadsen, G.E.; Hvas, C.L.; Bartels, L.E.; Kelsen, J.; Christensen, L.A.; Dahlerup, J.F. Clinical trial: vitamin D3 treatment in Crohn's disease - a randomized double-blind placebo-controlled study. *Aliment. Pharmacol. Ther.* **2010**, *32*, 377–383. [CrossRef]

102. Jun, J.C.; Yoon, H.; Choi, Y.J.; Shin, C.M.; Park, Y.S.; Kim, N.Y.; Lee, D.H.; Kim, J.S. Tu1715 - The Effect of Vitamin D Administration on Inflammatory Marker in Patients with Inflammatory Bowel Disease. *Gastroenterology* **2018**, *154*. [CrossRef]

103. Arihiro, S.; Nakashima, A.; Matsuoka, M.; Suto, S.; Uchiyama, K.; Kato, T.; Mitobe, J.; Komoike, N.; Itagaki, M.; Miyakawa, Y.; et al. Randomized Trial of Vitamin D Supplementation to Prevent Seasonal Influenza and Upper Respiratory Infection in Patients With Inflammatory Bowel Disease. *Inflamm. Bowel Dis.* **2019**. [CrossRef]

104. Govani, S.M.; Higgins, P.D.; Stidham, R.W.; Montain, S.J.; Waljee, A.K. Increased ultraviolet light exposure is associated with reduced risk of inpatient surgery among patients with Crohn's disease. *J. Crohns Colitis* **2015**, *9*, 77–81. [CrossRef]

105. Ananthakrishnan, A.N.; Cheng, S.C.; Cai, T.; Cagan, A.; Gainer, V.S.; Szolovits, P.; Shaw, S.Y.; Churchill, S.; Karlson, E.W.; Murphy, S.N.; et al. Association between reduced plasma 25-hydroxy vitamin D and increased risk of cancer in patients with inflammatory bowel diseases. *Clin. Gastroenterol. Hepatol.* **2014**, *12*, 821–827. [CrossRef]

106. Baron, J.A.; Barry, E.L.; Mott, L.A.; Rees, J.R.; Sandler, R.S.; Snover, D.C.; Bostick, R.M.; Ivanova, A.; Cole, B.F.; Ahnen, D.J.; et al. A Trial of Calcium and Vitamin D for the Prevention of Colorectal Adenomas. *New Engl. J. Med.* **2015**, *373*, 1519–1530. [CrossRef]

107. Syed, S.; Michalski, E.S.; Tangpricha, V.; Chesdachai, S.; Kumar, A.; Prince, J.; Ziegler, T.R.; Suchdev, P.S.; Kugathasan, S.; Ms, S.S.M. Vitamin D status is Associated with Hepcidin and Hemoglobin concentrations in Children with Inflammatory Bowel Disease. *Inflamm. Bowel Dis.* **2017**, *23*, 1650–1658. [CrossRef]

108. Moran-Lev, H.; Weisman, Y.; Cohen, S.; Deutsch, V.; Cipok, M.; Bondar, E.; Lubetzky, R.; Mandel, D. The interrelationship between hepcidin, vitamin D, and anemia in children with acute infectious disease. *Pediatr. Res.* **2018**, *84*, 62–65. [CrossRef]

109. Stio, M.; Treves, C.; Martinesi, M.; D'Albasio, G.; Bagnoli, S.; Bonanomi, A.G. Effect of Anti-TNF Therapy and Vitamin D Derivatives on the Proliferation of Peripheral Blood Mononuclear Cells in Crohn's Disease. *Am. J. Dig. Dis.* **2004**, *49*, 328–335. [CrossRef]

110. Winter, R.W.; Collins, E.; Cao, B.; Carrellas, M.; Crowell, A.M.; Korzenik, J.R. Higher 25-hydroxyvitamin D levels are associated with greater odds of remission with anti-tumour necrosis factor-alpha medications among patients with inflammatory bowel diseases. *Aliment. Pharmacol. Ther.* **2017**, *45*, 653–659. [CrossRef]

111. Zator, Z.A.; Cantu, S.M.; Konijeti, G.G.; Nguyen, D.D.; Sauk, J.; Yajnik, V.; Ananthakrishnan, A.N. Pretreatment 25-hydroxyvitamin D levels and durability of anti-tumor necrosis factor-alpha therapy in inflammatory bowel diseases. *JPEN* **2014**, *38*, 385–391. [CrossRef]

112. Fialho, A.; Fialho, A.; Kochhar, G.; Shen, B. Association between vitamin D deficiency and anemia in inflammatory bowel disease patients with ileostomy. *J. Coloproctology* **2015**, *35*, 139–145. [CrossRef]
113. Henderson, C.M.; Fink, S.L.; Bassyouni, H.; Argiropoulos, B.; Brown, L.; Laha, T.J.; Jackson, K.J.; Lewkonia, R.; Ferreira, P.; Hoofnagle, A.N.; et al. Vitamin D–Binding Protein Deficiency and Homozygous Deletion of the GC Gene. *New Engl. J. Med.* **2019**, *380*, 1150–1157. [CrossRef]
114. Chun, R.F.; Peercy, B.E.; Orwoll, E.S.; Nielson, C.M.; Adams, J.S.; Hewison, M. Vitamin D and DBP: The free hormone hypothesis revisited. *J. Steroid Biochem. Mol. Boil.* **2014**, *144*, 132–137. [CrossRef]

6

Chemopreventive Effects of Strawberry and Black Raspberry on Colorectal Cancer in Inflammatory Bowel Disease

Tong Chen [1,2,*], Ni Shi [1,2] and Anita Afzali [3,4]

[1]   Division of Medical Oncology, Department of Internal Medicine, The Ohio State University, Columbus, OH 43210, USA; ni.shi@osumc.edu

[2]   Comprehensive Cancer Center, The Ohio State University, Columbus, OH 43210, USA

[3]   Division of Gastroenterology, Hepatology and Nutrition, The Ohio State University, Columbus, OH 43210, USA; Anita.Afzali@osumc.edu

[4]   Inflammatory Bowel Disease Center, Wexner Medical Center, The Ohio State University, Columbus, OH 43210, USA

*   Correspondence: tong.chen@osumc.edu

Abstract: Colorectal cancer (CRC) remains the third most common cause of cancer-related death in the United States and the fourth globally with a rising incidence. Inflammatory bowel disease (IBD) is a chronic immunologically mediated disease that imposes a significant associated health burden, including the increased risk for colonic dysplasia and CRC. Carcinogenesis has been attributed to chronic inflammation and associated with oxidative stress, genomic instability, and immune effectors as well as the cytokine dysregulation and activation of the nuclear factor kappa B (NFκB) signaling pathway. Current anti-inflammation therapies used for IBD treatment have shown limited effects on CRC chemoprevention, and their long-term toxicity has limited their clinical application. However, natural food-based prevention approaches may offer significant cancer prevention effects with very low toxicity profiles. In particular, in preclinical and clinical pilot studies, strawberry and black raspberry have been widely selected as food-based interventions because of their potent preventive activities. In this review, we summarize the roles of strawberry, black raspberry, and their polyphenol components on CRC chemoprevention in IBD.

Keywords: colorectal cancer; inflammatory bowel disease; colorectal cancer; dysplasia; berries; chemoprevention

---

1. Introduction

Inflammatory bowel disease (IBD) (e.g., Crohn's disease and ulcerative colitis) is a chronic immunologically mediated disease that develops in interactions between genetics, immunology, the environment, and the microbiome [1,2]. IBD is highly prevalent in North America and Europe, affecting about 1.3 million people in the United States and 2.2 million people in Europe [1]. Moreover, the rising prevalence of IBD has been reported across other countries worldwide. Notably, patients with IBD are at the increased risk of developing colorectal cancer (CRC), which further increases the urgency of understanding and treating this disease [3].

In IBD, chronic inflammation induces oncogenic mutations, genomic instability, immune microenvironment changes, early tumor promotion, and angiogenesis. These factors are likely related to the increased risk of CRC in IBD [4]. Importantly, supporting the association between chronic inflammation in IBD and CRC risk, the results of studies employing 5-aminosalicylate (5-ASAs) to target and reduce inflammation identified some chemopreventive effects in IBD [5]. In population-based cohorts, the incidence of CRC in patients with ulcerative colitis was 2.4-fold higher than in the controls [6]. Furthermore, some results suggested that at 10 years after the initial onset of ulcerative colitis around 2% of patients with ulcerative colitis developed CRC: 8% after 20 years and 18% after 30 years of disease duration [7]. Previous data also showed that 2.9% of Crohn's disease patients developed CRC within 10 years after the initial onset of the disease, and that percentage increased to 5.6% after 20 years and 8.3% after 30 years. Due to multifocal tumors and cell histopathology, CRC that develops in IBD patients tends to have a worse prognosis and survival rate compared to sporadic CRC in the advanced stage [8]. Additionally, the mean age for developing CRC in IBD patients (40–50 years) tends to be lower than the mean age for sporadic CRC (60 years) [4].

Due to the increased risk and poorer prognosis associated with CRC in individuals with IBD, its early detection and prevention are essential. In adults aged 50–75 years with an average risk of CRC, the US Preventive Services Task Force recommends yearly CRC screening by a fecal occult blood test (FOBT), sigmoidoscopy every five years, and colonoscopy every 10 years. In patients with IBD, a colonoscopy is recommended every one to two years beginning at 8–10 years from the diagnosis of the disease as well as multiple colonic biopsy specimens for dysplasia detection to screen for dysplasia or CRC [9]. Although chemoprevention is another important goal for IBD-related CRC management, the current therapies used in IBD have shown little to no effect, and the long-term toxicity associated with these treatments limits their clinical application for this purpose.

Diets that are high in animal fat and low in fruit and vegetables can be important triggers of both IBD and cancers [10,11]. Based on the associations between diet and cancers, natural food-based prevention approaches may represent a promising strategy. Notably, food-based approaches involving components of fruits and vegetables, vitamins, minerals, probiotics, and herbal medicines have shown potential cancer prevention effects with low toxicity profiles. Flavonoids, which are a major class of polyphenols that occur naturally in fruit and vegetables, have shown promising in vitro anti-colon cancer effects. Additionally, several case-control and cohort studies have verified the inverse association between flavonoid intake and CRC [12–14]. In particular, berries are a good source of polyphenols, especially anthocyanins, micronutrients, and fiber, which suggests that these foods may be associated with benefits for cardiovascular and immune health as well as chemoprevention [15]. Moreover, strawberry and black raspberry have been widely selected for food-based interventions in preclinical and pilot clinical studies because of their potent activity in the prevention of oral, esophageal, colon, skin, and prostate cancer [16–20]. Strawberry is the most commonly consumed berry type on the current market. Our previous study showed the significant chemoprevention effects of strawberry in CRC mouse model and its role in inflammation inhibition [18]. We also demonstrate that black raspberry inhibits oxidative stress, the inflammation mediators, cyclooxygenase-2 (COX-2) and inducible nitric oxide synthase (iNOS) and exhibits superior anti-cancer effects than inhibitors of COX-2 and iNOS in an animal model [21,22]. In this review, we summarize the roles of strawberry, black raspberry, and their polyphenol components on CRC chemoprevention in IBD.

2. Animal Models of Inflammatory Bowel Disease and IBD-Related Colorectal Cancer

Genetic engineering models can produce IBD in animals, such as muc-2 deficiency, muc-2/C3GnT dual deletion, muc-2/Core 1-derived O-glycans deficiency, P-gp deficiency, T-bet knockout, IKK-γ or IKK-β deletion, STAT3 deficiency, STAT3/IL-22 dual deficiency, XBP1 deletion, IL-10 deficiency, and IL-7 overexpression [2,11]. These targeted genes are responsible for epithelial barrier function, intestinal permeability, oxidative stress, cytokine, inflammation and immune effector regulation signaling pathway, and gut microflora etc. Additionally, colonic epithelium injures, ectogenic immunogenic response, adoptive transfer of naïve CD4$^+$ T cells to immune deficiency animals are strategies to induce IBD in animals. In Dextran sulfate sodium (DSS) model, DSS in drinking water is toxic in the epithelial lining of the colon and produce severe colitis. DSS treatment combined with gene deficiency in immune effectors regulation, cytokine response and immune response signaling pathways can enhance the inflammation in animals. Intrarectal injection of the haptenating agent 2,4,6-trinitrobenzene sulfonic acid (TNBS) or 4-ethoxymethylene-2-phenyl-2-oxazolin-5-one (oxazolone) can cause ulcerative colitis with different features. The inflammation in the TNBS model is regulated by TH1-mediated immune response with CD4$^+$ T cells, neutrophils and macrophages infiltration showing symptoms including severe diarrhea, weight loss, and rectal prolapse similar to Crohn's disease. TNBS model is used for the immune-related studies for Crohn's disease. The oxazolone model driven by NKT cells and IL-13 is considered as a valuable model for ulcerative colitis. The regulatory T cell deficiency in naïve CD4$^+$ T cells is a critical factor for inflammation in the transfer model. This model is ideal for immunoregulation and regulatory T cell research.

In studies on colon carcinogenesis and chemopreventive screening interventions for CRC in IBD, gene engineering mouse model such as apc mutation, apc deletion, smad mutation, smad 3 knockout, rag2-deficiency, k-ras mutation have been used [23]. In chemically induced preclinical models, murine treated with azoxymethane (AOM)/DSS has been a commonly used model for IBD-related CRC research for over a decade. AOM is a metabolite of 1,2-dimethylhydrazine (DMH) and the carcinogen to induce CRC in murine. It is important to note that AOM-induced tumors showed histopathological characteristics similar to human CRC, such as frequent K-Ras, β-catenin mutation, and microsatellite instability [24]. When combined with AOM, DSS works as a promoter of colorectal carcinogenesis through an initial acute inflammation phase. To induce colon carcinogenesis in murine, a single intraperitoneal injection of AOM at 10 mg/kg body weight or less can be given, followed by one to three cycles of 2% or 3% DSS in drinking water. In this method, tumors typically form 14 weeks after the AOM injection. Multistep tumor histogenesis can be efficiently reproduced in the AOM/DSS murine model. As found in our former studies, intraepithelial neoplasia, including changes ranging from dysplasia to adenoma and adenocarcinoma, were observed (Figure 1) [18]. T lymphocytes and other immune cells typically found in CRC patients are also frequently observed in tumors developed in AOM/DSS murine models. Therefore, AOM/DSS murine models are important for the investigation of inflammation-induced colon carcinogenesis and chemoprevention strategy screening.

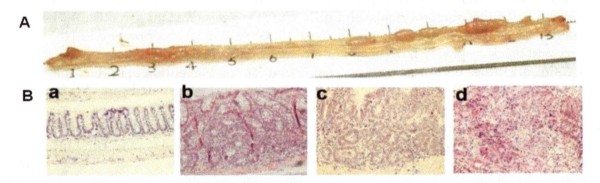

Figure 1. Histopathology of azoxymethane (AOM)/dextran sodium sulfate (DSS)-induced colorectal cancer (CRC) in mice. (**A**) The representative macroscopic appearance of a mouse colon treated with AOM/DSS; (**B**) The representative hematoxylin and eosin stained sections showing different histopathology of mouse colon, including normal (**a**), dysplasia (**b**), adenoma (**c**), and adenocarcinoma (**d**).

3. Molecular Mechanisms Associated with Chronic Inflammation and Colorectal Cancer

3.1. Inflammation-Dependent Oxidative Stress

Previous studies identified that carcinogenesis in IBD was related to reactive nitrogen intermediates (RNI) and reactive oxygen species (ROS) [3,25,26]. RNI and ROS are produced by neutrophils and macrophages, and they may cause oxidative damage to DNA, proteins, and lipids in the surrounding mucosal cells [3,23,24]. RNI, an indicator of nitrosative stress, is associated with nitrotyrosine, which is formed when peroxynitrite interacts with protein tyrosine. Hence, nitrotyrosine can serve as an important biomarker. In murine treated with AOM/DSS, more numerous and concentrated nitrotyrosine positive cells were observed as well as the greater expression of iNOS [18]. ROS are small oxygen-derived molecules produced by various biochemical and physiological oxidative processes, including superoxide (O_2^-), hydroxyl (OH), peroxyl (RO_2), and alkoxyl (RO), hypochlorous acid (HOCl), ozone (O_3), singlet oxygen (O_2), and hydrogen peroxide (H_2O_2) [21]. The imbalance in the generation and elimination of ROS and RNI was found to lead to oxidative stress. Hepatic malondialdehyde (MDA) levels, which are indicators of oxidative stress, were increased in murine treated with AOM/DSS [27]. Enzymatic and nonenzymatic antioxidants, such as superoxide dismutase, catalase, glutathione peroxidase and glutathione reductase, were decreased in an AOM/DSS mouse model [27]. Deficiencies in antioxidant genes, such as transcription factor NF-E2-related factor 2 (Nrf-2) and glutathione peroxidase 3 (Gpx3), were associated with increased numbers of aberrant crypt foci and tumors with higher dysplasia [28,29].

In patients with IBD-associated CRC, increased RNI and ROS concentrations were related to oxidative damage and active DNA damage response at cancer sites [30,31]. In AOM/DSS mouse models, knocking down genes that code for DNA damage repair-related enzymes, e.g., Alkyladenine DNA glycosylase (Aag), mutY DNA glycosylase (Mutyh), 8-oxoguanine DNA glycosylase 1 (Ogg1), may increase CRC incidence [9,30,32]. Overall, there is sufficient evidence from animal studies to support the carcinogenic role of inflammation-dependent oxidative stress in CRC developed from IBD.

3.2. Genomic Instability

Genomic instability includes base pair mutation, microsatellite instability, chromosome abnormality, gene fusion, gene copy number change, and other small or large structural variations. Inflammation-dependent oxidative stress is also related to high genomic instability in IBD. Genomic instability profiles were found significantly different between IBD-related CRC and sporadic CRC [33]. For example, mutations in IDH1 R132, BRAF V600E; the amplification of FGFR1, FGFR2, ERBB2; and the fusion protein EML4-ALK are more commonly found in IBD related CRC compared to sporadic CRC. Microsatellite instability formed by the malfunction of genes coding for DNA repair mismatch enzymes was found to be a clinical feature of Lynch syndrome and sporadic CRC, but not IBD-related CRC [34]. Little overlap between microsatellite instability in IBD-related CRC and sporadic CRC has been found [35,36]. Aneuploidy is higher in IBD-related CRC than in sporadic CRC, and it could function as an independent factor for the prediction of dysplasia and CRC developed in IBD patients [25,37]. Due to the higher inflammation-dependent oxidative stress and genomic instability in IBD, the critical molecular events in CRC development in sporadic CRC differ from those in IBD-related CRC. For example, the loss of heterozygosity in chromosome 17p, the locus of TP53 (a well-known tumor suppressor) and mutations of TP53 occurred earlier in IBD-related CRC than in sporadic CRC [3,38]. Other study found that the frequency of TP53 mutation in inflamed, non-dysplastic colonic epithelia was correlated with increased oxidative stress [39]. TP53 mutation may be caused by oxidative stress and inflammation in IBD, which promote carcinogenesis of IBD-related CRC. Inflammation-dependent oxidative stress and genomic instability play critical roles in IBD-related carcinogenesis.

3.3. Cytokines

A pro-inflammatory microenvironment also contributes to carcinogenesis in IBD. Studies on IBD-associated CRC patients and AOM/DSS mouse models showed that activated neutrophils, fibroblasts, dendritic cells, macrophages, and T cells were present in IBD related CRC tissue [40–43]. The cytokines released by these effectors in a pro-inflammatory microenvironment also showed distinct roles in carcinogenesis in IBD. For instance, the tumor necrosis factor (TNF), which is released by monocyte/macrophage lineages and plays an important role in cell proliferation, differentiation and death, was shown to be increased in an AOM/DSS mouse model [44]. Hence, TNF-α antagonists could significantly reduce the number and size of tumors in this model [18,45]. Interleukin 1 (IL-1)/interleukin 6 (IL-6) axis activation was found to be involved in IBD related CRC carcinogenesis. In IBD, IL-6 is mainly released by monocytes, macrophages, and by T and B lymphocytes. IL-1 produced by neutrophils has also been shown to promote the development of CRC in IBD by inducing IL-6 production in intestine-resident mononuclear phagocytes [43]. High expressions of IL-1β and IL-6 were found in an AOM/DSS mouse model [18]. Knocking down IL-6 in AOM/DSS mouse models reduced the number of tumors developed [46,47]. The IL-23/IL-17 axis, including IL-17A, IL-17F, IL-22, and IL-23, are also important cytokines in IBD. The elevated IL-17A and IL-17F in IBD patients are released by Th17 cells. The successful development of Th17 cells to induce chronic inflammation was found to be dependent on the high levels of IL-21, IL-23, IL-6, and TGF [48,49]. IL-23 was found to be essential for the expression of TNFα, IL-6, and TNFγ in the pro-inflammatory microenvironment. These cytokines have the potential to bind to receptors or transcriptional factors in order to activate related signaling pathways to promote carcinogenesis.

3.4. NFκB

A key molecular component in the pro-inflammation molecular network is nuclear factor kappa B (NFκB). Under normal circumstances, NFκB dimers remain in the cytoplasm by binding to the specific inhibitors of NFκB (IκBs). Cell stimulation activates IκB kinase (IKK) subunits (α, β and γ) to induce the degradation of IκB proteins. The unbound NFκB then translocates to the nucleus and initiates transcription of several hundred target genes to promote the carcinogenesis of CRC. Lipopolysaccharide (LPS), and pro-inflammatory cytokines TNFα, IL-1, and CD40 ligand can activate the NFκB pathway. In inflammatory cells, NFκB is generally activated by reacting to bacteria, virus, and necrotic cell production as well as some inflammatory cytokines. The activation of NFκB could induce its downstream pathways including growth and survival signals as well as angiogenic factors. In malignant cells, NFκB reacts to inflammatory cytokine, growth, and survival signals and angiogenic factors released from inflammatory cells and regulate cell cycle related genes, thus, induce apoptosis inhibition effects and promote invasion and metastasis. Specifically, in AOM/DSS mouse models, studies found that in myeloid cells, IKK-β-driven NFκB promoted the production of cytokines that acted as growth factors in pre-malignant enterocytes. In enterocytes, IKK-β-driven NFκB was found to activate anti-apoptotic genes, thereby suppressing the apoptotic elimination of pre-neoplastic cells.

3.5. Microbiome

The alteration in composition and function of bacterial microbiota and fungal microbiota are considered as significant factors for IBD development [50,51]. The gut microbiome is linked to chronic inflammation in IBD [52]. The cytokines and increased ROS production induced by inflammation favors the outgrowth of some bacteria or kill others, and shape the gut microbiome. The gut microbiome plays an important role in the host immune system. Gut microbiome regulates the function of T help cell profile, CD4+ Treg cell, the production of several interleukins, such as (IL)-17A, IL-17F, IL-21, and IL-22. Compared to healthy people, IBD patients have more bacteria with inflammatory function and fewer bacteria with anti-inflammatory function [50,51,53,54]. Bacteria with anti-inflammatory effects such as *Faecalibacterium prausnitzii*, *Blautia faecis*, *Roseburia inulinivorans*, *Ruminococcus torques*, *and Clostridium lavalense* decreased and adhesion-invasive *Escherichia coli* with pro-inflammatory effects increased in IBD patients.

4. Chemoprevention of Colorectal Cancer in Inflammatory Bowel Disease with Anti-Inflammation Pharmaceuticals

One of the first therapies used to treat IBD is 5-ASA, which inhibits the production of cyclo-oxygenase and prostaglandin, thromboxane synthetase, platelet activating factor synthetase, and IL-1 to reduce the acute inflammatory response [5,52]. However, a systematic review and meta-analysis conducted by Velayos and colleagues that assessed 5-ASA for CRC chemoprevention showed only a slight preventative role of 5-ASA in CRC development [52]. The chemopreventive effects of corticosteroid are not clear, as toxicities from long-term use have limited its implementation as a chemopreventive agent [5]. A major trial that was conducted to assess the roles of immunomodulators, such as azathioprine, 6-mercaptopurine, and methotrexate, showed no significant protective effects on CRC [5]. Both azathioprine and 6-mercaptopurine can inhibit purine nucleotide synthesis, metabolism and the DNA/RNA production in immune effectors, and methotrexate can inhibit DNA/RNA production by competitively inhibiting dihydrofolate reductase during tetrahydrofolate synthesis. Thus, these drugs may inhibit DNA/RNA productions in other somatic cells and increase the risk of gene structure change and genomic instability. The side effects of immunomodulators have been associated with increased risks of lymphoma and non-melanomatous skin cancers, thus, limit the use of these medications in IBD patients in the clinical setting. NSAIDs, which inhibit the conversion of arachidonic acid to prostaglandins in the cyclo-oxygenase-2 pathway, have some chemoprevention effects on CRC. The U.S. Preventive Services Task Force (USPSTF) recommends aspirin for adults aged 50–59 to prevent CRC. However, most of the IBD patients are diagnosed in their 20 s and 30 s [55], and USPSTF didn't recommend aspirin for adults younger than 50 to take aspirin for colon cancer prevention. The role of aspirin in chemoprevention of IBD related CRC is limited. Moreover, several pieces of evidence showed that NSAIDs promote IBD development [2]. Overall, agents that target inflammation have shown modest results in preventing CRC development in IBD patients.

The complexity of the inflammatory pathways and multiple processes involved in CRC carcinogenesis indicates that a multitude of targets exist; hence, new chemoprevention agents are needed to address this issue. The additive and synergistic activities of multiple bioactive phytochemicals in natural food products may have greater overall efficacy and safety in cancer prevention. Hence, in the following section, we discuss the chemoprevention effects of black raspberry and strawberry on CRC.

5. Chemoprevention of Colorectal Cancer in Inflammatory Bowel Disease with Berries

5.1. Efficiency of Strawberry and Black Raspberry in Cell Lines and Animal Models

The major investigational models and findings on the chemoprevention effects associated with strawberry and black raspberry are summarized in Table 1. The black raspberry extract showed anti-cancer activity in HT-29 colon cancer cells by regulating the cell cycle and apoptosis signaling pathways [56,57]. In the DSS-treated ulcerative colitis mouse model, the short-term black raspberry intervention reduced the degree of mucosal ulceration, suppressed the levels of pro-inflammation cytokines TNF-α and IL-1β, and inhibited the COX-2 and NFκB signaling pathways [58]. When the berry intervention was extended for a longer period of time, the number of macrophages and neutrophils infiltrating the colon tissue decreased and the hypermethylation of tumor suppressor genes increased [59]. In another model of ulcerative colitis using IL-10 knockout mice, a diet of 5% black raspberry was shown to significantly reduce ulceration in colonic mucosa and submucosa, which are associated with aberrant epigenetic dysregulation in the Wingless/Integrated (Wnt) signaling pathway [60].

Table 1. Preventive effects of black raspberry and strawberry on Inflammatory Bowel Disease (IBD) and CRC.

Systems	Major Findings	Ref.
Black Raspberry		
1. CRC Cell Lines		
HT-29 /HT-116 cell lines	Regulating cell cycle and apoptosis	[56,57]
2. Animal Models of IBD		
DSS treated mouse	Colonic epithelium acute injury↓, ulceration↓, TNF-α and IL-1β↓, COX2 and NFκB↓	[58]
DSS treated mouse	Ulceration↓, macrophages and neutrophils infiltrated the colon tissue↓, NFκB↓, Dkk3↑, β-Catenin nuclear localization↓,c-Myc, DNMT3B, HDAC1, HDAC2, MBD2↓	[59]

Table 1. *Cont.*

Systems	Major Findings	Ref.
IL-10 knockout mice	Ulceration↓, Wnt pathway↓, wif1, sox17, and qki↑,dnmt3b, hdac1, hdac2, and mbd2↓	[60]
3. Animal Models of IBD-Related CRC		
Mouse epidermal JB6Cl41 cells	AP-1, NFκB, and COX-2↓	[61,62]
AOM induced rat model	ACF multiplicity↓, total tumor multiplicity↓, urinary 8-OHdG↓	[63]
Muc2−/− mice	COX-2, TNF-α, IL-1, IL-6, and IL-10 ↓	[64]
4. Clinical Studies of CRC		
CRC patients	GM-CSF and IL-8↓, Ki-67↓, apoptosis↓	[65]
CRC patients	Wnt pathway↓ (SFRP2, WIF1, β-catenin, E-cadherin), DNMT1↓	[66]
Strawberry		
1. CRC Cell Lines		
HT-29 cell lines	Proliferation↓, cell apoptosis and p21WAF1↑	[57,67]
CaCo-2	Proliferation↓	[68]
HCT-116	Proliferation↓	[69]
2. Animal Models of IBD		
Gum acacia induced IBD rats	Disease activity index↓, lesion scores↓, antioxidant enzymes myeloperoxidase↑, tissue catalase↑, superoxide dismutase↑	[70]
3. Animal Models of IBD-Related CRC		
AOM/DSS mouse	Tumor incidence↓, nitrosative stress↓, TNF-α, IL-1β, IL-6, COX-2 and iNOS ↓, PI3K, Akt, ERK and NFκB↓	[18]

Note: ↓, decrease; ↑, increase.

In mouse epidermal JB6Cl41 cells, carcinogen BaP diol-epoxide (BPDE) treatment activated the activator protein 1 (AP-1), NFκB, and COX-2, which were then inhibited by the methanol extract of black raspberry [61,62]. In an AOM-induced aberrant crypt foci rat model, black raspberry diets significantly reduced the aberrant crypt foci multiplicity, total tumor multiplicity, and urinary 8-hydroxy-2′-deoxyguanosine (8-OHdG) levels [63]. A black raspberry diet was also significantly associated with reduced expression of COX-2 and pro-inflammatory cytokines TNF-α, IL-1, IL-6, and IL-10. Interestingly, when it was compared to the mechanism associated with tumor development in Apc1638+/− mice, the inhibition of β-catenin was found only in Apc1638+/− mice [64].

Strawberry extracts were shown to inhibit HT-29 proliferation by stimulating cell apoptosis and p21WAF1 [57,67]. Strawberries also showed significant anti-tumor effects on CRC cells CaCo-2 and HCT-116 [68,69]. In a gum acacia-induced IBD rat model, ethanolic extract of *Fragaria vesca*, a wild strawberry, decreased the disease activity index and lesion scores and increased antioxidant enzymes including myeloperoxidase, tissue catalase and superoxide dismutase [70]. In the AOM/DSS mouse model, 2.5%, 5%, or 10% (wt%) lyophilized strawberry significantly decreased tumor incidence, suppressed nitrosative stress, decreased the inflammation mediators TNF-α, IL-1β, IL-6, COX-2 and iNOS, and inhibited the phosphorylation of phosphatidylinositol 3-kinase (PI3K), Akt (Protein Kinase B), extracellular signal-regulated kinase (ERK), and NFκB [18].

In comparison to other berries, black raspberry and strawberry showed the potential for superior effects in CRC cell lines. In a study that compared the pro-apoptosis effects of six popularly consumed berries (blackberry, black raspberry, blueberry, cranberry, red raspberry, and strawberry), black raspberry and strawberry showed the most significant pro-apoptotic effects in CRC cell lines [57]. In another study that compared different berry extracts, strawberries showed the best anti-proliferation effects with an EC50 value of 20 ug/mL [68].

5.2. Efficiency of Black Raspberry in Clinical Studies

It is reported that a phase I study with black raspberry has been conducted in patients with CRC. The overall objective of this study is to identify measurable genetic and epigenetic biomarkers modulated by black raspberry in patients with CRC. This study demonstrates that 60 g of black raspberry powder per day for nine weeks significantly modulate the Wnt pathway through demethylating tumor suppressor genes SFRP2 and WIF1, and decrease the expression of β-catenin and E-cadherin. Black raspberry also decreases the expression of DNMT1, GM-CSF and IL-8 as well as the proliferation of biomarker Ki-67 and apoptosis [65,66]. The reports on the effects of strawberry on CRC or IBD are not available.

5.3. Major Bioactive Components in Berries

Anthocyanins are flavonoid compounds that are responsible for the colors of most fruits and vegetables, and they contribute to the protective effects of fruits and vegetables against chronic diseases and cancer (Figure 2). According to our previous studies, anthocyanins are the main components in strawberry and black raspberry (Table 2) [18,22]. Among the anthocyanins, cyanidin rutinoside is the most abundant in black raspberry, whereas pelargonidin glucoside is the most abundant in strawberry. Pelargonidin rutinoside is the only anthocyanin that has been identified in both black raspberry and strawberry. Following anthocyanins, ellagic acid and derivatives are the second most abundant components of strawberry although they are rare in black raspberry. Among ellagic acid and its derivatives, agrimoniin is the main component of strawberry. Additionally, ellagitannins account for about 10% of the phytochemical components in black raspberry and strawberry. Flavonols have also been identified in both black raspberry and strawberry, but in much lower concentrations than anthocyanins.

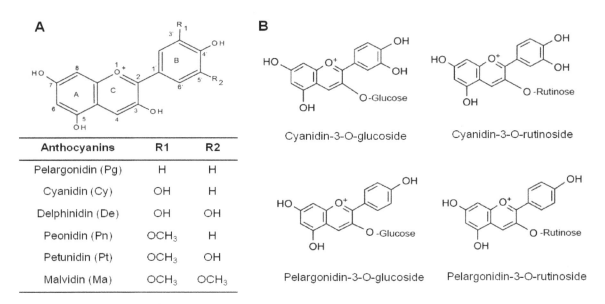

Figure 2. Structure of anthocyanins. (**A**) The structural classification of the six most common anthocyanins; (**B**) The structural classification of the four most common anthocyanins identified in strawberry and black raspberry.

Table 2. Major components in strawberry and black raspberry.

Strawberry	mg/ 100 mg	% by mg	Black Raspberry	mg/ 100 mg	% by mg
Anthocyanins			**Anthocyanins**		
pelargonidin glucoside	367.7	41.1	cyanidin rutinoside	2924.7	58.2
pelargonidin malonyl glucoside	83.9	9.4	cyanidin xylorutinoside	916.3	18.2
pelargonidin rutinoside	55.3	6.2	cyanidin glucoside	245.1	4.9
cyanidin glucoside	14.9	1.7	cyanidin sambubioside	103.5	2.1
			pelargonidin rutinoside	38.3	0.8
	130.4	**58.4%**		**4227.9**	**84.2%**
Ellagitannins			**Ellagitannins**		
ellagitannin	64.1	7.2	sanguiin H6	173.2	3.4
ellagitannin	11.4	1.3	ellagitannin 783-1	101.1	2.0
ellagitannin	23.1	2.6	ellagitannin 933-2	75.8	1.5
Lambertianin	20.3	2.3	elagitannin 783-2	75.8	1.5
			ellagitannin 935-1	62.8	1.3
			ellagitannin 933-1	50.5	1.0
			Lambertiannin	31.3	0.6
			ellagitannin 935-2	7.9	0.2
	118.9	**13.3%**		**578.5**	**11.5%**
Ellagic acid and derivatives			**Ellagic acid and derivatives**		
Agrimoniin	144.5	16.2	methyl ellagic acid pentoside	16.0	0.3
ellagic acid rhamnoside	23.1	2.6	ellagic acid	9.3	0.2
ellagic acid	7.3	0.8	ellagic acid rhamnoside	5.8	0.1
			myricetin hexoside, EA derivative (coelution)	3.8	0.1
	174.9	**19.5%**		**34.8**	**0.7%**
Flavonols			**Flavonols**		
quercetin hexuronide	58.8	6.6	quercetin hexuronide	82.2	1.6
kaempferol glucoside/hexuronide	14.5	1.6	rutin (quercetin rutinoside)	75.4	1.5
kaempferol malonyl hexoside	5.1	0.6	quercetin xylorutinoside	24.2	0.5
	78.4	**8.8%**		**181.8**	**3.6%**

Berry extracts and anthocyanin compounds have been studied both in vivo and in vitro. Table 4 provides a summary of the role of anthocyanins in CRC cell lines or animal models. Anthocyanin-enriched fractions from black raspberry inhibited cell growth in HT-29 and HCT-119 cells [57,67,69,71–93]. In CRC, an anthocyanin-enriched extract of black raspberry showed effects similar to black raspberry powder on CRC cell lines in suppressing cell proliferation, inducing apoptosis, decreasing the activity of DNMT1 and DNMT3B and of demethylate CDKN2A, SFRP2, SFRP5 and WIF1 in the Wnt pathway [60,71]. Cyanidin-3-glycoside, which is the anthocyanin found in black raspberry, decreased DNA strand breakage in human colon epithelial cells (HCEC), and it reduced cytotoxicity induced by peroxyl radicals by suppressing apoptosis and decreasing the sub-G1 phase of the cell population in Caco-2 CRC cells [72,73]. Cyanidin-3-O-beta glucopyranoside and its aglycon form, cyanidin chloride, was shown to have the potential to function in inhibiting cell growth and proliferation and in decreasing the ROS level in Caco-2 cells [74]. Strawberry extracts also showed cell growth and proliferation inhibition effects, antioxidative effects, and p21WAF1 suppression effects in HT-29, HCT-116 cells [57,66,70]. The anthocyanins identified in other fruit and vegetables that showed anti-cancer effects in CRC cells lines included the anthocyanins found in black raspberry and strawberry.

Table 3. Effects of anthocyanins in IBD and IBD-related CRC.

Original Sources	Models	Major Findings	Anthocyanin Profiles	Ref.
Cell Lines				
1. Black Raspberry				
Black raspberry extract	Cell line HT-29 HCT-116	Inhibited cell growth HT-29 IC50 = 89.11, HCT-116, IC50 = 89.00	cyanidin-3-sophoroside rhamnoside, cyanidin-3-sambubioside rhamnoside, cyanidin-3-rutinoside	[57]
Black raspberry anthocyanin-enriched extract	Cell line HCT116	Decreased DNMT activity; decreased methylation of CDKN2A, SFRP5, SFRP2 and WIF1; suppressed cell proliferation; induced apoptosis	cyanidin-3-O-glucoside, cyanidin-3-O-rutinoside, cyanidin-3-O-xylosylrutinoside, cyanidin-3-O-sambubioside	[58]
2. Strawberry				
Strawberry extract	Cell line HT-29 HCT-116	Inhibited cell growth HT-29 IC_{50} = 114.30, HCT-116, IC_{50} = 62.00	cyanidin-3-glucoside, pelargonidin-3-glucoside, pelargonidin-3-rutinoside	[57]
Strawberry extract	Cell line HT29 HCT-116	Antioxidative effects.	cyanidin-3-glucoside, pelargonidin, cyanidin-3-glucoside, pelargonidin, pelargonidin-3-rutinoside	[66]
Strawberry extract	Cell line HT29	Inhibited proliferation; reduced expression of p21WAF1	cyanidin derivative; pelargonidin derivative	[67]
3. Anthocyanins				
cyanidin-3-glycoside	Cell line HCEC	Decreased DNA strand breakage	cyanidin-3-glycoside	[72]
Cyanidin-3-glycoside	Cell line Caoco-2	Reduced cytotoxicity induced by AAPH; suppressed apoptosis; decreased sub-G1 phase cell population	cyanidin-3-glycoside	[73]
Cyanidin-3-O-beta glucopyranoside, cyanidin chloride	Cell line Caoco-2	Inhibited cell growth and proliferation; decreased reactive oxygen species (ROS) level	cyanidin-3-O-beta glucopyranoside, cyanidin chloride	[74]
4. Protocatechuic Acid (PCA)				
Brown rice extracted PCA	Cell line SW480	Inhibited cell growth and colony formation	PCA	[75]
5. Other Fruit and Vegetables				
Blueberry	Cell line Caoco-2	IC_{50} 0.53 ± 0.04	delphinidin 3-galactoside, delphinidin 3-glucoside, cyanidin 3-galactoside, delphinidin 3-arabinoside, cyanidin 3-glucoside, petunidin 3-galactoside, cyanidin 3-arabinoside, petunidin 3-glucoside, peonidin 3-galactoside, petunidin 3-arabinoside, peonidin 3-glucoside, malvidin 3-galactoside, peonidin 3-arabinoside, malvidin 3-glucoside, malvidin 3-arabinoside	[76]
Blueberry extract	Cell lines HT-29	Inhibited cell growth; induced apoptosis	delphinidin 3-O-β-glucopyranoside; cyanidin 3-O-β-galactopyranoside; cyanidin 3-O-β-glucopyranoside; petunidin 3-O-β-glucopyranoside; peonidin 3-O-β-galactopyranoside; peonidin 3-O-β-glucopyranoside; malvidin 3-O-β-glucopyranoside.	[77]
Bilberry purified anthocyanins	Cell line HCT-116	Decreased cell viability	pelargonidin, cyanidin, peonidin, delphinidin, and malvidin	[78]
Cocoplum anthocyanins exert	Cell line HT-29	Cell proliferation was suppressed; increased intracellular ROS production; increased intracellular ROS production	delphinidin-3-glucoside, cyanidin 3-glucoside, petunidin 3-glucoside, delphinidin 3-(6-acetoyl) galactoside, delphinidin 3-(6-oxaloyl) arabinoside, peonidin 3-glucoside, petunidin 3-(6-acetoyl) galactoside, petunidin 3-(6-oxaloyl) arabinoside, peonidin 3-(6-acetoyl) glucoside, peonidin 3-(6-oxaloyl) arabinoside	[79]
Eugenia jambolana (Java Plum) fruit extract	Cell lines HCT-116 colon cancer stem cells	Inhibited proliferation; induced apoptosis	delphinidin-3,5-diglucoside, cyanidin-3,5-diglucoside, ptunidin-3,5-diglucosid, dtunidin-3,5-diglucosid, peonidin-3,5-diglucoside, monidin-3,5-diglucosid, cyanidin-3-glucoside, petunidin-3-glucoside, etunidin-3-glucosi	[80]

Table 4. Effects of anthocyanins in IBD and IBD-related CRC.

Original Sources	Models	Major Findings	Anthocyanin Profiles	Ref.
Cell Lines				
Anthocyanin-containing baked purple-fleshed potato extract	Colon cancer stem cells	Suppressed proliferation; elevated apoptosis; decreased β-catenin, c-Myc and Cyclin D1	pet-3-rut-5-glc, mal-3-rut-5-glc, cya-3-O(6-O-malonyl-β-D-glc), peo-3-(p-coum)-isophoro-5-glc, peo-3-rut-5-glc, pet-3-(p-coum)-rut-5-glc, peo-3-caffeyl-rut-5-glc, pel-3-(p-coum)-rut-5-glc, pel-3-(4-ferul-rut)-5-glc, peo-3-(p-coum)-rut-5-glc, mal-3-(p-coum)-rut-5-glc	[81]
Blue maize extract	Cell line Caco2 and HT29	Suppressed proliferation	cyanidin 3-glucoside, cyanidin 3-glucoside, cyanidin malonyl-glucoside, cyanidin succinyl-glucoside, pelargonidin 3-glucoside, pelargonidin malonyl-glucoside	[82]
Eggplant extract	Cell lines HT-29	Decreased DNA damage	delphinidin-3-rhamnosyl-glucoside-5-glucoside, delphinidin-3-rutinoside-5-glucoside	[83]
anthocyanin-enriched purple-fleshed sweet potato	Cell line SW480	Decreased cell number, G1 phase arrest	peonidin-3-glucoside	[84]
Vitis coignetiae Pullia extract		Inhibited cell invasion; suppressed MMP-2, MMP-9, NFkB	delphinidin-3,5-diglucoside, cyanidin-3,5-diglucoside, petunidin-3,5-diglucoside, delphinidin-3-glucoside, malvdin-3,5-diglucoside, peonidin-3,5-diglucoside, cyanidin-3-glucoside, petunidin-3-glucoside, peonidin-3-glucoside, malvidin-3-glucoside	[85]
Blackberry extract	Cell lines HT-29	Inhibited cell growth; inhibited IL-12 release	cyanidin-3-glucoside, cyanidin-3-arabinoside, delphinidin-3-xyloside, cyanidin-3-xyloside, cyanidin-3-malonylglucoside, cyanidin-3-dioxalylglucoside	[86]
Tart cherry anthocyanin	Cell line HT 29, HCT16	Inhibited cell growth	3-cyanidin 2″-O-β-D-glucopyranosyl-6″-O-α-L-rhamnopyransyl-β-D-glucopyranoside	[87]
Animal Models				
1. PCA				
PCA	AOM-treated rat	Decreased the number of aberrant crypt foci, ornithine decarboxylase activity and AgNOR	PCA	[88,89]
PCA	DSS-treated rat	Prevented diarrhea and bleeding; decreased pro-inflammatory cytokines; nitric oxide concentration, oxidative damage, and expression of COX-2 and iNOS	PCA	[90]
2. Other fruit and vegetables				
Anthocyanin-rich extracts from bilberry, chokeberry, and grape	AOM-treated rat	Reduced total ACF and the number of large ACF Suppressed cell proliferation reduces COX-2		[91]
Anthocyanin derived from purple sweet potato color in their basal diet	AOM/DSS rats	Decreased MDF, colon weight, low-grade dysplasia and total histopathology changes; decreased the expression of β-catenin, Ki67and Cyclin D1		[92]
anthocyanin-enriched purple-fleshed sweet potato	Animal AOM mice	Suppressed formation of aberrant crypt foci; decreased PCNA; increased caspase-3	peonidin-3-glucoside	[84]
Tart cherry anthocyanin	Apc^Min mice	Decreased the number and volume of adenomas	3-cyanidin 6″-O-α-L-rhamnopyranosyl-β-D-glucopyranoside	[87]
Tomato	DSS mice	Increased bacterial *Parabacteroides* and *Lactobacilli*		[93]

The distribution of anthocyanins has been found in almost all tissues. The black raspberry phytochemicals, cyanidin-3-rutinoside and cyanidin-3-xylosylrutinoside, have been detected in oral cancer tissues in patients after the administration of oral troches containing freeze-dried black raspberry powder as well as in prostate tissue in mice models after a diet of black raspberry powder [94,95]. Importantly, bioavailability and pharmacokinetic studies of strawberry anthocyanins showed that only modest amounts of ingested anthocyanins were absorbed from the upper small intestine. Most phytochemicals enter the colon where the substantial microbial metabolism and interaction with the colonic epithelium take place [18]. Protocatechuic acid (PCA) is one of the main metabolites of anthocyanins that can be absorbed by animals and humans. PCA significantly inhibited cell proliferation and colony formation in colon cancer SW 480 cells [75]. PCA also prevented diarrhea and bleeding in DSS-treated rats, and it decreased pro-inflammatory cytokines, nitric oxide concentration, and oxidative damage as well as the expression of COX-2 and iNOS [90]. Additionally, PCA diets may decrease the number of aberrant crypt foci, ornithine decarboxylase activity and the expression of AgNOR in AOM-induced CRC rat models [88,89]. In strawberries, 4-hydroxybenzoic acid (4HBA) was considered a metabolite of pelargonidin-3-glucoside, but it did not show anti-cancer activity in colon cancer in a limited number of studies [96,97].

The growth and spread of cancer depended not only on the biological characteristics of the tumor cells but also on the host immunology response. Black raspberry extracts and the single anthocyanins component cyanidin-3-rutinoside and quercitin-3-rutinoside were shown to inhibit T cell proliferation, limit myeloid-derived suppressor cells (MDSC) expansion, and suppress MDSC capacity [98]. Cyanidin-3-glucoside and cyanidin-3-rutinoside also reduced the inflammation cytokines TNF-α, IL-6, IL-1 β in lipopolysaccharide (LPS)-treated murine macrophage RAW264.7 cells [99].

In contrast to the consistent effects of anthocyanins in black raspberry and strawberry on chemoprevention, the results of studies that assessed the ellagitannin components of berries in chemoprevention have varied. Some studies found that ellagitannins were the most responsible for the anti-cancer activity of berry extracts [56,67]. However, the findings of other studies suggested that berry ellagitannins may not be sufficient for the prevention of many cancers, such as esophageal squamous cell carcinoma, because various concentrations of ellagitannins showed no differences in chemoprevention [100].

A recent study that used a high-resolution 1H NMR-based multivariate statistical model showed that anthocyanins, cyanidin 3-rutinoside, and cyanidin 3-xylosylrutinoside were the predominant contributors to the anti-cancer effects of black raspberry. However, in the same study, salicylic acid derivatives (salicylic acid glucosyl ester), quercetin 3-glucoside, quercetin 3-rutinoside, p-coumaric acid, epicatechin, methyl ellagic acid derivatives (methyl ellagic acetyl pentose), and citric acid derivatives were also shown to contribute significantly to anti-cancer effects [101].

Anthocyanins have brought the research community's attention in the field of IBD [102,103]. In our opinion, anthocyanins are the major components responsible for the chemoprevention effects of black raspberry and strawberry. This opinion is based on five main lines of evidence: (1) anthoycanins are the most abundant components in black raspberry and strawberry; (2) the anti-cancer effects of anthocyanins and the role of anthocyanins in immune modification are well-documented; (3) PCA, the metabolites of anthocyanins in black raspberry, show chemoprevention effects similar to those of black raspberry; (4) anthocyanins are found in cancer tissues; (5) the colon is the major site of the metabolism of anthocyanins. However, because other components also significantly contribute to anti-cancer effects, it is clear that further studies are needed to assess the chemopreventive compounds in black raspberry and strawberry.

5.4. Mechanisms Associated with Preventative Effects of Berries on Colon Cancer

The benefits of berries in reducing antioxidative stress are well known. In a study that compared the antioxidant role of 10 phenolic compounds in strawberry extracts, the most potent antioxidants identified by a trolox equivalent antioxidant capacity (TEAC) assay were cyanidin-3-glucoside, cyanidin-3-pelargonidin, and kaempferol [66]. Moreover, urinary 8-OHdG levels and tissue nitrosative stress are important biomarkers of oxidative stress, which were reduced by the intake of black raspberry and strawberry [18,63]. Overall, several studies using cell lines, animal models, and human clinical trials of strawberry and black raspberry reported significantly decreased oxidative and inflammatory signals, such as COX-2 and NFκB. However, not all related signals were shown to be regulated by either black raspberry or strawberry, including the following: DNA repair-related enzymes, such as Aag, Mutyh, Ogg1; enzymatic and nonenzymatic antioxidants, such as SOD; and the antioxidant genes Nrf-2, Gpx3. Therefore, these molecular processes should be examined in future studies.

One form of genomic instability is the loss of heterozygosity, which in previous studies was reduced by the topical application of the black raspberry gel on oral intraepithelial neoplasia lesions (17p13 location containing TP53 genes are included in the loss of heterozygosity). Hypermethylation, or the increased number of methyl groups added to the promoter region, were shown to function to inhibit the transcription of target genes. Similar to the loss of heterozygosity, hypermethylation was shown to be an important approach in deactivating tumor suppressor genes during carcinogenesis. As previously mentioned in this review, black raspberry powder and anthocyanin-enriched extract of black raspberry worked to demethylate CDKN2A, SFRP2, SFRP5, and WIF1 in the Wnt pathway through suppressing DNMT1 and DNMT3B [60,71]. In a phase Ib study on the effects of black raspberries on rectal polyps in patients with familial adenomatous polyposis, a greater number of the demethylated transcription start sites and the increased expression of DNMT1 was found in patients who received a black raspberry intervention compared to those that did not [104]. Combined with the demonstrated antioxidant effects of black raspberry and strawberry, the above evidence suggests the potential of black raspberry and strawberry to prevent inflammation-dependent oxidative stress and genomic instability in colon epithelial cells.

In a DSS-treated ulcerative colitis mouse model, an intervention employing a long-term black raspberry diet resulted in the decreased infiltration by macrophages and neutrophils in colon tissue [61]. Black raspberry and strawberry were both associated with the reduced expression of COX-2 and the pro-inflammatory mediators, COX-2, iNOS, TNF-α, IL-1, IL-6, and IL-10 in cell studies, animal models, and clinical trials [17–22]. Cytokine GM-CSF and IL-8 were also found to be decreased by black raspberry powder in untreated colon cancer patients [67]. Black raspberry also altered innate immune cell trafficking in NMBA-induced esophageal squamous cell carcinoma in a rat model [105]. Single anthocyanins cyanidin-3-rutinoside and quercitin-3-rutinoside inhibited MDSC expansion and modulated T lymphocyte proliferation [98]. Hence, another interesting area for further research is the regulation of immune effectors by black raspberry and strawberry.

NFκB is present in almost all cell types, and it is involved in inflammation, cell differentiation, and carcinogenesis. The cyclin-dependent kinase inhibitor, p21WAF1/Cip1, was induced by black raspberry in a Muc2−/− mice CRC model [64]. In addition, the cell proliferation markers Ki-67, c-Jun, p27, Erk1/2, MAPK, and AKT were regulated by treatment with black raspberry or strawberry [18,103,104,106]. Oxidative stress activates MAPK family members, including p38 MAPK and JNK, which subsequently activated genes involved in cellular proliferation. MAPK is activated by a range of stimuli, and it mediates several physiological processes, which are observed during carcinogenesis. AKT signaling plays an important role in multiple cellular processes, including cell proliferation, survival, motility, and angiogenesis. The induction of cell survival by AKT is mediated through NFκB signaling. The activation of the AKT and ERK pathways acts synergistically to promote the mechanistic target of rapamycin signaling, which controls NFκB activity [18,20]. NFκB was also found to regulate cell apoptosis during carcinogenesis. Black raspberry and strawberry increased apoptosis markers, TUNNEL staining, and the Bcl-2/Bax ratio in both animal models and human patients [16,105–108]. NFκB is required for the stabilization of snail, which is the transcription factor involved in regulating the expression of E-cadherin to induce cell migration and invasion induced by inflammatory cytokines. The inhibition of NFκB was found to potentially induce the degradation of Snail, which increased the expression of E-cadherin and hence inhibited cell migration and invasion. NFκB signaling was an important molecular event associated with the chemoprevention effects of black raspberry and strawberry on IBD-induced CRC. The mechanisms associated with the chemoprevention effects of black raspberry and strawberry are summarized in Figure 3.

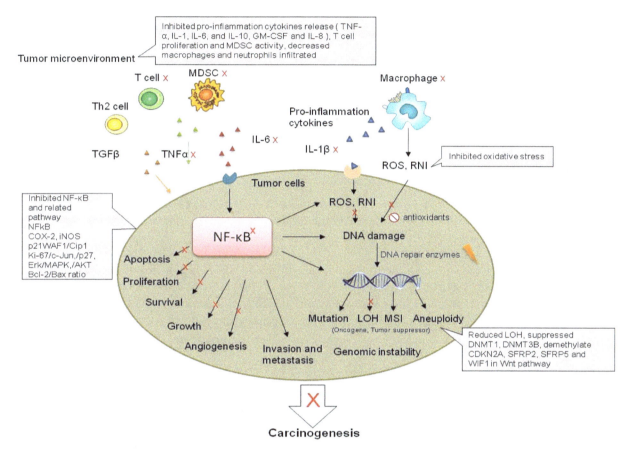

Figure 3. Possible mechanisms of the inhibition of IBD-related CRC by strawberry and black raspberry. MDSC: myeloid-derived suppressor cells; RNI: reactive nitrogen intermediates; LOH: Loss of heterozygosity; MSI: microsatellite instability.

6. Conclusions

Strawberry and black raspberry have been shown to have potential cancer prevention effects with low toxicity profiles in IBD-related CRC. Inflammation-induced carcinogenesis has been associated with oxidative stress, genomic instability, immune effectors, cytokine dysregulation, and the NFκB signaling pathway. In contrast to anti-inflammation pharmaceuticals, strawberry and black raspberry interventions have shown to have a synergistic role in multiple molecular events, including suppressing cytokines release, decreasing oxidative stress, reducing genomic instability, and inhibiting NFκB and related signaling pathways. The chemopreventive activity of strawberry and black raspberry is likely due to multiple nutrients and bioactives, especially anthocyanins. The clinical translational application of berries in IBD patients for CRC prevention is limited, which may suggest that this "low-hanging fruit" should be assessed in future clinical trials on colon cancer prevention in IBD. The evidence to date is a step toward the development of specific phytochemicals and metabolites as chemopreventive agents based on the principles of pharmacognosy.

Author Contributions: Conceptualization, T.C. and N.S.; writing—original draft preparation, T.C. and N.S.; writing—review and editing, T.C., N.S. and A.A.; supervision, T.C.; project administration, T.C.; funding acquisition, T.C.

Acknowledgments: The authors would like to thank Stephanie Fortier, MSc (The Ohio State University, Division of Medical Oncology) for her help in editing this manuscript.

References

1. Ananthakrishnan, A.N. Epidemiology and risk factors for ibd. *Nat. Rev. Gastroenterol. Hepatol.* **2015**, *12*, 205–217. [CrossRef] [PubMed]
2. Ananthakrishnan, A.N.; Bernstein, C.N.; Iliopoulos, D.; Macpherson, A.; Neurath, M.F.; Ali, R.A.R.; Vavricka, S.R.; Fiocchi, C. Environmental triggers in IBD: A review of progress and evidence. *Nat. Rev. Gastroenterol. Hepatol.* **2018**, *15*, 39–49. [CrossRef] [PubMed]
3. Feagins, L.A.; Souza, R.F.; Spechler, S.J. Carcinogenesis in ibd: Potential targets for the prevention of colorectal cancer. *Nat. Rev. Gastroenterol. Hepatol.* **2009**, *6*, 297–305. [CrossRef] [PubMed]
4. Mattar, M.C.; Lough, D.; Pishvaian, M.J.; Charabaty, A. Current management of inflammatory bowel disease and colorectal cancer. *Gastrointest. Cancer Res.* **2011**, *4*, 53–61.
5. Subramanian, V.; Logan, R.F. Chemoprevention of colorectal cancer in inflammatory bowel disease. *Best Pract. Res. Clin. Gastroenterol.* **2011**, *25*, 593–606. [CrossRef]
6. Jess, T.; Rungoe, C.; Peyrin-Biroulet, L. Risk of colorectal cancer in patients with ulcerative colitis: A meta-analysis of population-based cohort studies. *Clin. Gastroenterol. Hepatol.* **2012**, *10*, 639–645. [CrossRef]
7. Eaden, J.A.; Abrams, K.R.; Mayberry, J.F. The risk of colorectal cancer in ulcerative colitis: A meta-analysis. *Gut* **2001**, *48*, 526–535. [CrossRef]
8. Liao, J.; Seril, D.N.; Lu, G.G.; Zhang, M.; Toyokuni, S.; Yang, A.L.; Yang, G.Y. Increased susceptibility of chronic ulcerative colitis-induced carcinoma development in DNA repair enzyme ogg1 deficient mice. *Mol. Carcinog.* **2008**, *47*, 638–646. [CrossRef]
9. Kornbluth, A.; Sachar, D.B. Ulcerative colitis practice guidelines in adults (update): American college of gastroenterology, practice parameters committee. *Am. J. Gastroenterol.* **2004**, *99*, 1371–1385. [CrossRef]
10. Lewis, J.D.; Abreu, M.T. Diet as a trigger or therapy for inflammatory bowel diseases. *Gastroenterology* **2017**, *152*, 398–414.e6. [CrossRef]
11. Khalili, H.; Chan, S.S.M.; Lochhead, P.; Ananthakrishnan, A.N.; Hart, A.R.; Chan, A.T. The role of diet in the aetiopathogenesis of inflammatory bowel disease. *Nat. Rev. Gastroenterol. Hepatol.* **2018**, *15*, 525–535. [CrossRef] [PubMed]
12. Woo, H.D.; Kim, J. Dietary flavonoid intake and risk of stomach and colorectal cancer. *World J. Gastroenterol.* **2013**, *19*, 1011–1019. [CrossRef]
13. Arts, I.C.; Jacobs, D.R., Jr.; Gross, M.; Harnack, L.J.; Folsom, A.R. Dietary catechins and cancer incidence among postmenopausal women: The iowa women's health study (united states). *Cancer Causes Control* **2002**, *13*, 373–382. [CrossRef] [PubMed]
14. Simons, C.C.; Hughes, L.A.; Arts, I.C.; Goldbohm, R.A.; van den Brandt, P.A.; Weijenberg, M.P. Dietary flavonol, flavone and catechin intake and risk of colorectal cancer in the netherlands cohort study. *Int. J. Cancer* **2009**, *125*, 2945–2952. [CrossRef] [PubMed]
15. Stoner, G.D. Foodstuffs for preventing cancer: The preclinical and clinical development of berries. *Cancer Prev. Res.* **2009**, *2*, 187–194. [CrossRef]
16. Zhu, X.R.; Xiong, L.F.; Zhang, X.Y.; Shi, N.; Zhang, Y.T.; Ke, J.; Sun, Z.; Chen, T. Lyophilized strawberries prevent 7,12-dimethylbenz[alpha]anthracene (dmba)-induced oral squamous cell carcinogenesis in hamsters. *J. Funct. Foods* **2015**, *15*, 476–486. [CrossRef]
17. Chen, T.; Yan, F.; Qian, J.; Guo, M.; Zhang, H.; Tang, X.; Chen, F.; Stoner, G.D.; Wang, X. Randomized phase ii trial of lyophilized strawberries in patients with dysplastic precancerous lesions of the esophagus. *Cancer Prev. Res.* **2012**, *5*, 41–50. [CrossRef]
18. Shi, N.; Clinton, S.K.; Liu, Z.; Wang, Y.; Riedl, K.M.; Schwartz, S.J.; Zhang, X.; Pan, Z.; Chen, T. Strawberry phytochemicals inhibit azoxymethane/dextran sodium sulfate-induced colorectal carcinogenesis in crj: Cd-1 mice. *Nutrients* **2015**, *7*, 1696–1715. [CrossRef]
19. Duncan, F.J.; Martin, J.R.; Wulff, B.C.; Stoner, G.D.; Tober, K.L.; Oberyszyn, T.M.; Kusewitt, D.F.; Van Buskirk, A.M. Topical treatment with black raspberry extract reduces cutaneous uvb-induced carcinogenesis and inflammation. *Cancer Prev. Res.* **2009**, *2*, 665–672. [CrossRef]
20. Mallery, S.R.; Tong, M.; Shumway, B.S.; Curran, A.E.; Larsen, P.E.; Ness, G.M.; Kennedy, K.S.; Blakey, G.H.; Kushner, G.M.; Vickers, A.M.; et al. Topical application of a mucoadhesive freeze-dried black raspberry gel induces clinical and histologic regression and reduces loss of heterozygosity events in premalignant oral

intraepithelial lesions: Results from a multicentered, placebo-controlled clinical trial. *Clin. Cancer Res.* **2014**, *20*, 1910–1924.

21. Shi, N.; Chen, F.; Zhang, X.; Clinton, S.K.; Tang, X.; Sun, Z.; Chen, T. Suppression of oxidative stress and nfkappab/mapk signaling by lyophilized black raspberries for esophageal cancer prevention in rats. *Nutrients* **2017**, *9*, 413. [CrossRef]

22. Shi, N.; Riedl, K.M.; Schwartz, S.J.; Zhang, X.L.; Clinton, S.K.; Chen, T. Efficacy comparison of lyophilised black raspberries and combination of celecoxib and pbit in prevention of carcinogen-induced oesophageal cancer in rats. *J. Funct. Foods* **2016**, *27*, 84–94. [CrossRef]

23. Fu, S.K.; Lawrance, I.C. Anima model of IBD-associated CRC and colorectal cancer tumorigenesis. *Clin. Med. Insight* **2015**, *7*, 1–9.

24. De Robertis, M.; Massi, E.; Poeta, M.L.; Carotti, S.; Morini, S.; Cecchetelli, L.; Signori, E.; Fazio, V.M. The aom/dss murine model for the study of colon carcinogenesis: From pathways to diagnosis and therapy studies. *J. Carcinog.* **2011**, *10*, 9.

25. Pozza, A.; Scarpa, M.; Ruffolo, C.; Polese, L.; Erroi, F.; Bridda, A.; Norberto, L.; Frego, M. Colonic carcinogenesis in ibd: Molecular events. *Ann. Ital. Chir.* **2011**, *82*, 19–28.

26. Grivennikov, S.I.; Greten, F.R.; Karin, M. Immunity, inflammation, and cancer. *Cell* **2010**, *140*, 883–899. [CrossRef]

27. Pandurangan, A.K.; Saadatdoust, Z.; Esa, N.M.; Hamzah, H.; Ismail, A. Dietary cocoa protects against colitis-associated cancer by activating the nrf2/keap1 pathway. *Biofactors* **2015**, *41*, 1–14. [CrossRef]

28. Osburn, W.O.; Karim, B.; Dolan, P.M.; Liu, G.; Yamamoto, M.; Huso, D.L.; Kensler, T.W. Increased colonic inflammatory injury and formation of aberrant crypt foci in nrf2-deficient mice upon dextran sulfate treatment. *Int. J. Cancer* **2007**, *121*, 1883–1891. [CrossRef]

29. Barrett, C.W.; Ning, W.; Chen, X.; Smith, J.J.; Washington, M.K.; Hill, K.E.; Coburn, L.A.; Peek, R.M.; Chaturvedi, R.; Wilson, K.T.; et al. Tumor suppressor function of the plasma glutathione peroxidase gpx3 in colitis-associated carcinoma. *Cancer Res.* **2013**, *73*, 1245–1255. [CrossRef]

30. Kawanishi, S.; Hiraku, Y.; Pinlaor, S.; Ma, N. Oxidative and nitrative DNA damage in animals and patients with inflammatory diseases in relation to inflammation-related carcinogenesis. *Biol. Chem.* **2006**, *387*, 365–372. [CrossRef]

31. Sohn, J.J.; Schetter, A.J.; Yfantis, H.G.; Ridnour, L.A.; Horikawa, I.; Khan, M.A.; Robles, A.I.; Hussain, S.P.; Goto, A.; Bowman, E.D.; et al. Macrophages, nitric oxide and micrornas are associated with DNA damage response pathway and senescence in inflammatory bowel disease. *PLoS ONE* **2012**, *7*, e44156. [CrossRef]

32. Grasso, F.; Di Meo, S.; De Luca, G.; Pasquini, L.; Rossi, S.; Boirivant, M.; Biffoni, M.; Bignami, M.; Di Carlo, E. The mutyh base excision repair gene protects against inflammation-associated colorectal carcinogenesis. *Oncotarget* **2015**, *6*, 19671–19684. [CrossRef]

33. Yaeger, R.; Shah, M.A.; Miller, V.A.; Kelsen, J.R.; Wang, K.; Heins, Z.J.; Ross, J.S.; He, Y.; Sanford, E.; Yantiss, R.K.; et al. Genomic alterations observed in colitis-associated cancers are distinct from those found in sporadic colorectal cancers and vary by type of inflammatory bowel disease. *Gastroenterology* **2016**, *151*, 278–287. [CrossRef]

34. Boland, C.R.; Goel, A. Microsatellite instability in colorectal cancer. *Gastroenterology* **2010**, *138*, 2073–2087 e2073. [CrossRef]

35. van Dieren, J.M.; Wink, J.C.; Vissers, K.J.; van Marion, R.; Hoogmans, M.M.; Dinjens, W.N.; Schouten, W.R.; Tanke, H.J.; Szuhai, K.; Kuipers, E.J.; et al. Chromosomal and microsatellite instability of adenocarcinomas and dysplastic lesions (dalm) in ulcerative colitis. *Diagn. Mol. Pathol.* **2006**, *15*, 216–222. [CrossRef]

36. Willenbucher, R.F.; Aust, D.E.; Chang, C.G.; Zelman, S.J.; Ferrell, L.D.; Moore, D.H., 2nd; Waldman, F.M. Genomic instability is an early event during the progression pathway of ulcerative-colitis-related neoplasia. *Am. J. Pathol.* **1999**, *154*, 1825–1830. [CrossRef]

37. Tsai, J.H.; Rabinovitch, P.S.; Huang, D.; Small, T.; Mattis, A.N.; Kakar, S.; Choi, W.T. Association of aneuploidy and flat dysplasia with development of high-grade dysplasia or colorectal cancer in patients with inflammatory bowel disease. *Gastroenterology* **2017**, *153*, 1492–1495. [CrossRef]

38. Itzkowitz, S.H. Molecular biology of dysplasia and cancer in inflammatory bowel disease. *Gastroenterol. Clin. N. Am.* **2006**, *35*, 553–571. [CrossRef]

39. Hussain, S.P.; Amstad, P.; Raja, K.; Ambs, S.; Nagashima, M.; Bennett, W.P.; Shields, P.G.; Ham, A.J.;

Swenberg, J.A.; Marrogi, A.J.; et al. Increased p53 mutation load in noncancerous colon tissue from ulcerative colitis: A cancer-prone chronic inflammatory disease. *Cancer Res.* **2000**, *60*, 3333–3337.

40. Garrett, W.S.; Punit, S.; Gallini, C.A.; Michaud, M.; Zhang, D.; Sigrist, K.S.; Lord, G.M.; Glickman, J.N.; Glimcher, L.H. Colitis-associated colorectal cancer driven by t-bet deficiency in dendritic cells. *Cancer Cell* **2009**, *16*, 208–219. [CrossRef]

41. Neufert, C.; Becker, C.; Tureci, O.; Waldner, M.J.; Backert, I.; Floh, K.; Atreya, I.; Leppkes, M.; Jefremow, A.; Vieth, M.; et al. Tumor fibroblast-derived epiregulin promotes growth of colitis-associated neoplasms through erk. *J. Clin. Investig.* **2013**, *123*, 1428–1443. [CrossRef]

42. Neurath, M.F. Cytokines in inflammatory bowel disease. *Nat. Rev. Immunol.* **2014**, *14*, 329–342. [CrossRef]

43. Wang, Y.; Wang, K.; Han, G.C.; Wang, R.X.; Xiao, H.; Hou, C.M.; Guo, R.F.; Dou, Y.; Shen, B.F.; Li, Y.; et al. Neutrophil infiltration favors colitis-associated tumorigenesis by activating the interleukin-1 (il-1)/il-6 axis. *Mucosal. Immunol.* **2014**, *7*, 1106–1115. [CrossRef]

44. Francescone, R.; Hou, V.; Grivennikov, S.I. Cytokines, ibd, and colitis-associated cancer. *Inflamm. Bowel. Dis.* **2015**, *21*, 409–418. [CrossRef]

45. Popivanova, B.K.; Kitamura, K.; Wu, Y.; Kondo, T.; Kagaya, T.; Kaneko, S.; Oshima, M.; Fujii, C.; Mukaida, N. Blocking tnf-alpha in mice reduces colorectal carcinogenesis associated with chronic colitis. *J. Clin. Investig.* **2008**, *118*, 560–570.

46. Grivennikov, S.; Karin, E.; Terzic, J.; Mucida, D.; Yu, G.Y.; Vallabhapurapu, S.; Scheller, J.; Rose-John, S.; Cheroutre, H.; Eckmann, L.; et al. Il-6 and stat3 are required for survival of intestinal epithelial cells and development of colitis-associated cancer. *Cancer Cell* **2009**, *15*, 103–113. [CrossRef]

47. Matsumoto, S.; Hara, T.; Mitsuyama, K.; Yamamoto, M.; Tsuruta, O.; Sata, M.; Scheller, J.; Rose-John, S.; Kado, S.; Takada, T. Essential roles of il-6 trans-signaling in colonic epithelial cells, induced by the il-6/soluble-il-6 receptor derived from lamina propria macrophages, on the development of colitis-associated premalignant cancer in a murine model. *J. Immunol.* **2010**, *184*, 1543–1551. [CrossRef]

48. McGovern, D.P.; Rotter, J.I.; Mei, L.; Haritunians, T.; Landers, C.; Derkowski, C.; Dutridge, D.; Dubinsky, M.; Ippoliti, A.; Vasiliauskas, E.; et al. Genetic epistasis of il23/il17 pathway genes in crohn's disease. *Inflamm. Bowel. Dis.* **2009**, *15*, 883–889. [CrossRef]

49. Zenewicz, L.A.; Antov, A.; Flavell, R.A. Cd4 t-cell differentiation and inflammatory bowel disease. *Trends Mol. Med.* **2009**, *15*, 199–207. [CrossRef]

50. Ni, J.; Wu, G.D.; Albenberg, L.; Tomov, V.T. Gut microbiota and IBD: Causation or correlation? *Nat. Rev. Gastroenterol. Hepatol.* **2017**, *14*, 573–584. [CrossRef]

51. Zhou, M.; He, J.; Shen, Y.; Zhang, C.; Wang, J.; Chen, Y. New Frontiers in Genetics, Gut Microbiota, and Immunity: A Rosetta Stone for the Pathogenesis of Inflammatory Bowel Disease. *Biomed. Res. Int.* **2017**, *2017*, 8201672. [CrossRef]

52. Velayos, F.S.; Terdiman, J.P.; Walsh, J.M. Effect of 5-aminosalicylate use on colorectal cancer and dysplasia risk: A systematic review and metaanalysis of observational studies. *Am. J. Gastroenterol.* **2005**, *100*, 1345–1353. [CrossRef]

53. Nishida, A.; Inoue, R.; Inatomi, O.; Bamba, S.; Naito, Y.; Andoh, A. Gut microbiota in the pathogenesis of inflammatory bowel disease. *Clin. J. Gastroenterol.* **2018**, *11*, 1–10. [CrossRef]

54. Santino, A.; Scarano, A.; De Santis, S.; De Benedictis, M.; Giovinazzo, G.; Chieppa, M. Gut Microbiota Modulation and Anti-Inflammatory Properties of Dietary Polyphenolsin IBD: New and Consolidated Perspectives. *Curr. Pharm. Des.* **2017**, *23*, 2344–2351. [CrossRef]

55. Duricova, D.; Burisch, J.; Jess, T.; Gower-Rousseau, C.; Lakatos, P.L.; ECCO-EpiCom. Age-related differences in presentation and course of inflammatory bowel disease: An update on the population-based literature. *J. Crohns Colitis* **2014**, *8*, 1351–1361. [CrossRef]

56. Cho, H.; Jung, H.; Lee, H.; Yi, H.C.; Kwak, H.K.; Hwang, K.T. Chemopreventive activity of ellagitannins and their derivatives from black raspberry seeds on ht-29 colon cancer cells. *Food Funct.* **2015**, *6*, 1675–1683. [CrossRef]

57. Seeram, N.P.; Adams, L.S.; Zhang, Y.; Lee, R.; Sand, D.; Scheuller, H.S.; Heber, D. Blackberry, black raspberry, blueberry, cranberry, red raspberry, and strawberry extracts inhibit growth and stimulate apoptosis of human cancer cells in vitro. *J. Agric. Food Chem.* **2006**, *54*, 9329–9339. [CrossRef]

58. Montrose, D.C.; Horelik, N.A.; Madigan, J.P.; Stoner, G.D.; Wang, L.S.; Bruno, R.S.; Park, H.J.; Giardina, C.; Rosenberg, D.W. Anti-inflammatory effects of freeze-dried black raspberry powder in ulcerative colitis. *Carcinogenesis* **2011**, *32*, 343–350. [CrossRef]

59. Wang, L.S.; Kuo, C.T.; Stoner, K.; Yearsley, M.; Oshima, K.; Yu, J.; Huang, T.H.; Rosenberg, D.; Peiffer, D.; Stoner, G.; et al. Dietary black raspberries modulate DNA methylation in dextran sodium sulfate (dss)-induced ulcerative colitis. *Carcinogenesis* **2013**, *34*, 2842–2850. [CrossRef]

60. Wang, L.S.; Kuo, C.T.; Huang, T.H.; Yearsley, M.; Oshima, K.; Stoner, G.D.; Yu, J.; Lechner, J.F.; Huang, Y.W. Black raspberries protectively regulate methylation of wnt pathway genes in precancerous colon tissue. *Cancer Prev. Res.* **2013**, *6*, 1317–1327. [CrossRef]

61. Huang, C.; Huang, Y.; Li, J.; Hu, W.; Aziz, R.; Tang, M.S.; Sun, N.; Cassady, J.; Stoner, G.D. Inhibition of benzo(a)pyrene diol-epoxide-induced transactivation of activated protein 1 and nuclear factor kappab by black raspberry extracts. *Cancer Res.* **2002**, *62*, 6857–6863.

62. Lu, H.; Li, J.; Zhang, D.; Stoner, G.D.; Huang, C. Molecular mechanisms involved in chemoprevention of black raspberry extracts: From transcription factors to their target genes. *Nutr. Cancer* **2006**, *54*, 69–78. [CrossRef]

63. Harris, G.K.; Gupta, A.; Nines, R.G.; Kresty, L.A.; Habib, S.G.; Frankel, W.L.; LaPerle, K.; Gallaher, D.D.; Schwartz, S.J.; Stoner, G.D. Effects of lyophilized black raspberries on azoxymethane-induced colon cancer and 8-hydroxy-2'-deoxyguanosine levels in the fischer 344 rat. *Nutr. Cancer* **2001**, *40*, 125–133. [CrossRef]

64. Bi, X.; Fang, W.; Wang, L.S.; Stoner, G.D.; Yang, W. Black raspberries inhibit intestinal tumorigenesis in apc1638+/− and muc2−/− mouse models of colorectal cancer. *Cancer Prev. Res.* **2010**, *3*, 1443–1450. [CrossRef]

65. Wang, L.S.; Arnold, M.; Huang, Y.W.; Sardo, C.; Seguin, C.; Martin, E.; Huang, T.H.; Riedl, K.; Schwartz, S.; Frankel, W.; et al. Modulation of genetic and epigenetic biomarkers of colorectal cancer in humans by black raspberries: A phase i pilot study. *Clin. Cancer Res.* **2011**, *17*, 598–610. [CrossRef]

66. Wang, L.S.; Kuo, C.T.; Cho, S.J.; Seguin, C.; Siddiqui, J.; Stoner, K.; Weng, Y.I.; Huang, T.H.; Tichelaar, J.; Yearsley, M.; et al. Black raspberry-derived anthocyanins demethylate tumor suppressor genes through the inhibition of dnmt1 and dnmt3b in colon cancer cells. *Nutr. Cancer* **2013**, *65*, 118–125. [CrossRef]

67. Wu, Q.K.; Koponen, J.M.; Mykkanen, H.M.; Torronen, A.R. Berry phenolic extracts modulate the expression of p21(waf1) and bax but not bcl-2 in ht-29 colon cancer cells. *J. Agric. Food Chem.* **2007**, *55*, 1156–1163. [CrossRef]

68. McDougall, G.J.; Ross, H.A.; Ikeji, M.; Stewart, D. Berry extracts exert different antiproliferative effects against cervical and colon cancer cells grown in vitro. *J. Agric. Food Chem.* **2008**, *56*, 3016–3023. [CrossRef]

69. Zhang, Y.; Seeram, N.P.; Lee, R.; Feng, L.; Heber, D. Isolation and identification of strawberry phenolics with antioxidant and human cancer cell antiproliferative properties. *J. Agric. Food Chem.* **2008**, *56*, 670–675. [CrossRef]

70. Kanodia, L.; Borgohain, M.; Das, S. Effect of fruit extract of Fragaria vesca L. on experimentally induced inflammatory bowel disease in albino rats. *Indian J. Pharm.* **2011**, *43*, 18–21. [CrossRef]

71. Mentor-Marcel, R.A.; Bobe, G.; Sardo, C.; Wang, L.S.; Kuo, C.T.; Stoner, G.; Colburn, N.H. Plasma cytokines as potential response indicators to dietary freeze-dried black raspberries in colorectal cancer patients. *Nutr. Cancer* **2012**, *64*, 820–825. [CrossRef]

72. Duthie, S.J.; Gardner, P.T.; Morrice, P.C.; Wood, S.G.; Pirie, L.; Bestwick, C.C.; Milne, L.; Duthie, G.G. DNA stability and lipid peroxidation in vitamin e-deficient rats in vivo and colon cells in vitro–modulation by the dietary anthocyanin, cyanidin-3-glycoside. *Eur. J. Nutr.* **2005**, *44*, 195–203. [CrossRef]

73. Elisia, I.; Kitts, D.D. Anthocyanins inhibit peroxyl radical-induced apoptosis in caco-2 cells. *Mol. Cell. Biochem.* **2008**, *312*, 139–145. [CrossRef]

74. Renis, M.; Calandra, L.; Scifo, C.; Tomasello, B.; Cardile, V.; Vanella, L.; Bei, R.; La Fauci, L.; Galvano, F. Response of cell cycle/stress-related protein expression and DNA damage upon treatment of $CaCO_2$ cells with anthocyanins. *Br. J. Nutr.* **2008**, *100*, 27–35. [CrossRef]

75. Hudson, E.A.; Dinh, P.A.; Kokubun, T.; Simmonds, M.S.; Gescher, A. Characterization of potentially chemopreventive phenols in extracts of brown rice that inhibit the growth of human breast and colon cancer cells. *Cancer Epidemiol. Biomark. Prev.* **2000**, *9*, 1163–1170.

76. Bornsek, S.M.; Ziberna, L.; Polak, T.; Vanzo, A.; Ulrih, N.P.; Abram, V.; Tramer, F.; Passamonti, S. Bilberry and blueberry anthocyanins act as powerful intracellular antioxidants in mammalian cells. *Food Chem.* **2012**, *134*, 1878–1884. [CrossRef]

77. Katsube, N.; Iwashita, K.; Tsushida, T.; Yamaki, K.; Kobori, M. Induction of apoptosis in cancer cells by bilberry (vaccinium myrtillus) and the anthocyanins. *J. Agric. Food Chem.* **2003**, *51*, 68–75. [CrossRef]

78. Lala, G.; Malik, M.; Zhao, C.; He, J.; Kwon, Y.; Giusti, M.M.; Magnuson, B.A. Anthocyanin-rich extracts inhibit multiple biomarkers of colon cancer in rats. *Nutr. Cancer* **2006**, *54*, 84–93. [CrossRef]

79. Kangawa, Y.; Yoshida, T.; Maruyama, K.; Okamoto, M.; Kihara, T.; Nakamura, M.; Ochiai, M.; Hippo, Y.; Hayashi, S.M.; Shibutani, M. Cilostazol and enzymatically modified isoquercitrin attenuate experimental colitis and colon cancer in mice by inhibiting cell proliferation and inflammation. *Food Chem. Toxicol.* **2017**, *100*, 103–114. [CrossRef]

80. Charepalli, V.; Reddivari, L.; Radhakrishnan, S.; Vadde, R.; Agarwal, R.; Vanamala, J.K. Anthocyanin-containing purple-fleshed potatoes suppress colon tumorigenesis via elimination of colon cancer stem cells. *J. Nutr. Biochem.* **2015**, *26*, 1641–1649. [CrossRef]

81. Urias-Lugo, D.A.; Heredia, J.B.; Muy-Rangel, M.D.; Valdez-Torres, J.B.; Serna-Saldivar, S.O.; Gutierrez-Uribe, J.A. Anthocyanins and phenolic acids of hybrid and native blue maize (Zea mays L.) extracts and their antiproliferative activity in mammary (MCF7), liver (HepG2), colon (Caco2 and HT29) and prostate (PC3) cancer cells. *Plant Foods Hum. Nutr.* **2015**, *70*, 193–199. [CrossRef] [PubMed]

82. Jing, P.; Qian, B.; Zhao, S.; Qi, X.; Ye, L.; Monica Giusti, M.; Wang, X. Effect of glycosylation patterns of chinese eggplant anthocyanins and other derivatives on antioxidant effectiveness in human colon cell lines. *Food Chem.* **2015**, *172*, 183–189. [CrossRef] [PubMed]

83. Lim, S.; Xu, J.; Kim, J.; Chen, T.Y.; Su, X.; Standard, J.; Carey, E.; Griffin, J.; Herndon, B.; Katz, B.; et al. Role of anthocyanin-enriched purple-fleshed sweet potato p40 in colorectal cancer prevention. *Mol. Nutr. Food Res.* **2013**, *57*, 1908–1917. [CrossRef] [PubMed]

84. Yun, J.W.; Lee, W.S.; Kim, M.J.; Lu, J.N.; Kang, M.H.; Kim, H.G.; Kim, D.C.; Choi, E.J.; Choi, J.Y.; Lee, Y.K.; et al. Characterization of a profile of the anthocyanins isolated from vitis coignetiae pulliat and their anti-invasive activity on ht-29 human colon cancer cells. *Food Chem. Toxicol.* **2010**, *48*, 903–909. [CrossRef]

85. Dai, J.; Patel, J.D.; Mumper, R.J. Characterization of blackberry extract and its antiproliferative and anti-inflammatory properties. *J. Med. Food* **2007**, *10*, 258–265. [CrossRef]

86. Yi, W.; Fischer, J.; Krewer, G.; Akoh, C.C. Phenolic compounds from blueberries can inhibit colon cancer cell proliferation and induce apoptosis. *J. Agric. Food Chem.* **2005**, *53*, 7320–7329. [CrossRef]

87. Kang, S.Y.; Seeram, N.P.; Nair, M.G.; Bourquin, L.D. Tart cherry anthocyanins inhibit tumor development in apc(min) mice and reduce proliferation of human colon cancer cells. *Cancer Lett.* **2003**, *194*, 13–19. [CrossRef]

88. Kawamori, T.; Tanaka, T.; Kojima, T.; Suzui, M.; Ohnishi, M.; Mori, H. Suppression of azoxymethane-induced rat colon aberrant crypt foci by dietary protocatechuic acid. *Jpn. J. Cancer Res.* **1994**, *85*, 686–691. [CrossRef]

89. Tanaka, T.; Kojima, T.; Suzui, M.; Mori, H. Chemoprevention of colon carcinogenesis by the natural product of a simple phenolic compound protocatechuic acid: Suppressing effects on tumor development and biomarkers expression of colon tumorigenesis. *Cancer Res.* **1993**, *53*, 3908–3913.

90. Farombi, E.O.; Adedara, I.A.; Awoyemi, O.V.; Njoku, C.R.; Micah, G.O.; Esogwa, C.U.; Owumi, S.E.; Olopade, J.O. Dietary protocatechuic acid ameliorates dextran sulphate sodium-induced ulcerative colitis and hepatotoxicity in rats. *Food Funct.* **2016**, *7*, 913–921. [CrossRef]

91. Venancio, V.P.; Cipriano, P.A.; Kim, H.; Antunes, L.M.; Talcott, S.T.; Mertens-Talcott, S.U. Cocoplum (chrysobalanus icaco l.) anthocyanins exert anti-inflammatory activity in human colon cancer and non-malignant colon cells. *Food Funct.* **2017**, *8*, 307–314. [CrossRef]

92. Charepalli, V.; Reddivari, L.; Vadde, R.; Walia, S.; Radhakrishnan, S.; Vanamala, J.K. Eugenia jambolana (java plum) fruit extract exhibits anti-cancer activity against early stage human hct-116 colon cancer cells and colon cancer stem cells. *Cancers (Basel)* **2016**, *8*, 29. [CrossRef] [PubMed]

93. Scarano, A.; Butelli, E.; De Santis, S.; Cavalcanti, E.; Hill, L.; De Angelis, M.; Giovinazzo, G.; Chieppa, M.; Martin, C.; Santino, A. Combined Dietary Anthocyanins, Flavonols, and Stilbenoids Alleviate Inflammatory Bowel Disease Symptoms in Mice. *Front. Nutr.* **2018**, *4*, 75. [CrossRef] [PubMed]

94. Pojer, E.; Mattivi, F.; Johnson, D.; Stockley, C.S. The case for anthocyanin consumption to promote human health. *Compr. Rev. Food Sci. Food Saf.* **2013**, *12*, 24.

95. Knobloch, T.J.; Uhrig, L.K.; Pearl, D.K.; Casto, B.C.; Warner, B.M.; Clinton, S.K.; Sardo-Molmenti, C.L.; Ferguson, J.M.; Daly, B.T.; Riedl, K.; et al. Suppression of proinflammatory and prosurvival biomarkers in oral cancer patients consuming a black raspberry phytochemical-rich troche. *Cancer Prev. Res.* **2016**, *9*, 159–171. [CrossRef]

96. Teoh, W.Y.; Tan, H.P.; Ling, S.K.; Abdul Wahab, N.; Sim, K.S. Phytochemical investigation of gynura bicolor leaves and cytotoxicity evaluation of the chemical constituents against hct 116 cells. *Nat. Prod. Res.* **2016**, *30*, 448–451. [CrossRef] [PubMed]

97. Femia, A.P.; Caderni, G.; Buzzigoli, C.; Cocca, E.; Salvadori, M.; Dolara, P. Effect of simple phenolic compounds on azoxymethane-induced aberrant crypt foci in rat colon. *Nutr. Cancer* **2001**, *41*, 107–110.

98. Mace, T.A.; King, S.A.; Ameen, Z.; Elnaggar, O.; Young, G.; Riedl, K.M.; Schwartz, S.J.; Clinton, S.K.; Knobloch, T.J.; Weghorst, C.M.; et al. Bioactive compounds or metabolites from black raspberries modulate t lymphocyte proliferation, myeloid cell differentiation and jak/stat signaling. *Cancer Immunol. Immunother.* **2014**, *63*, 889–900. [CrossRef] [PubMed]

99. Jo, Y.H.; Park, H.C.; Choi, S.; Kim, S.; Bao, C.; Kim, H.W.; Choi, H.K.; Lee, H.J.; Auh, J.H. Metabolomic analysis reveals cyanidins in black raspberry as candidates for suppression of lipopolysaccharide-induced inflammation in murine macrophages. *J. Agric. Food Chem.* **2015**, *63*, 5449–5458. [CrossRef]

100. Wang, L.S.; Hecht, S.; Carmella, S.; Seguin, C.; Rocha, C.; Yu, N.; Stoner, K.; Chiu, S.; Stoner, G. Berry ellagitannins may not be sufficient for prevention of tumors in the rodent esophagus. *J. Agric. Food Chem.* **2010**, *58*, 3992–3995. [CrossRef] [PubMed]

101. Paudel, L.; Wyzgoski, F.J.; Giusti, M.M.; Johnson, J.L.; Rinaldi, P.L.; Scheerens, J.C.; Chanon, A.M.; Bomser, J.A.; Miller, A.R.; Hardy, J.K.; et al. Nmr-based metabolomic investigation of bioactivity of chemical constituents in black raspberry (rubus occidentalis l.) fruit extracts. *J. Agric. Food Chem.* **2014**, *62*, 1989–1998. [CrossRef]

102. Farzaei, M.H.; El-Senduny, F.F.; Momtaz, S.; Parvizi, F.; Iranpanah, A.; Tewari, D.; Naseri, R.; Abdolghaffari, A.H.; Rezaei, N. An update on dietary consideration in inflammatory bowel disease: Anthocyanins and more. *Expert Rev. Gastroenterol. Hepatol.* **2018**, *10*, 1007–1024. [CrossRef] [PubMed]

103. Sodagari, H.R.; Farzaei, M.H.; Bahramsoltani, R.; Abdolghaffari, A.H.; Mahmoudi, M.; Rezaei, N. Dietary anthocyanins as a complementary medicinal approach for management of inflammatory bowel disease. *Expert Rev. Gastroenterol. Hepatol.* **2015**, *9*, 807–820. [CrossRef] [PubMed]

104. Wang, L.S.; Burke, C.A.; Hasson, H.; Kuo, C.T.; Molmenti, C.L.; Seguin, C.; Liu, P.; Huang, T.H.; Frankel, W.L.; Stoner, G.D. A phase ib study of the effects of black raspberries on rectal polyps in patients with familial adenomatous polyposis. *Cancer Prev. Res.* **2014**, *7*, 666–674. [CrossRef] [PubMed]

105. Wang, L.S.; Hecht, S.S.; Carmella, S.G.; Yu, N.; Larue, B.; Henry, C.; McIntyre, C.; Rocha, C.; Lechner, J.F.; Stoner, G.D. Anthocyanins in black raspberries prevent esophageal tumors in rats. *Cancer Prev. Res.* **2009**, *2*, 84–93. [CrossRef]

106. Peiffer, D.S.; Wang, L.S.; Zimmerman, N.P.; Ransom, B.W.; Carmella, S.G.; Kuo, C.T.; Chen, J.H.; Oshima, K.; Huang, Y.W.; Hecht, S.S.; et al. Dietary consumption of black raspberries or their anthocyanin constituents alters innate immune cell trafficking in esophageal cancer. *Cancer Immunol. Res.* **2016**, *4*, 72–82. [CrossRef]

107. Peiffer, D.S.; Zimmerman, N.P.; Wang, L.S.; Ransom, B.W.; Carmella, S.G.; Kuo, C.T.; Siddiqui, J.; Chen, J.H.; Oshima, K.; Huang, Y.W.; et al. Chemoprevention of esophageal cancer with black raspberries, their component anthocyanins, and a major anthocyanin metabolite, protocatechuic acid. *Cancer Prev. Res.* **2014**, *7*, 574–584. [CrossRef]

108. Chen, T.; Rose, M.E.; Hwang, H.; Nines, R.G.; Stoner, G.D. Black raspberries inhibit n-nitrosomethylbenzylamine (nmba)-induced angiogenesis in rat esophagus parallel to the suppression of cox-2 and inos. *Carcinogenesis* **2006**, *27*, 2301–2307. [CrossRef]

A Personalised Dietary Approach—A Way Forward to Manage Nutrient Deficiency, Effects of the Western Diet and Food Intolerances in Inflammatory Bowel Disease

Bobbi B Laing [1,2], Anecita Gigi Lim [1] and Lynnette R Ferguson [1,*]

[1]   Faculty of Medical and Health Sciences, University of Auckland, Auckland 1023, New Zealand
[2]   Nutrition Society of New Zealand, Palmerston North 4444, New Zealand
*   Correspondence: l.ferguson@auckland.ac.nz

Abstract: This review discusses the personalised dietary approach with respect to inflammatory bowel disease (IBD). It identifies gene–nutrient interactions associated with the nutritional deficiencies that people with IBD commonly experience, and the role of the Western diet in influencing these. It also discusses food intolerances and how particular genotypes can affect these. It is well established that with respect to food there is no "one size fits all" diet for those with IBD. Gene–nutrient interactions may help explain this variability in response to food that is associated with IBD. Nutrigenomic research, which examines the effects of food and its constituents on gene expression, shows that—like a number of pharmaceutical products—food can have beneficial effects or have adverse (side) effects depending on a person's genotype. Pharmacogenetic research is identifying gene variants with adverse reactions to drugs, and this is modifying clinical practice and allowing individualised treatment. Nutrigenomic research could enable individualised treatment in persons with IBD and enable more accurate tailoring of food intake, to avoid exacerbating malnutrition and to counter some of the adverse effects of the Western diet. It may also help to establish the dietary pattern that is most protective against IBD.

Keywords: inflammatory bowel disease; Westernisation; genotypes; nutrient deficiency; food intolerance; FODMAPs; gluten; fructose; lactose; brassica; mushrooms

1. Introduction

The personalised dietary approach in combination with the knowledge of the genotype and genetic variants of an individual who has nutrient deficiencies, follows the Western diet, or may have food intolerances may be helpful for people who have inflammatory bowel disease (IBD). Gene–nutrient interactions could help explain the variability in response to food that is associated with IBD, and using this knowledge with a personalised dietary approach may offer a way forward. Identification of individuals' genotypes is a first step to building up data sets which combine this information with data on individuals and their gut microbiome, dietary patterns, exercise routines, blood parameters and anthropometric measurements. This information can be used to build machine-learning algorithms to predict what foods/meals reduce inflammation and abdominal symptoms and maintain a healthy gut flora. Zeevi et al. have pioneered this approach in their work with diabetes [1]. They used this combination of information to successfully predict which foods/meals lowered postprandial blood glucose. Identifying genotypes associated with nutrient deficiencies or low nutrient absorption, the negative effects of the Western diet and the tolerance or intolerance of particular foods may also advise people on how to eat a greater variety of food. A wider range of food available to the gut microbiota enables their greater diversity, and this is associated with a healthy gut [2].

Pharmacogenetic research (the study of the variability in drug response due to genotype) is identifying gene variants with adverse reactions to drugs, and this is modifying clinical practice and allowing individualised treatment. The aim is to provide the right drug, at the right dose, at the right time, to the right patient [3]. Individual responses can be dependent on an individual's genotype. Genetic variants can alter the metabolism of drugs as well as responsiveness, and this may necessitate changes to standardised drug regimes. The standard dose may not maintain the required therapeutic level if individuals metabolise the drug more quickly; conversely, if they are slow metabolisers the standard dose maybe toxic. Knowledge of pharmacogenetics and its application to precision medicine to enhance treatment responses and minimize drug-related adverse events is one approach that has been suggested as the way forward for IBD [4]. Pharmacogenetics information facilitates the identification of responders and non-responders to drugs and guides the decision about optimal treatment [5]. Similarly, further nutrigenomic research could identify nutrient–gene interactions in people with IBD. This would enable the more accurate tailoring of food intake and could suggest dietary patterns which avoid exacerbating malnutrition, curtail the adverse effects of the Western diet and explain intolerance to particular foods. This could lead to the minimization of abdominal symptoms and disease activity in those who experience IBD.

In an extensive study of 366,351 European individuals in 2016 aiming to identify dietary patterns and risk of IBD, no dietary pattern was identified with the risk of either of the two main expressions of IBD (i.e., ulcerative colitis (UC) or Crohn's disease (CD)) [6]. However, when cases occurring within the first two years after dietary assessment were excluded, there was a positive association between a "high sugar and soft drinks" pattern and UC risk if they also had a low vegetable intake [6]. This study shows there are many challenges in determining the best dietary pattern for individuals with a particular chronic disease like IBD, given the genetic differences between people and their environments [7]. The current consensus is that no single nutrition recommendation can be made to modify this situation with respect to IBD—that is, there is no "one size fits all" solution for people with IBD [8]. However, using the personalised dietary approach combined with information on people's genotypes may offer a way to resolve this conundrum.

The aim of this narrative review (based on searching two data bases, PubMed and Google Scholar) is to discuss the personalised dietary approach with respect to IBD. First it will identify nutritional deficiencies which individuals with IBD commonly experience, and give an example of a key nutrient whose absorption is affected by genotype. Secondly it will review the role of the Western diet in contributing to nutrient deficiencies and IBD, and give examples of some of the genes involved. Thirdly it will review the various food intolerances and food avoidances associated with IBD which may also contribute to nutrient deficiencies, and how particular genotypes can contribute to these.

2. Nutrient Deficiencies Associated with IBD

2.1. Nutritional Status of People with Inflammatory Bowel Disease

Three studies which have assessed the nutritional status of people with IBD are illustrated in Table 1. Assessment of people with IBD often shows they are under weight, with specific vitamin and mineral imbalances, and this contributes to their ill health [9–14]. The three studies in this table illustrate the common nutritional findings. Vagianos and colleagues collected dietary information by questionnaires (including dietary supplements) and observed multiple and clinically significant vitamin and mineral deficiencies in adults with CD who attended a gastroenterology outpatient clinic [9]. Inadequate reported intake was defined as <66% of the dietary reference intake (RFI) for each micronutrient. These authors reported that when comparisons were made by disease type or disease activity, there were no significant differences in the percentage of subjects consuming inadequate amounts of micronutrients. Stein and Bott (2008) reported on nutrient deficiencies in hospitalised adults with CD [10]. Hartman et al. in 2016 [15] investigated the nutritional status of children and adolescents who were ambulatory outpatients at a gastroenterology clinic. They reported on the percentage median nutrient intake compared with the required daily allowance (RDA) and dietary intake of healthy children. The intake was considered low if it was less than 80% of the RDA. During this study, two thirds of participants had active disease. However, there was no significant difference in nutrient intake between those with active disease and those in remission, and no association of nutrient levels with disease activity.

Table 1. Nutrient deficiencies in adults and adolescents with inflammatory bowel disease (IBD).

Reference	Vagianos et al. [9]	Stein and Bott [10]	Hartman et al. [15]
	Outpatient	Inpatient	Outpatient
Year of Investigation	2007	2008	2016
Number of Participants	71	na	68
Gender (Male, Female)	32, 52	na	na
Age (years)	37.6 ± 14.3	Adult	13.9 ± 3.2
Country	Canada	Germany	Israel
Dietary Measurement	FFQ, 4-day records, Anthropometric	na	3-day records, Anthropometric
Laboratory Measurement	Biomarkers for nutrients (CD)	na	Biomarkers for nutrients
Dietary Deficiency			
Measures	% <66% RFI	% Inadequate Intake	% <80% of RDA
Vitamin B6	4.2	na	10
Vitamin B12	5.6	48	12
Folate	20	56–62	34
Vitamin C	9.9	na	31
Vitamin A	30	11–50	57
Vitamin D	38	23–75	25
Vitamin E	59	na	65
Calcium	25	13	79
Iron	14	25–50	22
Magnesium	na	14–33	69
Zinc	8.5	40	28

CD: Crohn's disease; FFQ: food frequency questionnaire; na: not available; RFI: dietary reference intake; RDA: required daily allowance.

All three studies showed low levels of vitamin A and D and folate in people with CD. Stein and Bott [10] and Hartman et al. [15] both found substantial risk for deficiencies of magnesium, zinc and iron (Table 1). Stein and Bott [10] also showed lower B_{12} concentrations for inpatients and Vagianos et al. commented that in those with CD (compared to those with UC, the other main expression of IBD) had lower B_{12} concentrations with their serum biomarkers. Also, among men with CD there was a significantly higher proportion who had haemoglobin below the normal range compared to men with UC. Hartman et al. reported that anaemia was the most common sign of nutrient deficiency in their adolescents (51%). These studies illustrate that people with different expressions of IBD (i.e., CD or UC) have different nutrient needs. It also illustrates that it is important to assess nutritional status (through laboratory measurement of nutrient biomarkers) to avoid exacerbating malnutrition if particular foods are removed from the diet.

For people with CD in particular, malnutrition may also occur because of the severity of oral lesions experienced, which results in difficulties with tasting, chewing and swallowing. This means that some foods are avoided (e.g., tomatoes because of their perceived acidity). Oral involvement in CD has been identified in 8%–29% of people, irrespective of disease activity [16]. Examples of oral symptoms include labial swelling (which also may include gingiva and mucosa), mucosal polyps, cracking at the edges of the lips (angular cheilitis), ulcers, fissures and granulomas [17,18]. The mucous membranes in the mouth normally have a rapid cell turnover of 3–7 days, in contrast to the skin which is up to 28 days [19]. Loss of cells without replacement can lead to the mouth showing early signs of systemic disease and early predisposition to nutritional deficiency. This is another reason why optimal nutrition is important for people with IBD.

Many vitamins and minerals are considered necessary for healthy mucous membranes (Table 2) [20]. A number of these essential nutrients are low in people with people with IBD (Table 1 [9,10,15]). These nutrient deficiencies, and a higher presence of bacteria associated with dental caries, undoubtedly contribute to the oral symptoms experienced by people with CD. Sufficient levels of these nutrients would need to be included in any food regime suggested for IBD.

Table 2. Nutrients associated with healthy mucous membranes [20].

Water Soluble Vitamins	Fat-Soluble Vitamins	Minerals
Vitamin B_2 (riboflavin)	A	Calcium
Vitamin B_3 (niacin)	D	Fluoride
Vitamin B_6 family	E	Zinc
Vitamin B_{12} (cobalamin)		Iron
Folic acid (folate)		
Vitamin C (ascorbic acid)		

2.2. Nutrient Absorption Impacted by Genotype

One example of a nutrient whose absorption can be impacted by genotype is beta-carotene. The gene that affects its absorption is the beta-carotene 15,15′-monooxygenase gene (*BCMO1*). This gene encodes a protein which is an important enzyme in the metabolism of the nutrient beta-carotene to vitamin A [21]. It is expressed in a number of tissues (e.g., liver, lungs, skin, small intestine). Within the enterocytes of the mucous membranes, the enzyme cleaves beta-carotene into two retinal molecules. These are packaged with other dietary lipids into chylomicrons and then secreted into the lymphatic system. Fat in the diet enables optimal chylomicron formation [21,22]. According to the study by Leung et al., carrying one of the two polymorphisms (R267S: rs12934922 or A379V: rs7501331) of the *BCMO1* gene impedes the conversion of beta-carotene to retinol [23]. This study was based on a healthy population from the UK. Up to 45% of people in this study carried one of these two polymorphisms. Having one of the two polymorphisms of the *BCMO1* gene in conjunction with IBD could thus have an impact on the health status of the carrier. New Zealand (NZ) is a country with a high incidence of IBD (26/100,000 in 2016) [24], and in their most recent National Nutrition Survey (2008/9) reported that the NZ population sourced 58% of their vitamin A intake from carotenoids. The NZ population as a whole was also recorded as 22.7% and 12.1% deficient in vitamin A for males and females, respectively. For those aged 15-18 years, these percentages increased to 27.4% and 37.5% [25].

Adequate vitamin A intake is necessary for optimal activity of the innate and adaptive immune systems. Vitamin A is needed for the appropriate innate immune defence response. It affects neutrophil reactions to microbes, macrophage phagocytosis, and natural killer cell activity. Cultured human macrophages enriched with retinoic acid have been shown to have increased resistance to *M. tuberculosis* by down-regulating tryptophan–aspartate-containing coat protein (TACO) [26]. Vitamin A is also needed for the optimal formation of T and B cells in the adaptive immune system and the balanced type 1 and type 2 cytokine responses. Impairment of these functions through vitamin A deficiency leads to epithelial barrier dysfunction and inflammation—hallmarks of IBD [27]. Vitamin A deficiency in children increases the risk of signs and symptoms often associated with CD (i.e., impairment of iron use that aggravates anaemia, respiratory infections and diminished growth rates) [28]. If individuals with IBD also carry one of these at-risk alleles, they are at risk of being vitamin A deficient.

This may be a contributing factor to this nutrient deficiency reported in people with IBD. Using the personalised dietary approach and identifying if a person with IBD carries these variants linked to poor absorption of vitamin A would enable the tailoring of nutrient advice to ameliorate this. The Western diet may also contribute to nutrient deficiencies.

3. The Western Diet

The incidence of gastro-intestinal disorders like CD and UC has been increasing [29–32]. This has often been related to the current Western diet, which has changed substantially in the past seven decades [33–39]. This is because of changes in food production and technology, which provides easy access of urban based populations to cheap ultra-processed foods and foods high in refined grains, oil and sugar [40]. In Bangladesh, for example, the incidence of diagnosed IBD is very low. However, when Bangladeshis move to the United Kingdom where they are more highly exposed to Western culture and food choices, the incidence of IBD increases substantially within a generation [41]. This may also be associated with autoimmune disease developing as a result of increasing latitude, decreased exposure to sunlight and lower vitamin D intake [42]. They may also receive better health care which identifies their disease pathology more accurately. However, modern Western food is also becoming more available in the developing world. In the review of the global epidemiology of IBD by M'Koma, it was noted that there has been an increase in the incidence and prevalence of IBD in parts of Asia and Africa—particularly in urban areas and in higher socio-economic classes [43]. This Westernisation of the diet has resulted in lower intakes of dietary fibre, increased consumption of saturated fatty acids, and sugar. Westernisation has also introduced other factors such as changes in birthing methods, increased use of artificial formula instead of breast feeding, and the use of sugar substitutes, food additives and antibiotics. Many of these changes have been associated with a reduction in gut microbial diversity, which is a feature of IBD [44,45].

3.1. Lower Intakes of Dietary Fibre

As the diet becomes more Westernised and processed, "Western" food often contains less fibre. Current intakes of fibre associated with the Western diet are assessed to be about 20 g/day, compared to a fibre content of 70–120 g/day when diets rich in fruit, vegetables and grains are consumed, as is estimated for hunter-gathers and agriculturalists in human history [46]. The low consumption of fruit, vegetables and dietary fibre and the increased intake of animal fat and refined sugars have been observed in people with disorders like IBD [47], as are exclusion diets for IBD that are made popular in the media [48].

The risk of IBD has been negatively associated with the intake of fibre [34,49,50]. Fibre can be defined in a number of ways, as illustrated by the different definitions by the American Association of Cereal Chemists (AACC) [51] and The Codex Alimentarius Commission [52]. A recent AACC definition describes fibre as being a component of "edible plants or analogous carbohydrates that are resistant to digestion and absorption in the human small intestine, with complete or partial fermentation in the large intestine" [53]. They include in their definition polysaccharides, oligosaccharides, lignin and associated plant substances. Fibre has been further subdivided into rapidly digested starch, slowly digested starch and resistant starch (RS), and the latter is classified into five categories (RS1–RS5). High levels of resistant starch are found in unripe bananas, raw potatoes, maize, pulse grains and legumes. However, depending on their processing, the RS content can vary, and in legumes this can range from a few percent to 80% [54]. The RS3 category (retrograded starch) has been shown in wild type interleukin-10-deficient IBD murine studies to decrease ileal and colonic inflammatory lesions compared to a low-fat diet [55,56]. The authors suggested that soluble fibre and resistant starch suppress gut inflammation. The inclusion of soluble fibre and resistant starch in the diet of individuals with IBD may be helpful for this reason.

Fibre can also be described as soluble and insoluble [57]. The removal of insoluble fibre, a component of the skins of fruit, vegetables, whole grains, and seeds, is a current recommendation by the Crohn's and Colitis Foundation of America [58]. When people are experiencing disease activity (sometimes described as a flare or relapse), insoluble fibre may intensify bloating, pain, diarrhoea and gas. However, the consumption of soluble fibre in vegetables (e.g., the brassica family, dried peas and beans, parsnips, carrots, potatoes, spinach, squash, zucchini) and fruit (e.g., pip and stone fruit, berries, bananas, dates, cantaloupe, grapes and pineapple), oat cereals and barley is recommended. Soluble fibre promotes water absorption, enabling the gut contents to form a gel-like consistency, which delays emptying of the gut and reduces diarrhoea [58]. Soluble fibre also provides a substrate for bacterial fermentation in the colon [59]. The soluble plant fibres in plantain and broccoli reduce the movement of *E. coli* across M cells in Peyer's patches in CD patients [60]. In CD, *E. coli* is found in increased numbers in the mucosa [61,62]. This means it is important that appropriate fibre types are chosen if people with IBD are removing food or food groups (e.g., selecting gluten-free diets or foods low in FODMAPs (fermentable oligo-, di- and mono-saccharides and polyols)) so they do not inadvertently contribute to an increase in disease activity later in their health journey [63].

There are also identified gene–nutrient interactions associated with the role of fibre. One of these is the free fatty acid receptor 2 gene (*FFAR2*; previously known as G protein-coupled receptor 43—*GPR43*). This gene is a member of the largest gene family—the seven-transmembrane receptor group known as G-protein-coupled receptors (*GPCRs*) [64]. These are involved as mediators of cellular responses to many neurotransmitters and hormones [65]. *FFAR2* is highly expressed in neutrophils [66]. One pathological marker of CD is the migration of neutrophilic granulocytes into the mucosa of the intestine [67]. *FFAR2* also activates pathways involved in intracellular Ca^{2+} release and inhibits the build-up of cAMP [68].

The *FFAR2* receptors are present in fat tissues, inflammatory cells and the large intestine [69]. In the large intestine, the receptors are stimulated by short-chain fatty acids (SCFAs), which are produced by bacteria fermenting dietary fibre [21,70]. Lower intakes of dietary fibre decrease the production of SCFAs, which stimulates *FFAR2* signalling. The study by Sivaprakasam et al. showed the critical role of *FFAR2* in the maintenance of healthy gut microbiota, leading to the suppression of intestinal carcinogenesis [71].

The interaction of SCFAs and FFAR2 greatly affects inflammatory processes. SCFAs play an important role in colon homeostasis, as they promote pathways involved in cell differentiation, growth regulation, immune regulation and apoptosis [72]. SCFAs and butyrate in particular seem to be the favoured fuel source of the bacteria in the colon as well as of colonocytes, which are required for the functional integrity of the epithelium [73–76]. The source of SCFAs is the intake of highly fermentable fibres, the residues of which are converted by anaerobic bacteria into SCFAs upon reaching the large bowel [77]. SCFAs have been observed to increase the beneficial populations of *Bifidobacterium* and *Lactobacillus*, which have a role in anti-inflammatory outcomes and immune functions [38,78,79]. SCFAs appear to be important in epithelial barrier maintenance and immune system regulation. Maslowski and Mackay consider the SCFAs produced in the colon to be very important for immunoregulation. They propose that the lower dietary fibre intake associated with the modern Western diet is the driver behind the increased incidence of inflammatory diseases associated with this lifestyle factor [70].

However, there is currently no published literature about the significance of this gene with respect to people with IBD and their intake of fibre. People with IBD (whether with disease activity or in remission) have been observed to have a low intake of fruit, vegetables and dietary fibre [49,80]. Perhaps particular variants in the *FFAR2* gene may affect a person's response to fibre, and this in turn contributes to changes in microbiota composition. This may explain how those who follow a strict FODMAP diet experience a reduction in beneficial bacteria [81,82].

3.2. Increased Consumption of Saturated Fatty Acids

Some authors believe that the Western diet has also become pro-inflammatory as a result of the increased consumption of saturated fatty acids and decreased consumption of polyunsaturated fatty acids (PUFAs), especially long-chain PUFAs (LC-PUFAs) [83–87]. There has also been a decrease in the ratio of the omega-3 and omega-6 PUFAs ingested, partly because of a lower consumption of fish. Fish intolerance and allergy is well-recognised in childhood, being the third most frequent allergen after cow's milk and egg in European children [88–90]. There is less evidence implicating fish intolerance or allergy in CD. Untersmayr et al. observed that antacid medication plus fish consumption impeded the digestion of dietary proteins in their BALB/c mouse fish allergy model [91].

In earlier times, people consumed only small amounts of these PUFAs, and in about the same proportion. Today it is estimated that this ratio is now about 1:10–1:20–25 omega-3:omega-6. This has occurred from the increased intake of vegetable oils (e.g., soy, safflower, corn and sunflower) [83,92,93]. The genes and their variants linked to differences in fatty acid absorption include fatty acid desaturase genes (*FADS1, FADS2*), the peroxisome proliferator-activated receptor genes (*PPARA, PPARG*), the X-ray repair cross-complementing protein 1 gene (*XRCC1*) and stearoyl-CoA desaturase (*SCD1*). A number of studies have discussed the role that these genes play in the serum levels of LC-PUFA-omega-3 and omega-6 fatty acids, as well as the effects of various variants on metabolic pathways and how this impacts inflammation and cancer risk [94–104]. These studies show that the impact of these fatty acids—especially on inflammation—is also influenced by the person's genotype. This may have deleterious effects on individuals with IBD who exclude fish and fish oils from their diet and have a high omega-3:omega-6 PUFA ratio.

3.3. Fructose and Sugar Consumption

There is much debate in the literature about the effects of fructose consumption [105–116]. The rise in obesity, diabetes, metabolic syndrome, IBD, coronary heart disease, and whether the increased consumption of fructose or fructans has contributed to these disorders, has been widely discussed [105–116]. Over recent decades, increasing amounts of fructose have been consumed as part of the Western diet. This has been particularly associated with the addition of sugars to processed foods, particularly high-fructose corn syrup (HFCS, comprising ~60% fructose) in the USA or with cane sugar (50% fructose) in NZ. Both are cheap and ubiquitous sweeteners, especially in soft drinks and cereal products [117]. The effect of fructose in infant formulas on vascular inflammation has also been investigated in full-term babies. The study found that the fructose formula had a higher inflammatory response than the fructose-free formula, but the difference was not significant [118]. The authors commented that the result may become significant in a preterm infant [118]. According to recent USDA figures, the estimated calories of HFCS consumed daily has risen from 0.4 g/day in 1970, peaked at 44.3 g/day in 1997, and has gradually declined (31.0 g/day in 2015) [25,119,120]. However, total "sweetener" consumption has increased compared to the 1970 figures (from 87.3 g/day in 1970 to 94.1 g/day in 2015) [119]. In NZ, the Adult Nutrition surveys of 1997 and 2008–2009 report that the mean fructose intake and the mean total sugar consumption for European males and females has declined from 1997 (26 g/day and 139 g/day, respectively), to 2008 (23.4 g/day and 100.3 g/day respectively) [121]. Unfortunately, there are no recent national consumption figures to see whether that national trend has continued. A small regional study (n = 227) in 2014 on a Canterbury (NZ) population aged 50 years reported that the mean intake for fructose for men was 25.5 g and 20.6 g for females [122]. This suggests that the downward trend has not continued.

Once ingested, fructose is transported into the blood stream through sugar-transporting proteins GLUT2 and GLUT5, via the small intestine in limited amounts to the liver. The liver removes some of the fructose from circulation to maintain the correct proportion of glucose to fructose (10 times lower) [123–126], and converts fructose into other metabolites including triglycerides and uric acid. This latter function is thought to be a contributor to the rise in obesity, metabolic syndrome and diabetes [106,110,127,128]. Fructose intake also stimulates the thioredoxin-interacting protein gene (*TXNIP*), which can lead to higher fructose intake [129]. The *TXNIP* gene has been associated with promoting inflammation in endothelial cells, mediating hepatic inflammation, and regulating NF-κB [130–134]. *TXNIP* has been shown to be involved in the differentiation of epithelial cells in the intestine [135]. *TXNIP* mRNA, which negatively regulates the *TXNIP* gene, shows decreased expression in the inflamed mucosa of the colon in people with UC [136]. Interestingly, thioredoxin-1 produced by the gene *TXNIP* is also inhibited by the production of vitamin D3 up-regulated protein 1 (VDUP1) when vitamin D_3 is given [137,138].

The relationship between fructose uptake and the *TXNIP* gene may explain why fructose intake has been increasingly linked to intestinal symptoms of bloating, abdominal pain, diarrhoea and fructose intolerance in individuals with IBD [126,139–142]. This underlies the need to consider fructose intake when managing these symptoms. A recent NZ study by Spencer et al. on people with irritable bowel syndrome (IBS) ($n = 277$) based in Canterbury, NZ found that the participants' IBS score, constipation and diarrhoea were not associated with fructose intake. However, they found that greater mean daily fructose intakes ($p = 0.05$) were associated with a lower prevalence of IBS pain [122].

In adults, fructose intolerance is most commonly assessed by breath testing after swallowing 25 g of fructose dissolved in water. Breath measurements are made on a 30-min schedule for up to three hours. A value of ≥ 20 ppm H_2, accompanied by symptoms (e.g., bloating, diarrhoea), is an affirmation of fructose intolerance [139,143]. This is because the hydrogen produced by gut bacteria is reacting with the fructose which has not been absorbed in the small intestine. Breath testing is a common method of testing for fructose, and there are a variety of methodologies in its application, as well as questions about its reliability [144]. A North American consensus statement has been drawn up for hydrogen and methane-based breath testing in gastrointestinal disorders to address these issues [145].

When it is suggested that high-fructose-containing foods be eliminated in the diet, care must be taken in deciding which foods are excluded, as the assessment of what constitutes a high-fructose food varies [146]. If people stay on a low-fructose diet for too long, they may be in danger of nutrient deficiencies due to lack of fruit and vegetables in the diet. It also needs to be remembered that fructose taken as a bolus (e.g., after swallowing 25 g of fructose in a fructose intolerance test) is metabolized differently to when it is ingested in the presence of glucose. Many people absorb fructose easily along with sucrose or with glucose that is at similar levels [147].

3.4. Other Western Diet Factors

Westernisation has also introduced other factors into the diet, such as changes in birthing methods, using artificial infant formula instead of breast feeding, and the use of sugar substitutes, food additives and antibiotics (Table 3). Many of these changes have been associated with a reduction in gut microbial diversity as well as dysbiosis (i.e., microbial imbalances in the gut)—a feature of IBD [44,45]. This path to dysbiosis may start early, with lack of exposure to appropriate gut microbiota as an infant. The composition of an infant's gut bacteria is affected by the delivery method (i.e., whether infants are born by caesarean (C-section) or vaginally, and whether breast-fed or given infant formula. C-section babies have microbiota that resembles that on the mother's skin, and those born vaginally are seeded by the microbiota in the mother's vagina [148,149]. The microbiota seeded from the mother's vagina is thought to contribute to a normal infant microbiome, whereas having a C-section and all the factors associated with the reason for having a C-section does not [150].

The type of first foods also contributes to the composition of the microbiota. Breast feeding promotes immune development and protects against many diseases. In a small study on 3-month-old babies 1214 probe sets for epithelial cells were significantly differently expressed in exclusively breast-fed ($n = 12$) and formula-fed babies ($n = 10$) [151]. This may explain some of the differences that have been noted in clinical and epidemiological observations of these two groups. The two groups have different gut development, with the breast-fed babies being described as being "less leaky". Bacteroidetes species, which are important players in the commensal bacteria, were not found in the stools of the formula-fed infants [151]. Breast milk also contains human milk oligosaccharides (HMOs) which stimulate the growth of the intestinal flora, acting as prebiotics for beneficial bacteria [152]. Human bioactive milk proteins modulate the immune system, and this too would contribute to the enhancement of gut barrier function [153,154]. Formula feeding is becoming an increasingly common pattern of infant feeding in Western culture.

The increasing use of artificial sweeteners (ASs) may also contribute to dysbiosis [155]. A number of studies have been conducted on the effects of ASs on the gut. These have looked at their effects on secretion, absorption, gut motility, the microbiome and gastrointestinal symptoms [156–160]. Some studies imply that ASs have measurable effects on the oral/gut microbiota [155,161,162]. In one example, male rats were randomised into control and AS groups and were exposed to doses ranging from 1.1 to 11 mg/kg/day for 12 weeks (the USA Federal Drug Administration (FDA) acceptable daily intake for humans is 5 mg/kg/day). At the low dose of 1.1 mg/kg, the researchers reported that total anaerobes were reduced by approximately 50% in all sucralose plus maltodextrin groups. However, when this study was reviewed by an expert panel [163], it was criticised for not having an isocaloric carbohydrate control, and not correcting for the water content of the stools. Both these factors can affect the interpretation of the bacterial concentrations. This report also commented that the difference between control and treatment groups for bacterial counts given were also less than 10-fold. They concluded that this meant that the results could not be interpreted as indicative of adverse change, but reflected the normal range of variation in bacteria over this period of time. However, further research in healthy human subjects continues to suggest that microbiota are adversely affected by ASs. Suez and colleagues showed that with 11 weeks of exposure to three common ASs, saccharin altered gut microbiota and induced glucose intolerance [161]. This indicates the need for more studies—particularly in humans—to elucidate the effects of ASs on microbiota [164–166].

Table 3. Western diet food factors, effects related to IBD and associated genes. LC-PUFA: long-chain polyunsaturated fatty acid; SCFA: short-chain fatty acid.

Western Diet Food Factors	Effects Related to IBD	Associated Genes
Foods low in resistant starch and soluble dietary fibre [47]	• Increased risk of IBD [34,36,49,50] • Increased risk of *E. coli* in the mucosa [60] • Decreased production of SCFAs (important in epithelial barrier maintenance and immune system regulation) [69]	*FFAR2* (The interaction of SCFAs and *FFAR2* greatly affects inflammatory processes) [21,70]
Increased consumption of saturated fatty acids with decreased consumption of LC-PUFAs from the increased intake of soy, safflower, corn and sunflower oils and reduced consumption of fish [83,92,93]	• Inflammation and cancer risk impacted by gene variant influence on metabolic pathways [85–87]	*FADS1 and FADS2* *PPARA, PPARG* *XRCC1, SCD1* [94–104]
Increased fructose consumption [25,119,120]	• Associated with the rise in obesity, diabetes, metabolic syndrome, IBD, coronary heart disease [105–116] • Linked to intestinal symptoms of bloating, abdominal pain, diarrhoea and fructose intolerance in IBD [112] • Possible effect on vascular inflammation from infant formulas containing fructose [118]	*TXNIP* [128] (associated with promoting inflammation in endothelial cells, mediating hepatic inflammation, and regulating NF-κB) [129–133]
Increased use of infant formula, artificial sweeteners, food emulsifiers and antibiotics [167,168]	• Reduction in gut microbiotal diversity [44,45] • Increase in antibiotic resistance [168]	Genes in the microbiome [168]

Two other recent additions to the Western diet are emulsifiers in food to improve mouth feel in low-fat products, and antibiotics in animal feed [167,168]. Emulsifiers have been shown in murine studies to have an impact on the mouse gut microbiota that promotes colitis and decrease in (alpha) diversity [167]. Antibiotics are used to reduce disease in livestock kept in confined quarters. Repeated courses of antibiotics can lead to the development of what is termed "the resistome"—the collection of genes in bacteria that confers resistance to antibiotics [169]. Increased antibiotic exposure in humans through food sourced from animals that have had antibiotics may affect the human biome. When these products from these animals are consumed, they contribute to antibiotic resistance. The US Food and Drug Administration (2009) indicated that 80% of antimicrobial products in the USA were used in animal feed as growth stimulants, not for veterinary use [170]. In the highly pastoral country New Zealand it is reported that about 60% of antibiotics are administered to animals [171]. The Ministry for Primary Industries (NZ) states the use of antibiotics in cattle and sheep is low compared to the intensive rearing pig and poultry industries [172].

The issue for people with IBD is its effect on the genetics of their microbiome when they incorporate these products into their diet. For example, with antibiotics, antibiotic resistance genes are built up in the microbial community both in pathogenic and non-pathogenic bacteria, and this builds the resistome [169]. Genes in the resistome are readily transferred not only from one bacterial cell to another, but also by cassettes of multiple genes [173,174]. This has been shown to result in a build-up of multidrug resistance to *E. coli* in domestic animals [175,176]. These bacteria have also been identified as being in increased numbers in those with CD [177–179]. Collectively, all these Western diet factors impinge on the genetics of the biome and reduce microbiota diversity. Personalising the dietary approach for people with IBD and identifying the effects of genes associated with these changes (Table 3) would help reduce this adverse impact on the genes of the microbiome. It would help maintain microbiotal diversity and positively modulate disease activity.

4. Food Intolerances

IBD has been linked with a number of food intolerances, especially with foods containing gluten, dairy products/lactose or fructose (discussed earlier), or food high in FODMAPs. Many of these intolerances can also be linked to specific genes or genotypes. Other food intolerances linked with genotypes and IBD are brassica vegetables, mustard, wasabi, raw and cooked tomatoes, sweet potatoes, mushrooms, sulphur dioxide, sulphites and sulphur compounds. The specific genes or genotypes associated with these intolerances will be discussed further. This section begins with a discussion of the FODMAP approach, as this is the newest dietary strategy suggested as being helpful for IBD. It also links to a number of food intolerances associated with particular genotypes and/or gene variants.

4.1. FODMAPs

FODMAPs are fermentable oligo-, di- and mono-saccharides and polyols which, if lowered in the diet, have been shown to be effective in decreasing the abdominal symptoms associated with IBS. This approach is being proposed as being helpful also for people with IBD [2]. Foods that are identified as FODMAPs have been discussed extensively in the literature [111,180–184]. Table 4 gives examples of food sources of FODMAPs [185–191] and genes that are associated with them.

Table 4. Sources of foods high in fermentable oligo-, di- and mono-saccharides and polyols (FODMAPs) [185–191].

FODMAPs	Examples of Food Sources	Examples of Associated Genes
Fructose	Honey, mangoes, watermelon, grapes, fruit juices, high-fructose corn syrup	*TXNIP* with fructose that is linked to intestinal symptoms of bloating, abdominal pain, diarrhoea in IBD [125,138–141]
Lactose	Dairy products (e.g., milk, ice-cream, yoghurt, soft cheeses)	Lactose intolerance associated with variants of the *LCT* gene [191,192]
Fermentable oligosaccharides	Brussels sprouts, broccoli, cabbage, peas, beetroot, garlic, leeks, onions, wheat or rye bread, pasta, couscous, chickpeas, lentils	*GSTMl* and *GSTTl*, and *DIO1* variants, with tolerance of brassica vegetables [193–196]; *HLA-DQA1* and *HLA-DQB1* variants with gluten intolerance [197]
Polyols	Stone fruits, apples, pears, prunes, avocados, mushrooms; sweeteners: mannitol, sorbitol, xylitol, erythritol and isomalt.	*OCTN1* with mushrooms [198]

Foods high in FODMAPs have been characterized in a healthy population (i.e., those who do not experience inflammation) as not being well absorbed in the small intestine, having a laxative effect if taken in higher doses and fermented rapidly by bacteria [2]. Inflammation of the gut wall—a characteristic of IBD—also interrupts enzyme production by the brush border cells, and this also contributes to the sugars not being absorbed. Unabsorbed sugars go to the large intestine, where bacteria interact with them. When some metabolites (e.g., butan 2,3 diol, ketones, acids, aldehydes) are formed, they can result in an alteration of the signalling mechanisms of the bacteria and this causes gas, pain and diarrhoea [192]. Diarrhoea has a negative impact on water and electrolyte balance, and may lead to dehydration. Gas, pain and diarrhoea commonly occur in non-IBD gastro-intestinal tracts (i.e., healthy populations) if doses of oral fructose or polyols over 50 g are taken [113,193,194].

This physiological reaction is the rationale for using the FODMAP dietary regime in gastrointestinal disorders like IBD [111,195]. This is based on studies with irritable bowel syndrome (IBS), where the decreased consumption of these fermentable carbohydrates has decreased abdominal symptoms (i.e., pain, flatulence, bloating, constipation, diarrhoea). There is no question that the by-products of FODMAP digestion and absorption may be especially unpleasant, exacerbating the symptoms of individuals with gastrointestinal disorders. Thus, it might appear as self-evident that avoidance of this group of compounds could be therapeutic for individuals with IBD—especially if they also have IBS [111,195]. A number of trials with IBS have suggested that this approach shows potential for improving symptoms in IBD. However, to avoid compromising people's nutritional status, care must be taken so that any changes instigated in sources of fruits and vegetables do not reduce the total recommended intake of fruits, vegetables or fibres [196].

How does the FODMAP approach relate to genotypes? As will be discussed further on, intolerance to some vegetables (e.g., brassica, mushrooms, cooked tomatoes) whole grains and dairy products may be linked to specific genotypes and gene variants (Table 5). Recent research has also indicated that following a strict FODMAP diet can also have an effect on the genome of the microbiome and encourage harmful gut microbiota and a decrease in *Bifidobacterium* [183,184]. In people with disorders like IBD, their microbiotal composition is different from those found in healthy people [197–199]. Individuals with IBD have reduced numbers of microbiota, fewer divergent species with lower numbers of *Firmicutes*, and increased number of *Proteobacteria* species compared to healthy people [200–203]. This means that strict adherence to a low-FODMAP diet could contribute to this dysbiosis.

In addition, people with IBD may have a loss of function of the fucosyltransferase 2 (*FUT2*) gene, which identifies them as a "non-secretor". A non-secretor has a significant reduction in microbiotal diversity, richness and abundance [204]. The *FUT2* gene has been identified as increasing the susceptibility to CD [205–207]. Non-secretor individuals are also infrequently colonised by *Bifidobacterium bifidum* (important in the infant flora), *B. adolescentis* and *B. catenulatum/pseudocatenulatum* (important in adult intestinal flora) [204]. Bifidobacteria are an important part of the human intestinal microbiome. They are crucial to the development of a healthy infant microbiota, encouraging appropriate gut maturity and gut integrity, modulating immunity and negating the effects of pathogens [208,209]. This would suggest that people with IBD who are non-secretors have an increased risk of having a less-effective defence against a number of pathogens and are consequently more vulnerable to having an inflamed gut. Following a low-FODMAP diet may exacerbate this. Further research is needed on those who are a non-secretors, using the low-FODMAP approach to see how this affects their microbiota.

4.2. Gluten

Intolerance to foods containing gluten is associated with the autoimmune disease coeliac disease and with non-coeliac gluten sensitivity. These two have symptoms in common (e.g., bloating, diarrhoea, constipation, abdominal pain and weight loss). Unlike coeliac disease, gluten sensitivity is not associated with antibody formation and damage to the epithelium of the gut. Coeliac disease has genetic links. Gluten intolerance is associated with gene variants of the major histocompatibility complex, class II, DQ alpha 1 (*HLA-DQA1*) gene and the major histocompatibility complex, class II, DQ beta 1 (*HLA-DQB1*) gene [210]. Festen and colleagues in their meta-analysis of two genome-wide association studies GWAS also identified the genes interleukin 18 receptor accessory protein (*IL18RAP*); phosphatase, non-receptor type 2 (*PTPN2*); T cell activation RhoGTPase activating protein (*TAGAP*) and pseudouridine synthase 10 (*PUS10*) as having shared risk loci for CD and coeliac disease [211]. The gene *PTPN2* is involved in the regulation of the epithelial barrier function and is modulated by the vitamin D receptor gene (*VDR*) [212]. Current nutrition advice for people with IBD includes checking whether they have the autoimmune coeliac disease or if they have non-coeliac gluten sensitivity. The blood test to detect the presence of anti-tissue transglutaminase (tTG) antibodies can be taken. These antibodies are produced in the small intestine when inflammation occurs in response to gluten. Another test that has a high specificity for coeliac disease is the anti-endomysial antibody (EMA) test which detects villus atrophy—a feature of coeliac disease [213]. If IBD patients prove to have an adverse response to gluten from these tests, then avoiding these foods and products containing them is advised. These foods include wheat, oats, barley (which includes malt and malt vinegar) and rye. There is no definitive test for non-coeliac gluten sensitivity except for eliminating gluten from the diet to see if symptoms subside. The role of non-coeliac gluten or wheat sensitivity in the general population as well as in IBD has been debated extensively. A review of the topic suggests that it may be linked in IBD with those who also have IBS.

4.3. Dairy Products and Lactose

The sensitivity to dairy foods in people with IBD is about 10%–20% [214–216]. Some studies have also linked increased incidence of IBD with the increased intake of dairy foods [217], particularly cheese [218]. This may be because of the fat content of cheese [219]. Nolan-Clark and associates noted that in their study on CD, sensitivity to dairy products was not related to disease activity status [219]. In a year-long trial on UC conducted by Wright et al. it was noted that patients had fewer relapses on a milk-free diet [216].

This sensitivity to dairy products is often associated with the reduction of lactase enzyme in adulthood. Lactase is an enzyme located in the villus enterocytes that is required for the digestion of lactose in milk. Lactase catalyses lactose, the disaccharide in milk, to galactose and glucose (i.e., monosaccharides which can be absorbed into the blood stream). In most mammals, its activity declines shortly after weaning. In humans, the enzyme may persist with its activity into adulthood. This is known as lactase persistence, and it is a genetically determined trait. In Europe, a single allele—T-13910 of the lactase phlorizin hydrolase (*LCT*) gene—is the main one. However, in Africa and the Middle East many more mutations are associated with lactase persistence [220,221].

This lactase persistence has associations with CD. In an NZ-based study [222], lactase persistence in the Caucasian population was associated with an increased risk of CD for those with the lactase (*LCT*) gene who were homozygous for the T allele of rs4988235 as compared with those homozygous for the C allele (OR = 1.61, 95% CI: 1.03–2.51). Increasing lactase non-persistence in populations has also been linked to a decreased risk of CD [223]. In a study encompassing populations from 26 countries around the world, CD decreased as lactase non-persistence increased ($p < 0.01$), [223].

Not consuming dairy products raises the risk of having insufficient intakes of calcium in the diet, especially if few other sources of calcium are consumed. Calcium is not only essential for bone health, but Ca^{2+} is extensively used in biological messenger systems and cell functions [224]. Low calcium intake of people with Crohn's disease increases their risk of bone demineralisation and osteoporosis. These are well-known complications of this condition. Bernstein reported for people with IBD that "The overall relative risk of fractures is 40% greater than that in the general population and increases with age" [225]. Osteoporosis can also be exacerbated by the use of steroid medications (a common treatment in IBD), as they have a detrimental effect on calcium and phosphate metabolism [226]. Calcium intake is important with respect to IBD because, as discussed earlier, Vagianos et al. observed that 25% of their adult outpatients consumed less than the recommended intake of calcium. Further, the study of Hartman et al. showed that 79% of the adolescent outpatients consumed less than 80% of RDA [9,15]. If people are not tolerant to dairy foods, non-dairy sources of calcium are available, such as fortified soy, almond and rice milks, tofu, sardines, almonds, sesame seeds, broccoli and fortified breakfast cereals and juices [227].

4.4. Brassica

Vegetables such as broccoli, cabbage, Brussels sprouts and cauliflower are members of the brassica family of vegetables. These are known to be a good source of various micronutrients (e.g., selenium, iodine) [228] and various phytochemicals (e.g., glucosinolates and quercetin) [229]. Common members from this group of plants are recommended to be excluded from the low-FODMAP diet (Brussels sprouts, broccoli and cabbage) [195]. However, two randomized controlled diet studies conducted by Brauer et al. found different responses in individuals depending on their glutathione S-transferase Mu 1 (*GSTMl*) genotype with supplements of specific brassica vegetables (broccoli, cabbage, cauliflower and radish sprouts) [230]. Their study found that this combination of brassicas altered the circulating peptides transthyretin (TTR) and zinc alpha 2-glycoprotein (ZAG) fragments in a sensitive and identifiable manner. TTR declines in serum with early signs of inflammation. ZAG (an adipokine) is mainly involved in lipid mobilisation. In *GSTMl*+ individuals, ZAG and TTR declined with brassica intake. However, this did not occur in those with the *GSTMl-null* genotype.

GSTMl and genotypes of *GSTTl* are also significant with respect to individuals and their intakes of brassica. There have been over 500 studies on GST enzymes showing that genotypes of these *GSTMl* and *GSTTl* have an influence on cancer outcomes, contingent on the expression or non-expression of these genes [231]. *GSTT1* and *GSTMl* belong to the GST gene super family, which is an extensive group of enzymes. The *GST* family contains several classes (e.g., alpha, kappa, mu, omega, pi, sigma, theta and zeta) [232,233]. GST enzymes have significant roles in the metabolism of electrophilic compounds (e.g., drugs and carcinogens) [234].

At the *GSTMl* locus, four allelic variants have been discovered in humans, and the null allele is present in about 50% of individuals [235]. Where the *GSTMl* gene deletions or the null genotype exist, there is a total lack of the protein encoded by the gene [236]. People with deletions are thought to be more vulnerable to toxic xenobiotics (e.g., antibiotics and drugs) [237]. There is also a variation between different cultural groups in the frequency of the *GSTMl* deletion. In Caucasian and Asian populations, the frequency of the *GSTMl* null genotype genetic polymorphism is estimated to be about 53%. However, the frequency is lower in African- American populations, at 27% [231].

GST enzymes can also be acted on by isothiocyanates (found in brassicas) either as inducers or as substrates in liver detoxification pathways, so a deletion or lowered activity of a *GST* gene can result in a persistent or elevated level of isothiocyanates in the body [238]. Studies based in Asia suggest that the null or less-active genotypes for *GSTT1* and *GSTM1* are protective and lower the risk of colorectal cancer [239]. However, the opposite occurred in the USA-based studies. The active or expressed genotypes, not the null genotypes, were associated with higher risk reduction [240]. The disparity of these results may reflect the different glucosinolate content of the brassica consumed. In Asia, Chinese cabbage (bok choy) is the predominately eaten brassica, and its main glucosinolate is glucobrassicin, whereas in the USA where raw broccoli is the more favoured brassica, the glucosinolate contents differ [241]. The main glucosinolate in this vegetable is glucoraphanin [241]. Glucobrassicin is an indole, whereas glucoraphanin is a sulforaphane. Their distinct chemical structures as shown in Table 5 (adapted from Higdon et al.) may mean that they are metabolised differently as they pass through the intestine, and this would suggest that their influence on the GST genes could also be dissimilar.

Table 5. Differences in glucosinolate structures.

Glucobrassicin (in bok choy)	Glucoraphanin (in broccoli)
Indole-3-	Sulforaphane

A pilot study by Campbell et al. [242] was conducted on the *GSTT1* (-/-) deletion in people with CD, in a New Zealand cohort from the Auckland IBD study [243]. This also showed those consuming broccoli, cauliflower and Chinese greens were more likely to report experiencing a beneficial effect if they had the *GSTT1* deletion. This may well apply to people with other gastrointestinal disorders such as IBS [244]. Responses to another brassica, rocket (arugula), have also been found to be dependent on a variant in the single-nucleotide polymorphism (SNP) rs9469220 of the human leucocyte antigen gene (*HLA*) in people with CD [245]. An inflammatory colonic phenotype has also been associated with variants in the *HLA* gene region [246–248]. This polymorphism has been linked to total IgE levels, which have a key role in sensitivity type 1 reactions in allergies linked with rhinitis, dermatitis, asthma and urticaria [249–251]. This adverse reaction to rocket in people with CD suggests that consumption of this food initiates the immune response in a type I sensitivity reaction. Another variant in the SNP rs7515322 in the iodothyronine deiodinase 1 gene (*DIO1*) has also been associated with an adverse response to broccoli. *DIO1* is part of the selenoenzyme family, which are important as signalling molecules for thyroid hormones and pivotal to thyroid metabolism. Both selenium and iodine deficiencies exist in NZ, and this may heighten individuals' adverse response to broccoli if they have this variant [245]. This influence of micronutrients may also explain inter-country variation in responses to broccoli.

4.5. Mustard, Wasabi, Raw and Cooked Tomatoes and Sweet Potatoes

In another study by Marlow et al. [252], tolerance of mustard, wasabi, raw and cooked tomatoes and sweet potatoes was dependent on the G variant of the SNP rs12212067 in the *FOX03* gene. Seventeen foods were identified with beneficial effects, and four foods with detrimental effects. Sweet potatoes had the highest reported frequency of beneficial effects, and mustard, wasabi, raw and cooked tomatoes were detrimental for over 25% of the study population with the G allele (SNP rs12212067) associated with the *FOX03* gene. FODMAP guidelines suggest that tomato products such as canned tomatoes are not appropriate in the low-FODMAP diet, although plum tomatoes are [139]. This guidance could perhaps be tailored more for people using the low-FODMAP diet if their gene variants in the *FOX03* gene were identified.

4.6. Mushrooms

In a study on CD in an NZ population, a statistically significant association with a variant (the T allele) of the SNP rs1050152 of the organic cation transporter gene *OCTN1* was found. This variant is related to mushroom intolerance in those with CD, when compared with the general population. This indicates that NZ people with CD who have this variant have an increased risk of adverse symptoms associated with the intake of mushrooms [244].

4.7. Sulphur Dioxide, Sulphites and Sulphur Compounds

Sulphur dioxide and sulphites (at concentrations greater than 10 mg/kg or 10 mg/L) are now listed by the EU as a common cause of food intolerances and allergens [253]. Additive sulphites are often used in the food industry, as they have multiple functions. They are used as food preservatives, as they stop microbial growth and reduce the spoilage of food. They can act as antioxidants, inhibiting browning actions. They can modify texture in doughs. They are found in wine, soft drinks, sausages and burgers [254]. There is some evidence that they may aggravate IBD symptoms. Magee et al. report in their novel method of diet analysis that in UC, sulphites adversely affect symptoms through their anti-thiamine activity. Thiamine has a critical role in energy metabolism and cell function [255]. Low levels have been implicated in fatigue and IBD in those in remission (UC) or quiescent (CD) [256]. Those with very active disease who ate large quantities of food containing sulphites also had high food sigmoidoscopy scores [257].

Earlier studies linking sulphur compounds with IBD have described hydrogen sulphide as a bacterial toxin in people with UC [258]. This description was based on the experimental work where sulphated polysaccharides were ingested by guinea pigs and rabbits [259,260]. These sulphur products impaired butyrate oxidation—a characteristic of UC [261]. Butyrate, as a SCFA (as mentioned earlier), plays an important part in colon homeostasis by promoting the development of the intestinal barrier through enhancing tight-junction formation, which is impaired in people with IBD [262]. More recent work by Carbonero et al. has summarised the significance of microbiota in colonic sulphur metabolism and identified a number of gut microbiota taxa that participate in it [263]. These authors suggest that common variants in host genes involved in the sulphide oxidation pathways may be implicated in ineffective epithelial sulphide detoxification. This makes people with these variants predisposed to sulphide intolerance and consequent inflammation. The literature suggests that sulphur dioxide sulphites, and other ingested sulphur-containing products, are another example of where nutrient–gene interaction occurs. Particular variants are associated with their intolerance. Using the personalised nutrition approach and identifying these gene variants in people with IBD would identify those who are intolerant to sulphur dioxide, sulphites and sulphur compounds, and so remove foods containing these substances and reduce inflammation.

5. Ethical Issues

The willingness of individuals to engage in genetic testing that would enable a personalised diet/nutrition approach will depend on how they understand the benefits this would bring compared to their perceived privacy risk [264]. Genetic testing for individuals can now be readily accessed with a number of commercial applications available (e.g., Fitgenes, 23andMe) [265,266]. The availability of genetic testing also raises a number of questions: Who should hold and have access to this information? How safely is the information kept? How informed is the consent for consumers? [266]. The protection of an individual's genetic information and the validation of genetic tests needs to be guaranteed to ensure consumer safety. Health practitioners also need to be able to understand the role of genetic testing in their clinical practice so that they can integrate this information appropriately and offer a personalised nutrition approach.

6. Conclusions

This review gives examples of genotypes and genetic variants that have been associated with nutrient deficiencies, the Western diet, and food intolerances. Variation in genotypes could help explain the variability in response to food that is associated with IBD. We need to identify the variants associated with adverse reactions to food, as is currently being done in pharmacogenetic research with respect to drugs. Identification of gene variants would allow more precise tailoring of diets to avoid exacerbating malnutrition in vulnerable IBD groups. Use of the personalised nutrition approach can also more accurately identify individual food intolerances, help ameliorate abdominal symptoms and improve the quality of life for people with IBD. Further nutrigenomic research can continue to inform and improve the personalised nutrition approach in IBD. In the future, this information could be combined with data on individuals such as their gut microbiome, dietary patterns, exercise routines, blood parameters and anthropometric measurements. This combination of information could be used to build machine-learning algorithms to predict which foods/meals reduce inflammation and abdominal symptoms. This may also help to establish the dietary patterns and lifestyles that are most protective against IBD in those genetically susceptible to IBD. This combination of data may also help individuals with established IBD to tailor their diet and lifestyle to avoid exacerbating their signs and symptoms, and promote longer periods of remission. The protection of an individual's genetic information and the validation of genetic tests needs to be guaranteed to ensure consumers' safety when using this information with a personalised nutrition approach.

Author Contributions: Writing—original draft preparation, review and editing, B.B.L.; draft preparation, review and editing, A.G.L.; conceptualization, draft preparation, review and editing, L.R.F.

References

1. Zeevi, D.; Korem, T.; Zmora, N.; Israeli, D.; Rothschild, D.; Weinberger, A.; Ben-Yacov, O.; Lador, D.; Avnit-Sagi, T.; Lotan-Pompan, M. Personalized nutrition by prediction of glycemic responses. *Cell* **2015**, *163* 1079–1094. [CrossRef]
2. Ercolini, D.; Fogliano, V. Food design to feed the human gut microbiota. *J. Agric. Food Chem.* **2018**, *66'* 3754–3758. [CrossRef] [PubMed]
3. Grissinger, M. The five rights: A destination without a map. *Pharm. Ther.* **2010**, *35*, 542.
4. Halawi, H.; Camilleri, M. Pharmacogenetics and the treatment of functional gastrointestinal disorders. *Pharmacogenomics* **2017**, *18*, 1085–1094. [CrossRef] [PubMed]
5. Zhou, J.; Shen, J.; Seifer, B.J.; Jiang, S.; Wang, J.; Xiong, H.; Xie, L.; Wang, L.; Sui, X. Approaches and genetic determinants in predicting response to neoadjuvant chemotherapy in locally advanced gastric cancer. *Oncotarget* **2017**, *8*, 30477–30494. [CrossRef] [PubMed]
6. Racine, A.; Carbonnel, F.; Chan, S.S.; Hart, A.R.; Bueno-de-Mesquita, H.B.; Oldenburg, B.; van Schaik, F.D.; Tjonneland, A.; Olsen, A.; Dahm, C.C.; et al. Dietary patterns and risk of inflammatory bowel disease in europe: Results from the EPIC Study. *Inflamm. Bowel Dis.* **2016**, *22*, 345–354. [CrossRef] [PubMed]
7. Frazier-Wood, A.C. Dietary patterns, genes, and health: Challenges and obstacles to be overcome. *Curr. Nutr. Rep.* **2015**, *4*, 82–87. [CrossRef] [PubMed]
8. Ferguson, L.R. Nutrigenetics, nutrigenomics and inflammatory bowel diseases. *Expert Rev. Clin. Immunol.* **2013**, *9*, 717–726. [CrossRef] [PubMed]
9. Vagianos, K.; Bector, S.; McConnell, J.; Bernstein, C.N. Nutrition assessment of patients with inflammatory bowel disease. *J. Parenter. Enter. Nutr.* **2007**, *31*, 311–319. [CrossRef] [PubMed]
10. Stein, J.; Bott, C. *Diet and Nutrition in Crohn's Disease and Ulcerative Colitis 20 Questions 20 Answers*; Falk Foundation e.V.: Freiburg, Germany, 2008.
11. Basson, A. Nutrition management in the adult patient with Crohn's disease. *S. Afr. J. Clin. Nutr.* **2012**, *25* 164–172. [CrossRef]
12. Harries, A.; Rhodes, J. Undernutrition in Crohn's disease: An anthropometric assessment. *Clin. Nutr.* **1985'** *4*, 87–89. [CrossRef]
13. Gassull, M.A.; Cabré, E. Nutrition in inflammatory Bowel disease. *Curr. Opin. Clin. Nutr. Metab. Care* **2001'** *4*, 561–569. [CrossRef] [PubMed]
14. Lomer, M.C.; Kodjabashia, K.; Hutchinson, C.; Greenfield, S.M.; Thompson, R.P.; Powell, J.J. Intake of dietary iron is low in patients with Crohn's disease: A case–control study. *Br. J. Nutr.* **2004**, *91*, 141–148. [CrossRef [PubMed]
15. Hartman, C.; Marderfeld, L.; Davidson, K.; Mozer-Glassberg, Y.; Poraz, I.; Silbermintz, A.; Zevit, N.; Shamir, R. Food intake adequacy in children and adolescents with inflammatory Bowel disease. *J. Pediatr. Gastroenterol. Nutr.* **2016**, *63*, 437–444. [CrossRef] [PubMed]
16. Lourenço, S.; Hussein, T.; Bologna, S.; Sipahi, A.; Nico, M. Oral manifestations of inflammatory Bowel Disease: A review based on the observation of six cases. *J. Eur. Acad. Dermatol. Venereol.* **2010**, *24*, 204–207. [CrossRef]

17. Malins, T.; Wilson, A.; Ward-Booth, R. Recurrent buccal space abscesses: A complication of Crohn's disease. *Oral Surg. Oral Med. Oral Pathol.* **1991**, *72*, 19–21. [CrossRef]

18. Plauth, M.; Jenss, H.; Meyle, J. Oral manifestations of Crohn's Disease: An analysis of 79 cases. *J. Clin. Gastroenterol.* **1991**, *13*, 29–37. [CrossRef]

19. Schlosser, B.J.; Pirigyi, M.; Mirowski, G.W. Oral manifestations of hematologic and nutritional diseases. *Otolaryngol. Clin. N. Am.* **2011**, *44*, 183–203. [CrossRef]

20. Thomas, D.M.; Mirowski, G.W. Nutrition and oral mucosal diseases. *Clin. Dermatol.* **2010**, *28*, 426–431. [CrossRef]

21. Rebhan, M.; Chalifa-Caspi, V.; Prilusky, J.; Lancet, D. GeneCards: A novel functional genomics compendium with automated data mining and query reformulation support. *Bioinformatics* **1998**, *14*, 656–664. [CrossRef]

22. D'Ambrosio, D.N.; Clugston, R.D.; Blaner, W.S. Vitamin A metabolism: An update. *Nutrients* **2011**, *3*, 63–103. [CrossRef] [PubMed]

23. Leung, W.; Hessel, S.; Meplan, C.; Flint, J.; Oberhauser, V.; Tourniaire, F.; Hesketh, J.; Von Lintig, J.; Lietz, G. Two common single nucleotide polymorphisms in the gene encoding B-Carotene 15, 15'-monoxygenase alter B-carotene metabolism in female volunteers. *FASEB J.* **2009**, *23*, 1041–1053. [CrossRef] [PubMed]

24. Su, H.Y.; Gupta, V.; Day, A.S.; Gearry, R.B. Rising incidence of inflammatory Bowel Disease in Canterbury, New Zealand. *Inflamm. Bowel Dis.* **2016**, *22*, 2238–2244. [CrossRef] [PubMed]

25. University of Otago; Ministry of health New Zealand. *A Focus on Nutrition: Key Findings of the 2008/09 New Zealand Adult Nutrition Survey*; Ministry of Health: Wellington, New Zealand, 2011.

26. Anand, P.K.; Kaul, D. Downregulation of TACO gene transcription restricts mycobacterial entry/survival within human macrophages. *FEMS Microbiol. Lett.* **2005**, *250*, 137–144. [CrossRef] [PubMed]

27. Stephensen, C.B. Vitamin A, infection, and immune function. *Annu. Rev. Nutr.* **2001**, *21*, 167–192. [CrossRef] [PubMed]

28. Sommer, A. *Vitamin A Deficiency*; Wiley Online Library: Hoboken, NJ, USA, 2001.

29. Thia, K.T.; Loftus, E.V.; Sandborn, W.J.; Yang, S. An update on the epidemiology of inflammatory Bowel Disease in Asia. *Am. J. Gastroenterol.* **2008**, *103*, 3167–3182. [CrossRef] [PubMed]

30. Baumgart, D.C.; Bernstein, C.N.; Abbas, Z.; Colombel, J.F.; Day, A.S.; D'Haens, G.; Dotan, I.; Goh, K.L.; Hibi, T.; Kozarek, R.A. IBD around the world: Comparing the epidemiology, diagnosis, and treatment: Proceedings of the World Digestive Health Day 2010–Inflammatory bowel disease task force meeting. *Inflamm. Bowel Dis.* **2011**, *17*, 639–644. [CrossRef] [PubMed]

31. Gismera, C.S.; Aladren, B.S. Inflammatory Bowel diseases: A disease (s) of modern times? is incidence still increasing? *World J. Gastroenterol.* **2008**, *14*, 5491–5498. [CrossRef] [PubMed]

32. Logan, I.; Bowlus, C.L. The geoepidemiology of autoimmune intestinal diseases. *Autoimmun. Rev.* **2010**, *9*, A372–A378. [CrossRef] [PubMed]

33. Lomer, M.C.; Thompson, R.P.; Powell, J.J. Fine and ultrafine particles of the diet: Influence on the mucosal immune response and association with Crohn's disease. In *Proceedings-Nutrition Society of London*; Cambridge University Press: Cambridge, UK, 2002.

34. Persson, P.; Ahlbom, A.; Hellers, G. Diet and inflammatory bowel disease: A case-control study. *Epidemiology* **1992**, *3*, 47–52. [CrossRef] [PubMed]

35. Hou, J.K.; Abraham, B.; El-Serag, H. Dietary intake and risk of developing inflammatory bowel disease: A systematic review of the literature. *Am. J. Gastroenterol.* **2011**, *106*, 563–573. [CrossRef]

36. Chapman-Kiddell, C.A.; Davies, P.S.; Gillen, L.; Radford-Smith, G.L. Role of diet in the development of inflammatory bowel disease. *Inflamm. Bowel Dis.* **2010**, *16*, 137–151. [CrossRef] [PubMed]

37. Sartor, R.B. Mechanisms of disease: Pathogenesis of Crohn's disease and ulcerative colitis. *Nat. Rev. Gastroenterol. Hepatol.* **2006**, *3*, 390–407. [CrossRef] [PubMed]

38. Conterno, L.; Fava, F.; Viola, R.; Tuohy, K.M. Obesity and the gut microbiota: Does up-regulating colonic fermentation protect against obesity and metabolic disease? *Genes Nutr.* **2011**, *6*, 241–260. [CrossRef] [PubMed]

39. Myles, I.A. Fast food fever: Reviewing the impacts of the western diet on immunity. *Nutr. J.* **2014**, *13*, 1. [CrossRef] [PubMed]

40. Cordain, L.; Eaton, S.B.; Sebastian, A.; Mann, N.; Lindeberg, S.; Watkins, B.A.; O'Keefe, J.H.; Brand-Miller, J. Origins and evolution of the Western diet: Health implications for the 21st century. *Am. J. Clin. Nutr.* **2005**, *81*, 341–354. [CrossRef] [PubMed]

41. Tsironi, E.; Feakins, R.M.; Roberts, C.S.; Rampton, D.S. Incidence of inflammatory bowel disease is rising and abdominal tuberculosis is falling in bangladeshis in East London, United Kingdom. *Am. J. Gastroenterol.* **2004**, *99*, 1749–1755. [CrossRef] [PubMed]

42. Dankers, W.; Colin, E.M.; Van Hamburg, J.P.; Lubberts, E. Vitamin D in autoimmunity: Molecular mechanisms and therapeutic potential. *Front. Immunol.* **2017**, *7*, 697. [CrossRef] [PubMed]

43. M'koma, A.E. Inflammatory bowel disease: An expanding global health problem. *Clin. Med. Insights Gastroenterol.* **2013**, *6*, S12731. [CrossRef] [PubMed]

44. Segata, N. Gut microbiome: Westernization and the disappearance of intestinal diversity. *Curr. Biolog.* **2015**, *25*, R611–R613. [CrossRef] [PubMed]

45. Broussard, J.L.; Devkota, S. The changing microbial landscape of Western society: Diet, dwellings and discordance. *Mol. Metab.* **2016**, *5*, 737–742. [CrossRef] [PubMed]

46. Tuohy, K.M.; Conterno, L.; Gasperotti, M.; Viola, R. Up-regulating the human intestinal microbiome using whole plant foods, polyphenols, and/or fiber. *J. Agric. Food Chem.* **2012**, *60*, 8776–8782. [CrossRef] [PubMed]

47. Amre, D.K.; D'Souza, S.; Morgan, K.; Seidman, G.; Lambrette, P.; Grimard, G.; Israel, D.; Mack, D.; Ghadirian, P.; Deslandres, C. Imbalances in dietary consumption of fatty acids, vegetables, and fruits are associated with risk for Crohn's Disease in children. *Am. J. Gastroenterol.* **2007**, *102*, 2016–2025. [CrossRef] [PubMed]

48. Hou, J.K.; Lee, D.; Lewis, J. Diet and inflammatory bowel disease: Review of patient-targeted recommendations. *Clin. Gastroenterol. Hepatol.* **2014**, *12*, 1592–1600. [CrossRef] [PubMed]

49. Kelly, D.G.; Fleming, C.R. Nutritional considerations in inflammatory bowel diseases. *Gastroenterol. Clin. N. Am.* **1995**, *24*, 597–611.

50. Reif, S.; Klein, I.; Lubin, F.; Farbstein, M.; Hallak, A.; Gilat, T. Pre-illness dietary factors in inflammatory bowel disease. *Gut* **1997**, *40*, 754–760. [CrossRef] [PubMed]

51. DeVries, J.W. On defining dietary fibre. *Proc. Nutr. Soc.* **2003**, *62*, 37–43. [CrossRef]

52. Jones, J.M. CODEX-aligned dietary fiber definitions help to bridge the 'fiber gap'. *Nutr. J.* **2014**, *13*, 34. [CrossRef]

53. ACCC International Cereals & Grains association. Dietary Fiber. 2019. Available online: https://www.aaccnet.org/initiatives/definitions/Pages/DietaryFiber.aspx (accessed on 16 March 2019).

54. Ashwar, B.A.; Gani, A.; Shah, A.; Wani, I.A.; Masoodi, F.A. Preparation, health benefits and applications of resistant starch—A review. *Starch-Stärke* **2016**, *68*, 287–301. [CrossRef]

55. Higgins, J.A.; Brown, I.L. Resistant starch: A promising dietary agent for the prevention/treatment of inflammatory bowel disease and bowel cancer. *Curr. Opin. Gastroenterol.* **2013**, *29*, 190–194. [CrossRef]

56. Bassaganya-Riera, J.; DiGuardo, M.; Viladomiu, M.; De Horna, A.; Sanchez, S.; Einerhand, A.W.; Sanders, L.; Hontecillas, R. Soluble fibers and resistant starch ameliorate disease activity in interleukin-10–deficient mice with inflammatory bowel disease. *J. Nutr.* **2011**, *141*, 1318–1325. [CrossRef] [PubMed]

57. Pituch-Zdanowska, A.; Banaszkiewicz, A.; Albrecht, P. The role of dietary fibre in inflammatory bowel disease. *Prz Gastroenterol.* **2015**, *10*, 135–141. [CrossRef] [PubMed]

58. Crohn's & Colitis Foundation of America. *Diet, Nutrition, and Inflammatory Bowel Diseases*; Crohn's & Colitis Foundation of America: New York, NY, USA, 2013.

59. The role of vegetables in the cause remission and regression of Crohn's disease in an Auckland cohort. Available online: https://researchspace.auckland.ac.nz/handle/2292/19961 (accessed on 17 September 2018).

60. Roberts, C.L.; Keita, Å.V.; Duncan, S.H.; O'Kennedy, N.; Söderholm, J.D.; Rhodes, J.M.; Campbell, B.J. Translocation of Crohn's disease Escherichia coli across M-cells: Contrasting effects of soluble plant fibres and emulsifiers. *Gut* **2010**, *59*, 1331–1339. [CrossRef] [PubMed]

61. Miller, H.; Zhang, J.; Kuolee, R.; Patel, G.B.; Chen, W. Intestinal M cells: The fallible sentinels? *World J. Gastroenterol.* **2007**, *13*, 1477–1486. [CrossRef] [PubMed]

62. Siebers, A.; Finlay, B.B. M cells and the pathogenesis of mucosal and systemic infections. *Trends Microbiol.* **1996**, *4*, 22–29. [CrossRef]

63. Staudacher, H.M.; Kurien, M.; Whelan, K. Nutritional implications of dietary interventions for managing gastrointestinal disorders. *Curr. Opin. Gastroenterol.* **2018**, *34*, 105–111. [CrossRef] [PubMed]

64. Bockaert, J.; Pin, J.P. Molecular tinkering of G protein-coupled receptors: An evolutionary success. *EMBO J.* **1999**, *18*, 1723–1729. [CrossRef]

65. Stoddart, L.A.; Smith, N.J.; Milligan, G. International union of pharmacology. LXXI. free fatty acid receptors FFA1,-2, and-3: pharmacology and pathophysiological functions. *Pharmacol. Rev.* **2008**, *60*, 405–417. [CrossRef]

66. Senga, T.; Iwamoto, S.; Yoshida, T.; Yokota, T.; Adachi, K.; Azuma, E.; Hamaguchi, M.; Iwamoto, T. LSSIG is a novel murine leukocyte-specific GPCR that is induced by the activation of STAT3. *Blood* **2003**, *101*, 1185–1187. [CrossRef]

67. Fournier, B.; Parkos, C. The role of neutrophils during intestinal inflammation. *Mucosal Immunol.* **2012**, *5*, 354–366. [CrossRef]

68. Le Poul, E.; Loison, C.; Struyf, S.; Springael, J.; Lannoy, V.; Decobecq, M.; Brezillon, S.; Dupriez, V.; Vassart, G.; Van Damme, J. Functional characterization of human receptors for short chain fatty acids and their Role in polymorphonuclear cell activation. *J. Biol. Chem.* **2003**, *278*, 25481–25489. [CrossRef] [PubMed]

69. Bindels, L.B.; Dewulf, E.M.; Delzenne, N.M. GPR43/FFA2: physiopathological relevance and therapeutic prospects. Trends. *Pharmacol. Sci.* **2013**. [CrossRef] [PubMed]

70. Maslowski, K.M.; Vieira, A.T.; Ng, A.; Kranich, J.; Sierro, F.; Yu, D.; Schilter, H.C.; Rolph, M.S.; Mackay, F.; Artis, D. Regulation of inflammatory responses by gut microbiota and chemoattractant receptor. *GPR Nat.* **2009**, *461*, 1282–1286. [CrossRef] [PubMed]

71. Sivaprakasam, S.; Gurav, A.; Paschall, A.; Coe, G.; Chaudhary, K.; Cai, Y.; Kolhe, R.; Martin, P.; Browning, D.; Huang, L. An essential role of Ffar2 (Gpr43) in dietary fibre-mediated promotion of healthy composition of gut microbiota and suppression of intestinal carcinogenesis. *Oncogenesis* **2016**, *5*, e238. [CrossRef] [PubMed]

72. Bordonaro, M.; Mariadason, J.M.; Aslam, F.; Heerdt, B.G.; Augenlicht, L.H. Butyrate-induced apoptotic cascade in colonic carcinoma cells: modulation of the beta-catenin-Tcf pathway and concordance with effects of sulindac and trichostatin A but not curcumin. *Cell Growth Differ.* **1999**, *10*, 713–720. [PubMed]

73. Evans, W. Pharmacogenomics: Marshalling the human genome to individualise drug therapy. *Gut* **2003**, *52*, ii10–ii18. [CrossRef] [PubMed]

74. Eastwood, M.; Kritchevsky, D. Dietary fiber: How did we get where we are? *Annu. Rev. Nutr.* **2005**, *25*, 1–8. [CrossRef] [PubMed]

75. Maslowski, K.M.; Mackay, C.R. Diet, gut microbiota and immune responses. *Nat. Immunol.* **2010**, *12*, 5–9. [CrossRef] [PubMed]

76. Schneeman, B.O.; Gallaher, D. Effects of dietary fiber on digestive enzyme activity and bile acids in the small intestine. In *Proceedings of the Society for Experimental Biology and Medicine*; Society for Experimental Biology and Medicine: New York, NY, USA, 1985; pp. 409–414.

77. Lupton, J.R. Microbial degradation products influence colon cancer risk: The butyrate controversy. *J. Nutr.* **2004**, *134*, 479–482. [CrossRef] [PubMed]

78. Blaut, M.; Clavel, T. Metabolic diversity of the intestinal microbiota: Implications for health and disease. *J. Nutr.* **2007**, *137*, 751S–755S. [CrossRef]

79. National Academy Press. Dietary, Functional and Total Fibre. Available online: https://www.nap.edu/read/10490/chapter/9Accessed (accessed on 9 August 2018).

80. Silva, A.F.D.; Schieferdecker, M.E.M.; Amarante, H.M.B.d.S. Food intake in patients with inflammatory bowel disease. *ABCD Arq. Bras. Cir. Dig.* **2011**, *24*, 204–209. [CrossRef]

81. Staudacher, H.M.; Irving, P.M.; Lomer, M.C.; Whelan, K. Mechanisms and efficacy of dietary FODMAP Restriction in IBS. *Nat. Rev. Gastroenterol. Hepatol.* **2014**, *11*, 256. [CrossRef] [PubMed]

82. Halmos, E.P.; Christophersen, C.T.; Bird, A.R.; Shepherd, S.J.; Gibson, P.R.; Muir, J.G. Diets that differ in their FODMAP content alter the colonic luminal microenvironment. *Gut* **2015**, *64*, 93–100. [CrossRef] [PubMed]

83. Simopoulos, A.P. Omega-3 fatty acids in health and disease and in growth and development. *Am. J. Clin. Nutr.* **1991**, *54*, 438–463. [CrossRef] [PubMed]

84. Razack, R.; Seidner, D.L. Nutrition in inflammatory bowel disease. *Curr. Opin. Gastroenterol.* **2007**, *23*, 400–405. [CrossRef]

85. Patterson, E.; Wall, R.; Fitzgerald, G.; Ross, R.; Stanton, C. Health implications of high dietary omega-6 polyunsaturated fatty acids. *J. Nutr. Metab.* **2012**, *2012*, 1–16. [CrossRef] [PubMed]

86. Park, J.; Kwon, S.; Han, Y.; Hahm, K.; Kim, E. Omega-3 polyunsaturated fatty acids as potential chemopreventive agent for gastrointestinal cancer. *J. Cancer. Prev.* **2013**, *18*, 201. [CrossRef] [PubMed]

87. Thomas, J.; Thomas, C.; Radcliffe, J.; Itsiopoulos, C. Omega-3 fatty acids in early prevention of inflammatory neurodegenerative disease: A focus on Alzheimer's disease. *BioMed Res. Int.* **2015**, *2015*, 1–13. [CrossRef] [PubMed]

88. Pascual, C.Y.; Reche, M.; Fiandor, A.; Valbuena, T.; Cuevas, T.; Esteban, M.M. Fish allergy in childhood. *Pediatr. Allergy. Immunol.* **2008**, *19*, 573–579. [CrossRef] [PubMed]

89. Vitoria, J.C.; Camarero, C.; Sojo, A.; Ruiz, A.; Rodriguez-Soriano, J. Enteropathy related to fish, rice, and chicken. *Arch. Dis. Child.* **1982**, *57*, 44–48. [PubMed]

90. Dannaeus, A.; Johansson, S.; Foucard, T.; Öhman, S. Clinical and immunological aspects of food allergy in childhood I. Estimation of IgG, IgA and IgE antibodies to food antigens in children with food allergy and atopic dermatitis. *Acta Paediatrica* **1977**, *66*, 31–37. [CrossRef]

91. Untersmayr, E.; Schöll, I.; Swoboda, I.; Beil, W.J.; Förster-Waldl, E.; Walter, F.; Riemer, A.; Kraml, G.; Kinaciyan, T.; Spitzauer, S. Antacid medication inhibits digestion of dietary proteins and causes food allergy: A fish allergy model in BALB/C mice. *J. Allergy Clin. Immunol.* **2003**, *112*, 616–623. [CrossRef]

92. Leaf, A.; Weber, P.C. A new era for science in nutrition. *Am. J. Clin. Nutr.* **1987**. [CrossRef] [PubMed]

93. Eaton, S.B.; Konner, M. Paleolithic nutrition: A consideration of its nature and current implications. *N. Engl. J. Med.* **1985**, *312*, 283–289. [CrossRef] [PubMed]

94. Schaeffer, L.; Gohlke, H.; Muller, M.; Heid, I.M.; Palmer, L.J.; Kompauer, I.; Demmelmair, H.; Illig, T.; Koletzko, B.; Heinrich, J. Common genetic variants of the FADS1 FADS2 gene cluster and their reconstructed haplotypes are associated with the fatty acid composition in phospholipids. *Hum. Mol. Genet.* **2006**, *15*, 1745–1756. [CrossRef] [PubMed]

95. Fajas, L.; Auboeuf, D.; Raspé, E.; Schoonjans, K.; Lefebvre, A.; Saladin, R.; Najib, J.; Laville, M.; Fruchart, J.; Deeb, S. The organization, promoter analysis, and expression of the human PPARγ gene. *J. Biol. Chem.* **1997**, *272*, 18779–18789. [CrossRef]

96. Tai, E.S.; Corella, D.; Demissie, S.; Cupples, L.A.; Coltell, O.; Schaefer, E.J.; Tucker, K.L.; Ordovas, J.M. Polyunsaturated fatty acids interact with the PPARA-L162V polymorphism to affect plasma triglyceride and apolipoprotein C-III concentrations in the Framingham Heart Study. *J. Nutr.* **2005**, *135*, 397–403. [CrossRef]

97. De Keyser, C.E.; Becker, M.L.; Uitterlinden, A.G.; Hofman, A.; Lous, J.J.; Elens, L.; Visser, L.E.; Van Schaik, R.H.; Stricker, B.H. Genetic variation in the PPARA gene is associated with simvastatin-mediated cholesterol reduction in the Rotterdam Study. *Pharmacogenomics* **2013**, *14*, 1295–1304. [CrossRef]

98. Chen, M.; Wang, Y.; Zhang, W.; Han, X. Abstract PR428: Association of PparA Rs4253728 G> A gene polymorphisms with Cyp3A4 enzyme activity and fentanyl post-operative intravenous analgesic effect. *Anesth. Analg.* **2016**, *123*, 109–110. [CrossRef]

99. Ferreira, P.; Cravo, M.; Guerreiro, C.S.; Tavares, L.; Santos, P.M.; Brito, M. Fat intake interacts with polymorphisms of Caspase9, FasLigand and PPARgamma apoptotic genes in modulating Crohn's Disease activity. *Clin. Nutr.* **2010**, *29*, 819–823. [CrossRef]

100. Jiang, Z.; Li, C.; Xu, Y.; Cai, S. A meta-analysis on XRCC1 and XRCC3 polymorphisms and colorectal cancer risk. *Int. J. Colorectal Dis.* **2010**, *25*, 169–180. [CrossRef] [PubMed]

101. Stern, M.C.; Butler, L.M.; Corral, R.; Joshi, A.D.; Yuan, J.M.; Koh, W.P.; Yu, M.C. Polyunsaturated fatty acids, DNA repair single nucleotide polymorphisms and colorectal cancer in the Singapore Chinese Health Study. *J. Nutrigenet. Nutrigenomics* **2009**, *2*, 273–279. [CrossRef] [PubMed]

102. Stryjecki, C.; Roke, K.; Clarke, S.; Nielsen, D.; Badawi, A.; El-Sohemy, A.; Ma, D.W.; Mutch, D.M. Enzymatic activity and genetic variation in SCD1 modulate the relationship between fatty acids and inflammation. *Mol. Genet. Metab.* **2012**, *105*, 421–427. [CrossRef] [PubMed]

103. Larsson, S.C.; Kumlin, M.; Ingelman-Sundberg, M.; Wolk, A. dietary long-chain N-3 fatty acids for the prevention of cancer: A review of potential mechanisms. *Am. J. Clin. Nutr.* **2004**, *79*, 935–945. [CrossRef] [PubMed]

104. Nicholson, M.L.; Neoptolemos, J.P.; Clayton, H.A.; Talbot, I.C.; Bell, P.R. Inhibition of experimental colorectal carcinogenesis by dietary N-6 polyunsaturated fats. *Carcinogenesis* **1990**, *11*, 2191–2197. [CrossRef]

105. Bray, G.; Popkin, B.M. Calorie-sweetened beverages and fructose: What have we learned 10 years later. *Pediatr. Obes.* **2013**, *8*, 242–248. [CrossRef]

106. Elliott, S.S.; Keim, N.L.; Stern, J.S.; Teff, K.; Havel, P.J. Fructose, weight gain, and the insulin resistance syndrome1—3. *Am. J. Clin. Nutr.* **2002**, *76*, 911–922. [CrossRef]

107. Basu, S.; Yoffe, P.; Hills, N.; Lustig, R.H. The relationship of sugar to population-level diabetes prevalence: An econometric analysis of repeated cross-sectional data. *PloS ONE* **2013**, *8*, e57873. [CrossRef]

108. Goran, M.I.; Ulijaszek, S.J.; Ventura, E.E. High fructose corn syrup and diabetes prevalence: A global perspective. *Glob. Public Health* **2013**, *8*, 55–64. [CrossRef]

109. DiNicolantonio, J.J.; O'Keefe, J.H.; Lucan, S.C. Added fructose: A principal driver of type 2 diabetes mellitus and its consequences. *Mayo Clin. Proc.* **2015**, *90*, 372–381. [CrossRef]

110. Malik, V.S.; Schulze, M.B.; Hu, F.B. Intake of sugar-sweetened beverages and weight gain: A systematic review. *Am. J. Clin. Nutr.* **2006**, *84*, 274–288. [CrossRef] [PubMed]

111. Shepherd, S.J.; Gibson, P.R. Fructose malabsorption and symptoms of irritable bowel syndrome: Guidelines for effective dietary management. *J. Am. Diet. Assoc.* **2006**, *106*, 1631–1639. [CrossRef] [PubMed]

112. Gibson, P.; Shepherd, S. Personal view: Food for thought–western lifestyle and susceptibility to Crohn's Disease. the FODMAP hypothesis. *Aliment. Pharmacol. Ther.* **2005**, *21*, 1399–1409. [CrossRef] [PubMed]

113. Rumessen, J.J. Fructose and related food carbohydrates: Sources, intake, absorption, and clinical implications. *Scand. J. Gastroenterol.* **1992**, *27*, 819–828. [CrossRef] [PubMed]

114. Nguyen, S.; Choi, H.K.; Lustig, R.H.; Hsu, C. Sugar-sweetened beverages, serum uric acid, and blood pressure in adolescents. *J. Pediatr.* **2009**, *154*, 807–813. [CrossRef] [PubMed]

115. Rippe, J.M.; Angelopoulos, T.J. Fructose-containing sugars and cardiovascular disease. *Adv. Nutr.* **2015**, *6*, 430–439. [CrossRef] [PubMed]

116. DiNicolantonio, J.J.; Berger, A. Added sugars drive nutrient and energy deficit in obesity: A new paradigm. *Open Heart* **2016**, *3*, e000469. [CrossRef] [PubMed]

117. Brinton, E.A. The time has come to flag and reduce excess fructose intake. *Atherosclerosis* **2016**, *253*, 262–264. [CrossRef] [PubMed]

118. Schroeder, V.A.; Mattioli, L.F.; Kilkenny, T.A.; Belmont, J.M. Effects of lactose-containing vs lactose-free infant formula on postprandial superior mesenteric artery flow in term infants. *JPEN J. Parenter. Enteral Nutr.* **2014**, *38*, 236–242. [CrossRef] [PubMed]

119. USDA ERS. *Table High Fructose Corn Syrup: Estimated Number of Per Capita Calories Consumed Daily by Calendar Year*; USDA ERS: Washington, DC, USA, 2016.

120. Russell, D.; Parnell, W.; Wilson, N.; Faed, J.; Ferguson, E.; Herbison, P.; Horwath, C.; Nye, T.; Reid, P.; Walker, R. *NZ Food: NZ People. Key Results of the 1997 National Nutrition Survey*; Ministry of Health: Wellington, New Zealand, 1999; p. 71.

121. Spencer, R.; Gearry, R.; Pearson, J.; Skidmore, P. Relationship between fructose and lactose intakes and functional gastrointestinal symptoms in a sample of 50-year-old cantabrians in New Zealand. *NZ Med. J.* **2014**, *127*, 39.

122. Gould, G.W.; Thomas, H.M.; Jess, T.J.; Bell, G.I. Expression of human glucose transporters in xenopus oocytes: Kinetic characterization and substrate specificities of the erythrocyte, liver, and brain isoforms. *Biochemistry* **1991**, *30*, 5139–5145. [CrossRef] [PubMed]

123. Burant, C.F.; Takeda, J.; Brot-Laroche, E.; Bell, G.I.; Davidson, N.O. Fructose transporter in human spermatozoa and small intestine is GLUT5. *J. Biol. Chem.* **1992**, *267*, 14523–14526. [PubMed]

124. Douard, V.; Ferraris, R.P. Regulation of the Fructose Transporter GLUT5 in Health and Disease. *Am. J. Physiol. Endocrinol. Metab.* **2008**, *295*, E227–E237. [CrossRef] [PubMed]

125. Berni Canani, R.; Pezzella, V.; Amoroso, A.; Cozzolino, T.; Di Scala, C.; Passariello, A. Diagnosing and treating intolerance to carbohydrates in children. *Nutrients* **2016**, *8*, 157. [CrossRef] [PubMed]

126. Kolderup, A.; Svihus, B. Fructose metabolism and relation to atherosclerosis, type 2 diabetes, and obesity. *J. Nutr. Metab.* **2015**, *2015*, 823081. [CrossRef] [PubMed]

127. Stanhope, K.L.; Schwarz, J.M.; Keim, N.L.; Griffen, S.C.; Bremer, A.A.; Graham, J.L.; Hatcher, B.; Cox, C.L.; Dyachenko, A.; Zhang, W.; et al. Consuming fructose-sweetened, not glucose-sweetened, beverages increases visceral adiposity and lipids and decreases insulin sensitivity in overweight/obese humans. *J. Clin. Invest.* **2009**, *119*, 1322–1334. [CrossRef]

128. Dotimas, J.R.; Lee, A.W.; Schmider, A.B.; Carroll, S.H.; Shah, A.; Bilen, J.; Elliott, K.R.; Myers, R.B.; Soberman, R.J.; Yoshioka, J. Diabetes Regulates Fructose Absorption through Thioredoxin-Interacting Protein. *eLife* **2016**, *5*, e18313. [CrossRef]

129. Wang, X.Q.; Nigro, P.; World, C.; Fujiwara, K.; Yan, C.; Berk, B.C. Thioredoxin Interacting Protein Promotes Endothelial Cell Inflammation in Response to Disturbed Flow by Increasing Leukocyte Adhesion and Repressing Kruppel-Like Factor. *Circ. Res.* **2012**, *110*, 560–568. [CrossRef]

130. Liu, Y.; Lian, K.; Zhang, L.; Wang, R.; Yi, F.; Gao, C.; Xin, C.; Zhu, D.; Li, Y.; Yan, W. TXNIP Mediates NLRP3 Inflammasome Activation in Cardiac Microvascular Endothelial Cells as a Novel Mechanism in Myocardial Ischemia/Reperfusion Injury. *Basic Res. Cardiol.* **2014**, *109*, 1–14. [CrossRef]

131. Park, M.; Kim, D.; Lim, S.; Choi, J.; Kim, J.; Yoon, K.; Lee, J.; Lee, J.; Han, H.; Choi, I. Thioredoxin-Interacting Protein Mediates Hepatic Lipogenesis and Inflammation Via PRMT1 and PGC-1α Regulation in Vitro and in Vivo. *J. Hepatol.* **2014**, *61*, 1151–1157. [CrossRef]

132. Zhang, X.; Zhang, J.; Chen, X.; Hu, Q.; Wang, M.; Jin, R.; Zhang, Q.; Wang, W.; Wang, R.; Kang, L. Reactive Oxygen Species-Induced TXNIP Drives Fructose-Mediated Hepatic Inflammation and Lipid Accumulation through NLRP3 Inflammasome Activation. *Antioxid. Redox Signal* **2015**, *22*, 848–870. [CrossRef] [PubMed]

133. Kelleher, Z.T.; Sha, Y.; Foster, M.W.; Foster, W.M.; Forrester, M.T.; Marshall, H.E. Thioredoxin-Mediated Denitrosylation Regulates Cytokine-Induced Nuclear Factor kappaB (NF-kappaB) Activation. *J. Biol. Chem.* **2014**, *289*, 3066–3072. [CrossRef] [PubMed]

134. Takahashi, Y.; Ishii, Y.; Murata, A.; Nagata, T.; Asai, S. Localization of Thioredoxin-Interacting Protein (TXNIP) mRNA in Epithelium of Human Gastrointestinal Tract. *J. Histochem. Cytochem.* **2003**, *51*, 973–976. [CrossRef] [PubMed]

135. Takahashi, Y.; Masuda, H.; Ishii, Y.; Nishida, Y.; Kobayashi, M.; Asai, S. Decreased Expression of Thioredoxin Interacting Protein mRNA in Inflamed Colonic Mucosa in Patients with Ulcerative Colitis. *Oncol. Rep.* **2007**, *18*, 531–536. [CrossRef] [PubMed]

136. Billiet, L.; Furman, C.; Cuaz-Pérolin, C.; Paumelle, R.; Raymondjean, M.; Simmet, T.; Rouis, M. Thioredoxin-1 and its Natural Inhibitor, Vitamin D 3 Up-Regulated Protein 1, are Differentially Regulated by PPARα in Human Macrophages. *J. Mol. Biol.* **2008**, *384*, 564–576. [CrossRef] [PubMed]

137. Chung, J.W.; JEON, J.; YOON, S.; Choi, I. Vitamin D3 Upregulated Protein 1 (VDUP1) is a Regulator for Redox Signaling and Stress-mediated Diseases. *J. Dermatol.* **2006**, *33*, 662–669. [CrossRef]

138. Fedewa, A.; Rao, S.S. Dietary Fructose Intolerance, Fructan Intolerance and FODMAPs. *Curr. Gastroenterol. Rep.* **2014**, *16*, 1–8. [CrossRef]

139. Choi, Y.K.; Johlin, F.C.; Summers, R.W.; Jackson, M.; Rao, S.S. Fructose Intolerance: An Under-Recognized Problem. *Am. J. Gastroenterol.* **2003**, *98*, 1348–1353. [CrossRef]

140. Choi, Y.K.; Kraft, N.; Zimmerman, B.; Jackson, M.; Rao, S.S. Fructose Intolerance in IBS and Utility of Fructose-Restricted Diet. *J. Clin. Gastroenterol.* **2008**, *42*, 233–238. [CrossRef]

141. Buzas, G.M. Fructose and Fructose Intolerance. *Orv. Hetil.* **2016**, *157*, 1708–1716.

142. Rao, S.S.; Attaluri, A.; Anderson, L.; Stumbo, P. Ability of the Normal Human Small Intestine to Absorb Fructose: Evaluation by Breath Testing. *Clin. Gastroenterol. Hepatol.* **2007**, *5*, 959–963. [CrossRef] [PubMed]

143. Yao, C.K.; Tuck, C.J.; Barrett, J.S.; Canale, K.E.; Philpott, H.L.; Gibson, P.R. Poor Reproducibility of Breath Hydrogen Testing: Implications for its Application in Functional Bowel Disorders. *United Eur. Gastroenterol. J.* **2017**, *5*, 284–292. [CrossRef] [PubMed]

144. Rezaie, A.; Buresi, M.; Lembo, A.; Lin, H.; McCallum, R.; Rao, S.; Schmulson, M.; Valdovinos, M.; Zakko, S.; Pimentel, M. Hydrogen and Methane-Based Breath Testing in Gastrointestinal Disorders: The North American Consensus. *Am. J. Gastroenterol.* **2017**, *112*, 775. [CrossRef] [PubMed]

145. Campbell, B.; Han, D.Y.; Triggs, C.M.; Fraser, A.G.; Ferguson, L.R. Brassicaceae: Nutrient Analysis and Investigation of Tolerability in People with Crohn's Disease in a New Zealand Study. *Funct. Foods Health Dis.* **2012**, *2*, 460–486. [CrossRef]

146. Laughlin, M. Normal Roles for Dietary Fructose in Carbohydrate Metabolism. *Nutrients* **2014**, *6*, 3117–3129. [CrossRef] [PubMed]

147. Neu, J.; Rushing, J. Cesarean Versus Vaginal Delivery: Long-Term Infant Outcomes and the Hygiene Hypothesis. *Clin. Perinatol.* **2011**, *38*, 321–331. [CrossRef] [PubMed]

148. Dominguez-Bello, M.G.; Costello, E.K.; Contreras, M.; Magris, M.; Hidalgo, G.; Fierer, N.; Knight, R. Delivery Mode Shapes the Acquisition and Structure of the Initial Microbiota Across Multiple Body Habitats in Newborns. *Proc. Natl. Acad. Sci. USA* **2010**, *107*, 11971–11975. [CrossRef]

149. Stinson, L.F.; Payne, M.S.; Keelan, J.A. A Critical Review of the Bacterial Baptism Hypothesis and the Impact of Caesarean Delivery on the Infant Microbiome. *Front. Med.* **2018**, *5*, 135. [CrossRef]

150. Donovan, S.M.; Wang, M.; Li, M.; Friedberg, I.; Schwartz, S.L.; Chapkin, R.S. Host-Microbe Interactions in the Neonatal Intestine: Role of Human Milk Oligosaccharides. *Adv. Nutr.* **2012**, *3*, 450S–455S. [CrossRef]

151. Wu, S.; Tao, N.; German, J.B.; Grimm, R.; Lebrilla, C.B. Development of an Annotated Library of Neutral Human Milk Oligosaccharides. *J. Proteome Res.* **2010**, *9*, 4138–4151. [CrossRef]

152. Lönnerdal, B. Bioactive Proteins in Breast Milk. *J. Paediatr. Child Health* **2013**, *49*, 1–7. [CrossRef] [PubMed]

153. Andreas, N.J.; Kampmann, B.; Le-Doare, K.M. Human Breast Milk: A Review on its Composition and Bioactivity. *Early Hum. Dev.* **2015**, *91*, 629–635. [CrossRef]

154. Abou-Donia, M.B.; El-Masry, E.M.; Abdel-Rahman, A.A.; McLendon, R.E.; Schiffman, S.S. Splenda Alters Gut Microflora and Increases Intestinal P-Glycoprotein and Cytochrome P-450 in Male Rats. *J. Toxicol. Environ. Health A* **2008**, *71*, 1415–1429. [CrossRef] [PubMed]

155. Mattes, R.D.; Popkin, B.M. Nonnutritive Sweetener Consumption in Humans: Effects on Appetite and Food Intake and their Putative Mechanisms. *Am. J. Clin. Nutr.* **2009**, *89*, 1–14. [CrossRef] [PubMed]

156. Sylvetsky, A.; Rother, K.I.; Brown, R. Artificial Sweetener use among Children: Epidemiology, Recommendations, Metabolic Outcomes, and Future Directions. *Pediatr. Clin. North Am.* **2011**, *58*, 1467–1480. [CrossRef]

157. Sylvetsky, A.C.; Welsh, J.A.; Brown, R.J.; Vos, M.B. Low-Calorie Sweetener Consumption is Increasing in the United States. *Am. J. Clin. Nutr.* **2012**, *96*, 640–646. [CrossRef] [PubMed]

158. Bianchi, R.G.; Muir, E.T.; Cook, D.L.; Nutting, E.F. The Biological Properties of Aspartame. II. Actions Involving the Gastrointestinal System. *J. Environ. Pathol. Toxicol.* **1980**, *3*, 355–362. [PubMed]

159. Spencer, M.; Gupta, A.; Dam, L.V.; Shannon, C.; Menees, S.; Chey, W.D. Artificial Sweeteners: A Systematic Review and Primer for Gastroenterologists. *J. Neurogastroenterol. Motil.* **2016**, *22*, 168–180. [CrossRef]

160. Suez, J.; Korem, T.; Zeevi, D.; Zilberman-Schapira, G.; Thaiss, C.A.; Maza, O.; Israeli, D.; Zmora, N.; Gilad, S.; Weinberger, A. Artificial Sweeteners Induce Glucose Intolerance by Altering the Gut Microbiota. *Nature* **2014**, *514*, 181–186. [CrossRef]

161. Prashant, G.; Patil, R.B.; Nagaraj, T.; Patel, V.B. The Antimicrobial Activity of the Three Commercially Available Intense Sweeteners Against Common Periodontal Pathogens: An in Vitro Study. *J. Contemp. Dent. Pract.* **2012**, *13*, 749–752. [CrossRef]

162. Brusick, D.; Borzelleca, J.F.; Gallo, M.; Williams, G.; Kille, J.; Hayes, A.W.; Pi-Sunyer, F.X.; Williams, C.; Burks, W. Expert Panel Report on a Study of Splenda in Male Rats. *Regul. Toxicol. Pharmacol.* **2009**, *55*, 6–12. [CrossRef] [PubMed]

163. Schiffman, S.S. Rationale for further Medical and Health Research on High-Potency Sweeteners. *Chem. Senses* **2012**, *37*, 671–679. [CrossRef] [PubMed]

164. Suez, J.; Korem, T.; Zilberman-Schapira, G.; Segal, E.; Elinav, E. Non-Caloric Artificial Sweeteners and the Microbiome: Findings and Challenges. *Gut Microbes* **2015**, *6*, 149–155. [CrossRef] [PubMed]

165. Bian, X.; Chi, L.; Gao, B.; Tu, P.; Ru, H.; Lu, K. The Artificial Sweetener Acesulfame Potassium Affects the Gut Microbiome and Body Weight Gain in CD-1 Mice. *PLoS ONE* **2017**, *12*, e0178426. [CrossRef] [PubMed]

166. Chassaing, B.; Koren, O.; Goodrich, J.K.; Poole, A.C.; Srinivasan, S.; Ley, R.E.; Gewirtz, A.T. Dietary Emulsifiers Impact the Mouse Gut Microbiota Promoting Colitis and Metabolic Syndrome. *Nature* **2015**, *519*, 92. [CrossRef]

167. Zinöcker, M.; Lindseth, I. The Western Diet–microbiome-Host Interaction and its Role in Metabolic Disease. *Nutrients* **2018**, *10*, 365. [CrossRef] [PubMed]

168. Wright, G.D. The Antibiotic Resistome: The Nexus of Chemical and Genetic Diversity. *Nat. Rev. Microbiol.* **2007**, *5*, 175–186. [CrossRef]

169. United States Food and Drug Administration. *Summary Report on Antimicrobials Sold or Distributed for Use in Food-Producing Animals*; United States Food and Drug Administration: Silver Spring, MD, USA, 2009.

170. Kedgley, S. Parliament, press release. *Scoop Independent News*, 11 April 2011.

171. Ministry for Primary Industries NZ. *Antbiotic Resistance and Food*; Ministry for Primary Industries NZ: Wellington, New Zealand, 2013.

172. Ruiz-Garbajosa, P.; Bonten, M.J.; Robinson, D.A.; Top, J.; Nallapareddy, S.R.; Torres, C.; Coque, T.M.; Cantón, R.; Baquero, F.; Murray, B.E. Multilocus Sequence Typing Scheme for Enterococcus Faecalis Reveals Hospital-Adapted Genetic Complexes in a Background of High Rates of Recombination. *J. Clin. Microbiol.* **2006**, *44*, 2220–2228. [CrossRef]

173. Pray, L.; Pillsbury, L.; Tomayko, E. *The Human Microbiome, Diet and Health Workshop Summary*; The National Academies Press: Washington, DC, USA, 2012; pp. 5–7.

174. Silbergeld, E.K.; Graham, J.; Price, L.B. Industrial Food Animal Production, Antimicrobial Resistance, and Human Health. *Annu. Rev. Public Health* **2008**, *29*, 151–169. [CrossRef]

175. Lindsey, R.L.; Frye, J.G.; Thitaram, S.N.; Meinersmann, R.J.; Fedorka-Cray, P.J.; Englen, M.D. Characterization of Multidrug-Resistant Escherichia Coli by Antimicrobial Resistance Profiles, Plasmid Replicon Typing, and Pulsed-Field Gel Electrophoresis. *Microb. Drug Resist.* **2011**, *17*, 157–163. [CrossRef]

176. Knight, P.; Campbell, B.J.; Rhodes, J.M. Host-Bacteria Interaction in Inflammatory Bowel Disease. *Br. Med. Bull.* **2008**, *88*, 95–113. [CrossRef] [PubMed]

177. Martin, H.M.; Campbell, B.J.; Hart, C.A.; Mpofu, C.; Nayar, M.; Singh, R.; Englyst, H.; Williams, H.F.; Rhodes, J.M. Enhanced Escherichia Coli Adherence and Invasion in Crohn's Disease and Colon Cancer. *Gastroenterology* **2004**, *127*, 80–93. [CrossRef] [PubMed]

178. Darfeuille-Michaud, A.; Boudeau, J.; Bulois, P.; Neut, C.; Glasser, A.; Barnich, N.; Bringer, M.; Swidsinski, A.; Beaugerie, L.; Colombel, J. High Prevalence of Adherent-Invasive Escherichia Coli Associated with Ileal Mucosa in Crohn's Disease. *Gastroenterology* **2004**, *127*, 412–421. [CrossRef] [PubMed]

179. Gearry, R.B.; Irving, P.M.; Barrett, J.S.; Nathan, D.M.; Shepherd, S.J.; Gibson, P.R. Reduction of Dietary Poorly Absorbed Short-Chain Carbohydrates (FODMAPs) Improves Abdominal Symptoms in Patients with Inflammatory Bowel Disease—A Pilot Study. *J. Crohns Colitis* **2009**, *3*, 8–14. [CrossRef] [PubMed]

180. Barbalho, S.M.; Goulart, R.d.A. Aranão, Ana Luíza de Carvalho; de Oliveira, Pamela Grazielle Correa. Inflammatory Bowel Diseases and Fermentable Oligosaccharides, Disaccharides, Monosaccharides, and Polyols: An Overview. *J. Med. Food* **2018**, *21*, 633–640. [CrossRef] [PubMed]

181. Smith, M.A.; Smith, T.; Trebble, T.M. Nutritional Management of Adults with Inflammatory Bowel Disease: Practical Lessons from the Available Evidence. *Frontline Gastroenterol.* **2012**, *3*, 172–179. [CrossRef] [PubMed]

182. Hill, P.; Muir, J.G.; Gibson, P.R. Controversies and Recent Developments of the Low-FODMAP Diet. *Gastroenterol. Hepatol.* **2017**, *13*, 36–45.

183. Sloan, T.J.; Jalanka, J.; Major, G.A.; Krishnasamy, S.; Pritchard, S.; Abdelrazig, S.; Korpela, K.; Singh, G.; Mulvenna, C.; Hoad, C.L. A Low FODMAP Diet is Associated with Changes in the Microbiota and Reduction in Breath Hydrogen but Not Colonic Volume in Healthy Subjects. *PloS ONE* **2018**, *13*, e0201410. [CrossRef]

184. Mital, B.; Steinkraus, K. Utilization of Oligosaccharides by Lactic Acid Bacteria during Fermentation of Soy Milk. *J. Food Sci.* **1975**, *40*, 114–118. [CrossRef]

185. Naessens, M.; Cerdobbel, A.; Soetaert, W.; Vandamme, E.J. Leuconostoc Dextransucrase and Dextran: Production, Properties and Applications. *J. Chem. Technol. Biotechnol.* **2005**, *80*, 845–860. [CrossRef]

186. Van den Ende, W. Multifunctional Fructans and Raffinose Family Oligosaccharides. *Front. Plant Sci.* **2013**, *4*, 247. [PubMed]

187. Kuo, T.M.; VanMiddlesworth, J.F.; Wolf, W.J. Content of Raffinose Oligosaccharides and Sucrose in various Plant Seeds. *J. Agric. Food Chem.* **1988**, *36*, 32–36. [CrossRef]

188. Wang, Y.; Wang, L. Structures and Properties of Commercial Maltodextrins from Corn, Potato, and Rice Starches. *Starch-Stärke* **2000**, *52*, 296–304. [CrossRef]

189. Plaza-Díaz, J.; Martinez Augustin, O.; Gil Hernández, A. Foods as Sources of Mono and Disaccharides: Biochemical and Metabolic Aspects. *Nutr. Hosp.* **2013**, *28*, 5–16. [PubMed]

190. Calorie Control Council. Polyols. 2018. Available online: https://caloriecontrol.org/category/polyols/ (accessed on 5 November 2018).

191. Ingram, C.J.; Mulcare, C.A.; Itan, Y.; Thomas, M.G.; Swallow, D.M. Lactose Digestion and the Evolutionary Genetics of Lactase Persistence. *Hum. Genet.* **2009**, *124*, 579–591. [CrossRef] [PubMed]

192. Gerbault, P.; Liebert, A.; Itan, Y.; Powell, A.; Currat, M.; Burger, J.; Swallow, D.M.; Thomas, M.G. Evolution of Lactase Persistence: An Example of Human Niche Construction. Philos. *Trans. R. Soc. Lond. B. Biol. Sci.* **2011**, *366*, 863–877. [CrossRef] [PubMed]

193. Brauer, H.A.; Libby, T.E.; Mitchell, B.L.; Li, L.; Chen, C.; Randolph, T.W.; Yasui, Y.Y.; Lampe, J.W.; Lampe, P.D. Cruciferous Vegetable Supplementation in a Controlled Diet Study Alters the Serum Peptidome in a GSTM1-Genotype Dependent Manner. *Nutr. J.* **2011**, *10*, 11. [CrossRef]

194. Kristal, A.R.; Lampe, J.W. Brassica Vegetables and Prostate Cancer Risk: A Review of the Epidemiological Evidence. *Nutr. Cancer* **2002**, *42*, 1–9. [CrossRef]

195. Laing, B.; Han, D.Y.; Ferguson, L.R. Candidate Genes Involved in Beneficial or Adverse Responses to Commonly Eaten Brassica Vegetables in a New Zealand Crohn's Disease Cohort. *Nutrients* **2013**, *5*, 5046–5064. [CrossRef]

196. Higdon, J.V.; Delage, B.; Williams, D.E.; Dashwood, R.H. Cruciferous Vegetables and Human Cancer Risk: Epidemiologic Evidence and Mechanistic Basis. *Pharmacol. Res.* **2007**, *55*, 224–236. [CrossRef]

197. NIH. Celiac Disease. In *Genetics Home Reference*; NIH: Stapleton, NY, USA, 2013.

198. Petermann, I.; Triggs, C.M.; Huebner, C.; Han, D.Y.; Gearry, R.B.; Barclay, M.L.; Demmers, P.S.; McCulloch, A.; Ferguson, L.R. Mushroom Intolerance: A Novel Diet-Gene Interaction in Crohn's Disease. *Br. J. Nutr.* **2009**, *102*, 506. [CrossRef] [PubMed]

199. Campbell, A.K.; Matthews, S.B.; Vassel, N.; Cox, C.D.; Naseem, R.; Chaich, i.J.; Holland, I.B.; Green, J.; Wann, K.T. Bacterial Metabolic 'Toxins': A New Mechanism for Lactose and Food Intolerance, and Irritable Bowel Syndrome. *Toxicology* **2010**, *278*, 268–276. [CrossRef] [PubMed]

200. FAO/WHO. *Carbohydrates in Human Nutrition*; Report of a Joint FAO/WHO Expert Consultation; FAO Food and Nutrition Paper; FAO: Rome, Italy, 1998.

201. Hyams, J.S. Sorbitol Intolerance: An Unappreciated Cause of Functional Gastrointestinal Complaints. *Gastroenterology* **1983**, *84*, 30–33. [PubMed]

202. Gibson, P.R.; Shepherd, S.J. Evidence-based Dietary Management of Functional Gastrointestinal Symptoms: The FODMAP Approach. *J. Gastroenterol. Hepatol.* **2010**, *25*, 252–258. [CrossRef] [PubMed]

203. Catassi, G.; Lionetti, E.; Gatti, S.; Catassi, C. The Low FODMAP Diet: Many Question Marks for a Catchy Acronym. *Nutrients* **2017**, *9*, 292. [CrossRef] [PubMed]

204. Qin, J.; Li, R.; Raes, J.; Arumugam, M.; Burgdorf, K.S.; Manichanh, C.; Nielsen, T.; Pons, N.; Levenez, F.; Yamada, T. A Human Gut Microbial Gene Catalogue Established by Metagenomic Sequencing. *Nature* **2010**, *464*, 59–65. [CrossRef] [PubMed]

205. Ley, R.E.; Peterson, D.A.; Gordon, J.I. Ecological and Evolutionary Forces Shaping Microbial Diversity in the Human Intestine. *Cell* **2006**, *124*, 837–848. [CrossRef]

206. Turnbaugh, P.J.; Ley, R.E.; Mahowald, M.A.; Magrini, V.; Mardis, E.R.; Gordon, J.I. An Obesity-Associated Gut Microbiome with Increased Capacity for Energy Harvest. *Nature* **2006**, *444*, 1027–1131. [CrossRef]

207. Frank, D.N.; Robertson, C.E.; Hamm, C.M.; Kpadeh, Z.; Zhang, T.; Chen, H.; Zhu, W.; Sartor, R.B.; Boedeker, E.C.; Harpaz, N. Disease Phenotype and Genotype are Associated with Shifts in Intestinal-Associated Microbiota in Inflammatory Bowel Diseases. *Inflamm. Bowel Dis.* **2010**, *17*, 179–184. [CrossRef]

208. Frank, D.N.; St Amand, A.L.; Feldman, R.A.; Boedeker, E.C.; Harpaz, N.; Pace, N.R. Molecular-Phylogenetic Characterization of Microbial Community Imbalances in Human Inflammatory Bowel Diseases. *Proc. Natl. Acad. Sci. USA* **2007**, *104*, 13780–13785. [CrossRef]

209. Walker, A.W.; Sanderson, J.D.; Churcher, C.; Parkes, G.C.; Hudspith, B.N.; Rayment, N.; Brostoff, J.; Parkhill, J.; Dougan, G.; Petrovska, L. High-Throughput Clone Library Analysis of the Mucosa-Associated Microbiota Reveals Dysbiosis and Differences between Inflamed and Non-Inflamed Regions of the Intestine in Inflammatory Bowel Disease. *BMC Microbiol.* **2011**, *11*, 7. [CrossRef] [PubMed]

210. Nagalingam, N.A.; Lynch, S.V. Role of the Microbiota in Inflammatory Bowel Diseases. *Inflamm. Bowel Dis.* **2012**, *18*, 968–984. [CrossRef] [PubMed]

211. Wacklin, P.; Mäkivuokko, H.; Alakulppi, N.; Nikkilä, J.; Tenkanen, H.; Räbinä, J.; Partanen, J.; Aranko, K.; Mättö, J. Secretor Genotype (FUT2 Gene) is Strongly Associated with the Composition of Bifidobacteria in the Human Intestine. *PLoS ONE* **2011**, *6*, e20113. [CrossRef] [PubMed]

212. McGovern, D.P.; Jones, M.R.; Taylor, K.D.; Marciante, K.; Yan, X.; Dubinsky, M.; Ippoliti, A.; Vasiliauskas, E.; Berel, D.; Derkowski, C. Fucosyltransferase 2 (FUT2) Non-Secretor Status is Associated with Crohn's Disease. *Hum. Mol. Genet.* **2010**, *19*, 3468–3476. [CrossRef] [PubMed]

213. Miyoshi, J.; Yajima, T.; Okamoto, S.; Matsuoka, K.; Inoue, N.; Hisamatsu, T.; Shimamura, K.; Nakazawa, A.; Kanai, T.; Ogata, H. Ectopic Expression of Blood Type Antigens in Inflamed Mucosa with Higher Incidence of FUT2 Secretor Status in Colonic Crohn's Disease. *J. Gastroenterol.* **2011**, *46*, 1056–1063. [CrossRef]

214. Rausch, P.; Rehman, A.; Künzel, S.; Häsler, R.; Ott, S.J.; Schreiber, S.; Rosenstiel, P.; Franke, A.; Baines, J.F. Colonic Mucosa-Associated Microbiota is Influenced by an Interaction of Crohn Disease and FUT2 (Secretor) Genotype. *Proc. Natl. Acad. Sci. USA* **2011**, *108*, 19030–19035. [CrossRef] [PubMed]

215. Salminen, S.; Gueimonde, M. Gut Microbiota in Infants between 6 and 24 Months of Age. *Nestle Nutr. Workshop Ser. Pediatr. Program.* **2005**, *56*, 43–56.

216. Ebaid, H.; Hassanein, K.A. Comparative Immunomudulating Effects of Five Orally Administrated Bifidobacteria Species in Male Albino Rats. *Egypt. J. Biol.* **2007**, *9*, 14–23.

217. Festen, E.A.; Goyette, P.; Green, T.; Boucher, G.; Beauchamp, C.; Trynka, G.; Dubois, P.C.; Lagacé, C.; Stokkers, P.C.; Hommes, D.W. A Meta-Analysis of Genome-Wide Association Scans Identifies IL18RAP, PTPN2, TAGAP, and PUS10 as Shared Risk Loci for Crohn's Disease and Celiac Disease. *PLoS Genet.* **2011**, *7*, e1001283. [CrossRef]

218. Visser, R.; Barrett, K.; McCole, D. Regulation of Epithelial Barrier Function by Crohn's Disease Associated Gene PTPN. *BMC Proc.* **2012**, *6*, O41. [CrossRef]

219. Armstrong, D.; Don-Wauchope, A.C.; Verdu, E.F. Testing for Gluten-Related Disorders in Clinical Practice: The Role of Serology in Managing the Spectrum of Gluten Sensitivity. Can. *J. Gastroenterol.* **2011**, *25*, 193–197. [CrossRef] [PubMed]

220. Mishkin, S. Controversies regarding the Role of Dairy-Products in Inflammatory Bowel Disease. *Can. J. Gastroenterol.* **1994**, *8*, 205–212. [CrossRef]

221. Truelove, S.C. Ulcerative Colitis Provoked by Milk. Br. *Med. J.* **1961**, *1*, 154–160. [CrossRef] [PubMed]

222. Wright, R.; Truelove, S.C. A Controlled Therapeutic Trial of various Diets in Ulcerative Colitis. *Br. Med. J.* **1965**, *2*, 138–141. [CrossRef] [PubMed]

223. Mishkin, S. Dairy Sensitivity, Lactose Malabsorption, and Elimination Diets in Inflammatory Bowel Disease. *Am. J. Clin. Nutr.* **1997**, *65*, 564–567. [CrossRef]

224. Maconi, G.; Ardizzone, S.; Cucino, C.; Bezzio, C.; Russo, A.G.; Bianchi Porro, G. Pre-Illness Changes in Dietary Habits and Diet as a Risk Factor for Inflammatory Bowel Disease: A Case-Control Study. *World J. Gastroenterol.* **2010**, *16*, 4297–4304. [CrossRef] [PubMed]

225. Nolan-Clark, D.; Tapsell, L.C.; Hu, R.; Han, D.Y.; Ferguson, L.R. Effects of Dairy Products on Crohn's Disease Symptoms are Influenced by Fat Content and Disease Location but Not Lactose Content or Disease Activity Status in a New Zealand Population. *J. Am. Diet. Assoc.* **2011**, *111*, 1165–1172. [CrossRef]

226. Nolan, D.; Han, D.; Lam, W.; Morgan, A.; Fraser, A.; Tapsell, L.; Ferguson, L. Genetic Adult Lactase Persistence is Associated with Risk of Crohn's Disease in a New Zealand Population. *BMC Res. Notes* **2010**, *3*, 339. [CrossRef]

227. Shrier, I.; Szilagyi, A.; Correa, J.A. Impact of Lactose Containing Foods and the Genetics of Lactase on Diseases: An Analytical Review of Population Data. *Nutr. Cancer* **2008**, *60*, 292–300. [CrossRef]

228. Barbado, M.; Fablet, K.; Ronjat, M.; De Waard, M. Gene Regulation by Voltage-Dependent Calcium Channels. Biochim. *Biophys. Acta* **2009**, *1793*, 1096–1104. [CrossRef]

229. Bernstein, C.N.; Leslie, W.D.; Leboff, M.S. AGA Technical Review on Osteoporosis in Gastrointestinal Diseases. *Gastroenterology* **2003**, *124*, 795–841. [CrossRef] [PubMed]

230. Caniggia, A.; Nuti, R.; Lore, F.; Vattimo, A. Pathophysiology of the Adverse Effects of Glucoactive Corticosteroids on Calcium Metabolism in Man. *J. Steroid Biochem.* **1981**, *15*, 153–161. [CrossRef]

231. New Zealand Nutrition Foundation. Calcium. 2018. Available online: https://nutritionfoundation.org.nz/ nutrients-vitamins-and-minerals/calcium (accessed on 15 June 2019).

232. Burlingame, B.A.; Milligan, G.; Apimerika, D.; Arthur, J. *The Concise New Zealand Food Composition Tables*; New Zealand Institute for Crop & Food Research: Auckland, New Zealand, 2009.

233. Duke, J.; Beckstrom-Sternberg, S. *Phytochemical Database USDA-ARS-NGRL*; Beltsbille Agricultural Research Center: Beltsbille, MD, USA, 1998.

234. Parl, F.F. Glutathione S-Transferase Genotypes and Cancer Risk. *Cancer Lett.* **2005**, *221*, 123–129. [CrossRef] [PubMed]

235. Beckett, G.J.; Hayes, J.D. Glutathione S-Transferases: Biomedical Applications. *Adv. Clin. Chem.* **1993**, *30*, 282.

236. Wilce, M.C.; Parker, M.W. Structure and Function of Glutathione S-Transferases. *Biochim. Biophys. Acta* **1994**, *1205*, 1–18. [CrossRef]

237. Webb, G.; Vaska, V.; Coggan, M.; Board, P. Chromosomal Localization of the Gene for the Human Theta Class Glutathione Transferase (GSTT1). *Genomics* **1996**, *33*, 121–123. [CrossRef]

238. Sheehan, D.; Meade, G.; Foley, V.; Dowd, C. Structure, Function and Evolution of Glutathione Transferases: Implications for Classification of Non-Mammalian Members of an Ancient Enzyme Superfamily. *Biochem. J.* **2001**, *360*, 1–16. [CrossRef]

239. Hayes, J.D.; Strange, R.C. Glutathione S-Transferase Polymorphisms and their Biological Consequences. *Pharmacology* **2000**, *61*, 154–166. [CrossRef]

240. Inskip, A.; Elexperu-Camiruaga, J.; Buxton, N.; Dias, P.; MacIntosh, J.; Campbell, D.; Jones, P.; Yengi, L.; Talbot, J.; Strange, R. Identification of Polymorphism at the Glutathione S-Transferase, GSTM3 Locus: Evidence for Linkage with GSTM1* A. *Biochem. J.* **1995**, *312*, 713. [CrossRef]

241. Seow, A.; Yuan, J.; Sun, C.; Van Den Berg, D.; Lee, H.; Mimi, C.Y. Dietary Isothiocyanates, Glutathione S-Transferase Polymorphisms and Colorectal Cancer Risk in the Singapore Chinese Health Study. *Carcinogenesis* **2002**, *23*, 2055–2061. [CrossRef]

242. Steck, S.E.; Hebert, J.R. GST Polymorphism and Excretion of Heterocyclic Aromatic Amine and Isothiocyanate Metabolites After Brassica Consumption. *Environ. Mol. Mutagen.* **2009**, *50*, 238–246. [CrossRef]

243. Campbell, B.; Han, D.; Jiun, W.; Morgan, A.; Triggs, C.; Fraser, A.C.; Ferguson, L.R. Deletion of the *GSTT1* Genotype Linked to Tolerance of Brassicaceae in People with Crohn's Disease in a New Zealand Cohort. In Proceedings of the Annual Scientific Meeting of the Nutrition Society of New Zealand Auckland, Auckland, New Zealand, 21–22 November 2012.

244. Gentschew, L.; Bishop, K.S.; Han, D.Y.; Morgan, A.R.; Fraser, A.G.; Lam, W.J.; Karunasinghe, N.; Campbell, B.; Ferguson, L.R. Selenium, Selenoprotein Genes and Crohn's Disease in a Case-Control Population from Auckland, New Zealand. *Nutrients* **2012**, *4*, 1247–1259. [CrossRef] [PubMed]

245. Ahmad, T.; Marshall, S.E.; Jewell, D. Genetics of Inflammatory Bowel Disease: The Role of the HLA Complex. *World J. Gastroenterol.* **2006**, *12*, 3628. [CrossRef] [PubMed]

246. Lees, C.W.; Satsangi, J. Genetics of Inflammatory Bowel Disease: Implications for Disease Pathogenesis and Natural History. *Expert Rev. Gastroenterol. Hepatol.* **2009**, *3*, 513–534. [CrossRef] [PubMed]

247. Annese, V.; Piepoli, A.; Latiano, A.; Lombardi, G.; Napolitano, G.; Caruso, N.; Cocchiara, E.; Accadia, L.; Perri, F.; Andriulli, A. HLA-DRB1 Alleles may Influence Disease Phenotype in Patients with Inflammatory Bowel Disease: A Critical Reappraisal with Review of the Literature. *Dis. Colon. Rectum.* **2005**, *48*, 57–65. [CrossRef] [PubMed]

248. Moffatt, M.F.; Gut, I.G.; Demenais, F.; Strachan, D.P.; Bouzigon, E.; Heath, S.; Von Mutius, E.; Farrall, M.; Lathrop, M.; Cookson, W.O. A Large-Scale, Consortium-Based Genomewide Association Study of Asthma. *N. Engl. J. Med.* **2010**, *363*, 1211–1221. [CrossRef] [PubMed]

249. Levin, A.; Mathias, R.; Huang, L.R.; Roth, L.A.; Daley, D.; Myers, R.A.; Himes, B.E.; Romieu, I.; Yang, M.; Eng, C.; et al. *A Meta-Analysis of Genome Wide Association Studies for Serum Total IgE in Diverse Populations Groups*; American Academy of Allergy, Asthma and Immunology: Milwaukee, WI, USA, 2013; p. 1176.

250. Gould, H.J.; Sutton, B.J.; Beavil, A.J.; Beavil, R.L.; McCloskey, N.; Coker, H.A.; Fear, D.; Smurthwaite, L. The Biology of IgE and the Basis of Allergic Disease. *Annu. Rev. Immunol.* **2003**, *21*, 579–628. [CrossRef]

251. Marlow, G.; Han, D.Y.; Triggs, C.M.; Ferguson, L.R. Food Intolerance: Associations with the rs12212067 Polymorphism of FOXO3 in Crohn's Disease Patients in New Zealand. *J. Nutrigen. Nutrigen.* **2015**, *8*, 70–80. [CrossRef]

252. Food Safety Authority of Ireland. Food Ingredients that must be Declared as Allergens in the EU. Available online: https://www.fsai.ie/legislation/food_legislation/food_information/14_allergens.html (accessed on 2 February 2019).

253. Wedzicha, B.L. *Chemistry of Sulphur Dioxide in Foods*; Elsevier Applied Science Publishers Ltd.: Amsterdam, The Netherlands, 1984.

254. Coates, P.M.; Blackman, M.; Betz, J.; Cragg, G.M.; Levine, M.; Moss, J.; White, J.D. *Encyclopedia of Dietary Supplements*; Informa Healthcare: London, UK, 2010.

255. Costantini, A.; Pala, M.I. Thiamine and Fatigue in Inflammatory Bowel Diseases: An Open-Label Pilot Study. *J. Altern. Complement. Med.* **2013**, *19*, 704–708. [CrossRef]

256. Magee, E.A.; Edmond, L.M.; Tasker, S.M.; Kong, S.C.; Curno, R.; Cummings, J.H. Associations between Diet and Disease Activity in Ulcerative Colitis Patients using a Novel Method of Data Analysis. *Nutr. J.* **2005**, *4*, 7. [CrossRef]

257. Pitcher, M.C.; Cummings, J.H. Hydrogen Sulphide: A Bacterial Toxin in Ulcerative Colitis? *Gut* **1996**, *39*, 1–4. [CrossRef] [PubMed]

258. Marcus, R.; Watt, J. Seaweeds and Ulcerative Colitis in Laboratory Animals. *Lancet* **1969**, *2*, 489–490. [CrossRef]

259. Marcus, R.; Watt, J. Ulcerative Disease of the Colon in Laboratory Animals Induced by Pepsin Inhibitors. *Gastroenterology* **1974**, *67*, 473–483. [CrossRef]

260. Roediger, W. The Colonic Epithelium in Ulcerative Colitis: An Energy-Deficiency Disease? *Lancet* **1980**, *316*, 712–715. [CrossRef]

261. Peng, L.; Li, Z.; Green, R.S.; Holzman, I.R.; Lin, J. Butyrate Enhances the Intestinal Barrier by Facilitating Tight Junction Assembly Via Activation of AMP-Activated Protein Kinase in Caco-2 Cell Monolayers. *J. Nutr.* **2009**, *139*, 1619–1625. [CrossRef] [PubMed]

262. Carbonero, F.; Benefiel, A.C.; Alizadeh-Ghamsari, A.H.; Gaskins, H.R. Microbial Pathways in Colonic Sulfur Metabolism and Links with Health and Disease. *Front. Physiol.* **2012**, *3*, 448. [CrossRef] [PubMed]

263. Berezowska, A.; Fischer, A.R.; Ronteltap, A.; Lans, I.A.; Trijp, H.C. Consumer Adoption of Personalised Nutrition Services from the Perspective of a Risk–benefit Trade-Off. *Genes Nutr.* **2015**, *10*, 42. [CrossRef]

264. Nutrisearch. Fitgenes (DNA Testing). 2018. Available online: https://www.nutrisearch.co.nz/lab-diagnostics/fitgenes-dna-testing/ (accessed on 13 June 2018).

265. Zettler, P.J.; Sherkow, J.S.; Greely, H.T. 23 and Me, the Food and Drug Administration, and the Future of Genetic Testing. *JAMA Intern. Med.* **2014**, *174*, 493–494. [CrossRef]

266. Annas, G.J.; Elias, S. 23andMe and the FDA. *N. Engl. J. Med.* **2014**, *370*, 985–988. [CrossRef]

Cross-Sectional Analysis of Overall Dietary Intake and Mediterranean Dietary Pattern in Patients with Crohn's Disease

Lorian Taylor [1], Abdulelah Almutairdi [1], Nusrat Shommu [1], Richard Fedorak [2], Subrata Ghosh [3], Raylene A. Reimer [4], Remo Panaccione [1] and Maitreyi Raman [1,*]

[1] Department of Medicine, University of Calgary, Calgary, AB T2N 4N1, Canada; lorian.taylor@ucalgary.ca (L.T.); abdulelah.almutairdi@ucalgary.ca (A.A.); nsshommu@ucalgary.ca (N.S.); rpanacci@ucalgary.ca (R.P.)

[2] Faculty of Medicine & Dentistry, University of Alberta, Edmonton, AB T6G 2R7, Canada; richard.fedorak@ualberta.ca

[3] Institute of Translational Medicine, NIHR Biomedical Research Centre, University of Birmingham and Birmingham University Hospitals, Birmingham B15 2TT, UK; s.ghosh@bham.ac.uk

[4] Faculty of Kinesiology, University of Calgary, Calgary, AB T2N 4N1, Canada; reimer@ucalgary.ca

[*] Correspondence: mkothand@ucalgary.ca

Abstract: The primary objective of this study was to explore the macro- and micro-nutrient intakes and dietary patterns of patients with Crohn's disease (CD). Secondary objectives were to (a) compare the micronutrient intakes of CD patients with a representative sample of individuals, (b) describe the macro- and micronutrient intakes of male and female CD patients, and (c) describe Mediterranean diet scores (P-MDS) of male and female CD patients in remission that were recruited from an inflammatory bowel disease (IBD) clinic in Calgary, AB. Consecutive patients with ileal and/or colonic CD in endoscopic remission were recruited for participation in this cross-sectional study. Sixty-seven patients were enrolled with a mean age of 45, and a Body Mass Index (BMI) $\geq$ 25. Compared with the representative sample, patients with CD had similar energy, protein, carbohydrate, and total fat intake. However, polyunsaturated fats (PUFA), omega-6 and 3, and monounsaturated fats (MUFA) were lower in CD patients and dietary fiber intake was higher ($p < 0.05$). Vitamins C, D, thiamin, niacin, magnesium, phosphorus, zinc, and potassium were all significantly lower in all CD patients when compared to the representative sample ($p < 0.05$). Few patients with CD met the P-MDS criteria and overall scores were low (mean 4.5, Standard Deviation (SD) = 1.1 in males and 4.7, SD = 1.8 in females). The CD patients in this study had suboptimal dietary intakes and patterns and these data may be used to inform future dietary interventions in this population to improve intake.

Keywords: Crohn's disease; dietary intake; malnutrition; Mediterranean diet

---

1. Introduction

There is a compelling argument for environmental factors such as diet to play a role in the course of inflammatory bowel disease (IBD) [1]. Given the mounting evidence for the role of diet and gut microbial composition and function in IBD development and exacerbation, a richer understanding of the role of diet in disease pathogenesis is warranted. Perturbations related to dietary intake are thought to relate to the consumption of a dietary pattern that negatively alters gut microbiota composition [2,3], leading to functional changes in short chain fatty acid (SCFA) profiles affecting the inflammation process [4] and stimulating an inappropriate immune activation of the gut mucosa.

There are limited published data describing the dietary patterns and macro- and micronutrient intakes in patients with Crohn's disease (CD); in particular, the differences between males and females.

Nearly 50% of CD patients perceive diet to be an initiating factor in their disease, and over half of patients have reported diet exacerbates disease severity [5]. In IBD, deficiencies of micro- and macronutrients are observed and arise through multifactorial etiologies including disruptions in digestion, malabsorption, and disease activity, resulting in increased energy and nutrient requirements, anorexia, consumption of a nondiversified diet with food avoidance due to symptoms, and cachexia arising as a consequence of pro-inflammatory cytokines [6]. The reported prevalence of malnutrition is variable (12–85%) [7–9] and depends on disease activity and the definitions used to define malnutrition. Nutrient deficiencies usually develop over time and are linked to duration of illness. Macronutrient deficiencies leading to protein-energy malnutrition are less common in the biologic era, however, they are still of significant prevalence in patients admitted to hospital. Overt malnutrition may lead to complications such as frequent infections, poor immunity, and increased hospitalizations [10]. Micronutrient deficiencies occur for multiple reasons including chronic blood loss leading to iron deficiency; chronic diarrhea resulting in hypomagnesemia or zinc deficiency; malabsorption leading to B12, folate, and vitamin D deficiencies; and other deficiencies such as antioxidants [11,12]. No previous study has reported the prevalence of macro- and micronutrient deficiencies in Canadian CD patients compared to a representative population.

While single nutrients may play a role in the natural history of IBD [13,14], single nutrients are rarely consumed in isolation. Specific to IBD, epidemiological studies have described associations of increased risk of IBD and high dietary intake of refined sugar, grains, calories, animal fat from meat and dairy, and regular intake of processed foods, while a diet high in fruit, vegetables, and dietary fiber decreases risk [15,16]. A recent meta-analysis showed an inverse association between the intake of vegetables and fruit and CD, respectively (pooled odds ratio for the highest versus lowest consumption of fruit = 0.57; 95% Confidence Interval (CI) 0.44–0.74) [17]. Patients consuming a pro-inflammatory diet (e.g., high in animal protein, low in fruit and vegetables) have demonstrated a higher risk of ulcerative colitis [18]. Recently, the association between food intake and course of disease in patients with IBD was explored using fecal calprotectin and a protective role of legumes and potato, with a detrimental influence of meat in maintaining clinical remission in IBD was identified [19].

There is a large body of evidence showing Mediterranean dietary patterns regulate inflammation in chronic disease [20–22]. A Mediterranean dietary pattern is high in extra-virgin olive oil, vegetables, fruit, legumes, nuts, and seeds with a moderate consumption of fish, poultry, and milk products and is low in processed foods, baked goods, and red and processed meat. This dietary pattern is high in monounsaturated fats (MUFA), omega-3 polyunsaturated fats (PUFA), fermentable fibers and polyphenols, and adherence to a Mediterranean dietary pattern is associated with lower levels of inflammation biomarkers. A Mediterranean dietary pattern has shown positive effects in chronic disease [23], although it may impact men and women differently [24], and has been understudied in IBD.

The primary objective of this study was to examine the macro- and micro-nutrient intakes and dietary patterns of patients with CD to inform future dietary interventions. Secondary objectives were to (a) compare micronutrient intakes of CD patients to a representative sample of individuals, (b) describe macro- and micronutrient intakes of male and female CD patients, and (c) describe the Mediterranean diet scores (P-MDS) of male and female CD patients in a Canadian ambulatory care gastroenterology clinical setting.

2. Methods

2.1. Study Design and Recruitment

A single center cross-sectional study was undertaken at the University of Calgary, Foothills Medical Center, in Calgary, AB, Canada. Eligible patients were recruited consecutively from ambulatory gastrointestinal clinics at this site.

2.2. Eligibility Criteria

To be eligible for the study, patients were required to: (a) be ≥18 years of age; (b) have a documented diagnosis of ileal and/or colonic CD based on clinical, radiological and endoscopic criteria; (c) be in clinical and endoscopic remission, defined by a Harvey Bradshaw Index (HBI) <5 with evidence of mucosal healing by endoscopy defined by no large ulcers, inflammation, or strictures, within three months of recruitment; (d) been in steroid-free remission for three months prior to study entry; (e) achieved induction of remission either through anti-tumor necrosis factor (anti-TNF) agents or corticosteroids; and (f) provide informed consent. Patients were excluded if: (a) HBI >5, (b) had evidence of active endoscopic mucosal disease, (c) used corticosteroids within the preceding three months, (d) had >1 bowel resection, (d) presence of ostomy, (e) used laxatives in the past 3 months, (f) used prebiotic fiber supplements in the past three months, (f) used probiotic supplements in the past three months, and (g) used antibiotics in the past six months.

2.3. Ethics and Consent

The study protocol was approved by the University of Calgary Conjoint Health Research Ethics Board REB15-1805. All participants provided informed written consent prior to participating in the study.

2.4. Data Collection

Patient characteristics, medications, and symptoms were extracted from the patients' medical record and confirmed with the patient during their first study visit. The following data were collected: age, sex, HBI, recent endoscopic findings, current medication, previous IBD surgery, last use of antibiotics and/or probiotics, corticosteroids, and laxative use.

Dietary intake was collected using prospective 3-day weighed food records. Eligible patients met with the study coordinator to receive training on how to record an accurate 3-day weighed food record. Patients were instructed to document all food and drinks consumed and preparation method on two representative weekdays, and one weekend day. The food records were then reviewed by the study dietitian (RD) with the patient to identify any missing food or drink items.

Three-day dietary intake data were subsequently entered and analyzed using ESHA Food Analysis Software (Version 11.3 X, ESHA Food Processor Nutrition Analysis Software, Salem OR, USA) [25]. Intake data was reviewed for acceptable ranges of macro- and micronutrients. Adherence to a Mediterranean diet was measured using an adapted 13-item PREDIMED Mediterranean Diet Score (P-MDS) [26]; points were not given for red wine consumption considering the impact alcohol consumption may have on symptoms related to IBD. Each item in the P-MDS received a score of 0 or 1, and items were evenly weighted. Total P-MDS scores ranged from 0–13.

Macro- and micronutrient intakes of CD patients were compared to population usual nutrient intakes from the Canadian Community Health Survey (CCHS; Cycle 2.2) [27]. A complete description of the sampling frame is provided in the following documentation by Statistics Canada (www.statcan.ca/cgi-bin/imdb/p2SV.pl?FunctioN=getSurvey&SDDS=5049&lang=en&db=IMDB&dbg=f&adm=8&dis=2#b3). The sampling strategy was designed to provide a representative sample based on age, sex, geography, and socioeconomic status [28]. The CCHS used interviews to collect 24-h recall data with a subsample of respondents completing a second recall. To transfer daily intake into usual intake, a measurement error model was used to reduce the effect of within-individual variance and measure between-individual variance [27]. Data were compared for the following parameters: (a) total energy intake in kilocalories (kcal); (b) protein, carbohydrate, fiber, total fat, and PUFA including omega-6 and 3, MUFA and saturated fat (SFA) as proportions of total energy intake; and (c) select micronutrients (vitamins and minerals) reported as a percentage of daily recommended intakes (DRI) and mean daily/usual intakes.

2.5. Statistical Analysis

Statistical analysis was carried out using SPSS (IBM Corp. Version 24.0, Armonk, NY, USA). Data were expressed as means with standard deviation (SD) or standard errors (SE) where it facilitated a comparison with normative population data. Median and interquartile ranges (IQR) were presented for P-MDS due to the variability of the data. Comparisons were done using independent sample t-tests to identify mean differences between males and females and between CD patients' and population usual intakes. Chi-squared tests were conducted to identify gender differences in P-MDS for categorical variables and independent sample t-tests were used for mean P-MDS scores. Statistical significance was established at $p < 0.05$.

3. Results

3.1. Demographic and Health

Eighty-seven patients were originally recruited to participate, but complete dietary data were only completed by sixty-seven patients. These 67 patients had a mean age of 45, and a mean BMI characterized as overweight (Table 1). Most patients (female = 88%, male = 73%) were receiving anti-TNF maintenance therapy. Patients who were not receiving anti-TNF therapies were not on other IBD specific therapies including dietary therapies. Less than half of the study participants received immunomodulators. Close to one quarter of patients had one previous small bowel resection, none had colonic resections, and no patients had an ileostomy.

Table 1. Patient demographics and health information.

	Female N = 34	Male N = 33
Age in years (mean, SD)	44.7 (14.4)	49.7 (12.7)
BMI (kg/m^2; mean, SD)	27.8 (6.1)	26.7 (3.9)
Anti-TNF n, (%)	30 (88.2%)	24 (72.7%)
IMM n, (%)	15 (44.1%)	14 (42.4%)
Previous bowel surgery n, (%)	7 (20.6%)	11 (33.3%)

Abbreviations: SD: Standard Deviation, BMI: body mass index, Anti-TNF: Anti-tumor necrosis factor, IMM: Receiving immunomodulators.

3.2. Macronutrient Intake

Compared with the representative sample, male and female patients with CD had similar energy, protein, carbohydrate, and total fat intake (Table 2). However, fat intake from PUFA, omega-6, omega-3 in females only, and MUFA were significantly lower in patients with CD when compared to the representative sample of Albertans (Table 2). Dietary fiber intake was significantly higher in patients with CD when compared to the representative sample.

Table 2. Macronutrient composition compared to current guidelines.

Macronutrient	DRI Acceptable Macronutrient Distribution Range (AMDR) and Adequate Intake (AI) [29]	Academy of Nutrition and Dietetics [30]	Crohn's Patients (N = 67; Mean ± SE)		Representative Sample (N = 1547; Mean ± SE) [27]	
			M (N = 33)	F (N = 34)	M (N = 721)	F (N = 826)
Total energy intake (kcal/d)	Male = 662 − (9.53 × age (y)) + PA × {(15.91 × weight (kg)) + (539.6 × height (m))}, Female/Women = 354 − (6.91 × age (y)) + PA × {(9.36 × weight (kg)) + (726 × height (m))}		2358 (95.3)	1881 (86.5)	2346 (61)	1730 (42)
Protein (% total energy)	10–35% total energy		18.3 (1.0)	18.0 (0.7)	17.0 (0.4)	16.8 (0.3)
Carbohydrate (% total energy)	45–65% total energy		47.1 (1.5)	48.1 (1.1)	48.7 (0.9)	48.5 (0.6)
Fiber (g/day) ^	M: 30–38 F: 21–25		22.8 (1.4) *	20.9 (1.6) *	19.2 (0.6)	13.9 (0.5)
Total fat (% total energy)	20–35% total energy		33.7 (1.2)	34.3 (1.0)	31.0 (0.8)	32.4 (0.6)
PUFA (% total energy)	5–10% total energy	3–10% total energy	4.5 (0.4) *	3.9 (0.3) *	5.6 (0.2)	5.6 (0.1)
Omega-6 (linoleic)	5–10% total energy	3–10% total energy	3.3 (0.4) *	2.8 (0.2) *	4.5 (0.1)	4.5 (0.2)
Omega-3 (α-linolenic)	0.6–1.2% total energy	0.6–1.2% total energy	0.6 (0.15)	0.5 (0.09) *	0.8 (0.04)	0.8 (0.02)
MUFA (% total energy)	No AI level	15–20% total energy	8.2 (0.6)*	7.1 (0.5) *	12.6 (0.4)	12.8 (0.2)
SFA (% total energy)	As low as possible	7–10% of total energy <7% to reduce CVD risk 5–6% to lower lipids	10.7 (0.4)	11.1 (0.5)	9.8 (0.2)	10.7 (0.3)
TransFA (% total energy)	As low as possible	<1% total energy	0.4 (0.1)	0.3 (0.1)	unavailable	

Abbreviations: Dietary reference intakes (DRI), Male (M), Female (F), Polyunsaturated fatty acids (PUFA), Monounsaturated fatty acids (MUFA), Saturated Fatty Acids (SFA), Cardiovascular disease (CVD), Males (M), Females (F). TransFA, Trans Fatty Acids. * Indicates significant differences between patients with Crohn's compared to Albertan population, results are gender specific ($p < 0.05$). ^ Higher values are for adults 19–50 years.

3.3. Vitamin Intake

Vitamin comparisons are all listed in Table 3. Compared to the representative sample, vitamins C, D, thiamin, and niacin were significantly lower in male and female patients with CD, whereas a lower intake of riboflavin and pyridoxine was observed only in female patients with CD, and lower folate intake was noted only in males with CD. Males compared to female patients with CD had a significantly lower intake of vitamin K, and higher thiamin, niacin, pyridoxine, and biotin intakes. Compared to the DRIs, both male and female patients had inadequate intakes of vitamins A, D, E, pantothenic acid, biotin, folate, and choline, although there was a high level of variation around the mean scores. Representative sample data for some vitamins (E, K, pantothenic acid, biotin, and choline) and minerals (chromium, copper, manganese, and selenium) were not available for comparison.

3.4. Mineral Intake

Compared to the representative sample, intakes of magnesium, phosphorus, zinc, and potassium was lower for both male and female CD patients, whereas sodium intake was higher in female patients (Table 4). Compared to male patients with CD, female patients had lower intakes of iron, phosphorus, and sodium. Both male and female patients with CD did not meet the DRI adequacy for calcium, chromium, magnesium, zinc, or potassium.

3.5. P-MDS Adherence

Few patients with CD met the P-MDS criteria for olive oil, vegetable, legume intake or consumption of sofrito sauce (made from olive oil, onions, garlic, and tomatoes, and is similar to spaghetti sauce; Table 5). One quarter of male patients and one fifth of female patients met the P-MDS criteria for fruit servings, while 36% of males and 24% of females met the P-MDS criteria for nuts. Fish and/or shellfish intake had a median intake of 0 per week and 21% of males and 32% of females ate more than three or more servings a week. Over 70% of patients met the serving recommendations for limiting butter, sugar sweetened beverages, and red or processed meat, and approximately half of the patients limited baked goods and sweets to less than three times a week. Although patients reported limiting red meat according to the P-MDS criteria (<6 oz or 175 g/day), few chose poultry over red meat on a regular basis.

Table 3. Vitamin intake compared to a representative population.

Vitamins	DRI Adequate Intake/day (AI) [31]		Crohn's Patients (N = 67)				Representative Sample (N = 1547) [27]	
	Males	Females	M (N = 33)% of DRI (M ± SD)	F (N = 34)% of DRI (M ± SD)	M (N = 33) Daily intake (M ± SE)	F (N = 34) Daily intake (M ± SE)	M (N = 721) Usual intake (M ± SE)	F (N = 826)Usual intake (M ± SE)
Vitamin A RAE µg	900	700	69 (55)%	97 (162)%	609 (86)	682 (195)	667 (33)	577 (28)
Vitamin D µg [@]		15–20	21 (20)%	16 (17)%	3 (0.5) **	2.5 (0.4) **	5.9 (0.3)	5.0 (0.3)
Vitamin E α-tocopherol mg		15	48 (59)%	32 (28)%	5 (1.5)	7.1 (0.7)	n/a	n/a
Vitamin K µg	120	90	52 (46)% *	106 (101)% *	61 (9.7)	97 (15.7)	n/a	n/a
Vitamin C mg (N = 1484) Vitamin C smokers mg (N = 679)	90 125	75 110	121 (78)%	108 (84)%	106 (12) **	82 (11) **	143 (8) 92 (7)	113 (4) 102 (8)
Thiamin, B1 mg	1.2	1.1	115 (60)% *	82 (41)% *	1.4 (0.12) **	0.9 (0.08) **	2.0 (0.07)	1.4 (0.04)
Riboflavin, B2 mg	1.3	1.1	141 (67)%	113 (52)%	1.8 (0.15)	1.3 (0.10) **	2.1 (0.07)	1.6 (0.05)
Niacin, B3 NE	16	14	212 (113)% *	161 (76)% *	34 (2) **	23 (2) **	46 (2)	32 (1)
Pantothenic Acid, B5 mg		5	87 (46)%	68 (35)%	4.4 (0.4)	3.4 (0.3)	n/a	n/a
Pyridoxine, B6 mg [t]	1.3–1.7	1.3–1.5	119 (64)% *	86 (45)% *	1.8 (1.0)	1.2 (0.7) **	2.1 (0.1)	1.6 (0.1)
Biotin, B7 mg		30	47 (42)% *	25 (19)% *	14 (2.2)	8 (1.0)	n/a	n/a
Folate, B9 DFE µg		400	72 (32)%	61 (59)%	287 (34) **	244 (33)	488 (15)	325 (41)
Cobalamin, B12 µg		2.4	177 (123)%	130 (109)%	4.2 (0.5)	3.1 (0.5)	4.9 (0.3)	3.5 (0.2)
Choline mg ^	550	425	43 (26)%	39 (23)%	229 (25)	165 (17)	n/a	n/a

Abbreviations: Retinol Activity Equivalents (RAE), Dietary Folate Equivalents (DFE), Not available (n/a). [@] Higher values for greater than 70 years. Does not include values for children or pregnant females. [t] Higher values for 51 years and older. ^ Choline requirements may be met by endogenous production and food sources may not be required. * Indicates a significant difference in %DRI between males and females ($p < 0.05$). ** Indicates a significant difference between patients with Crohn's and representative sample intakes, specific to gender ($p < 0.05$).

Table 4. Mineral intake compared to a representative population.

Minerals	DRI Adequate Intake/Day (AI) [31]		Crohn's Patients, (N = 67)				Representative Sample (N = 1547) [27]	
	Males	Females	M (N = 33) % of DRI (M ± SD)	F (N = 34) % of DRI (M ± SD)	M (N = 33) Daily intake (M ± SE)	F (N = 34) Daily intake (M ± SE)	M (N = 721) Usual intake[2] (M ± SE)	F (N = 826) Usual intake[2] (M ± SE)
Calcium mg/d [@]		1000–1200	87 (49)%	73 (42)%	906 (97)	785 (76)	890 (38)	799 (35)
Chromium µg/d [t]	35–30	25–20	18 (50)%	8 (6)%	5.8 (3.1)	1.7 (0.3)	n/a	n/a
Copper µg/d		900	110 (63)%	93 (69)%	989 (99)	837 (106)	n/a	n/a
Iron mg/d ^	8	8–18	187 (102)% *	118 (86)% *	17 (1.6)	13 (1.1)	16 (0.5)	11 (0.3)
Magnesium mg/d [#]	400–420	310–320	63 (33)%	60 (34)%	256 (23) **	191 (19) **	352 (9)	274 (7)
Manganese mg/d	2.3	1.8	197 (306)%	114 (64)%	4.5 (1.2)	2.1 (0.2)	n/a	n/a
Phosphorus mg/d		700	144 (68)% *	111 (54)% *	1030 (79) **	777 (65) **	1500 (44)	1152 (33)
Selenium µg/d		55	151 (81)%	134 (78)%	83 (7.8)	74 (7.4)	n/a	n/a
Zinc mg/d	11	8	83 (38)%	72% (34)	9 (0.7) **	6 (0.5) **	13 (0.5)	10 (0.3)
Potassium mg/d		4700	54 (30)%	44 (31)%	2532 (246) **	1880 (157) **	3355 (103)	2657 (62)
Sodium mg/d		1200–1500 [+]	169 (74)% *	135 (51)% *	3880 (296)	3101 (203) **	3543 (120)	2550 (75)

Abbreviations: Not available (n/a); * Indicates a significant difference between males and females ($p < 0.05$). ** Indicates a significant difference between Crohn's patients and the Albertan population, gender specific ($p < 0.05$). [@] Higher values for greater than 70 years. Does not include values for children or pregnant females. [t] Higher values for 51 years and older. ^ Higher values are for menstruating females. [#] Higher values for 31 years and older. [+] Lower values for 51 years and older.

Table 5. Predimed Mediterranean Diet (P-MDS) adherence scores.

P-MDS Adherence Criteria [26]	Canada Food Guide 1-Serving Size and P-MDS Answers	Canada Food Guide Servings (Median ± IQR)		Percent Meeting P-MDS Criteria n (%)	
		Male	Female	Male	Female
• Olive oil as main culinary fat	• Yes, No answer	n/a	n/a	2 (6)	0 (0)
• ≥4 tbsp olive oil per day	• 1 Tbsp (15 mL)	n/a	n/a	0 (0)	0 (0)
• ≥5 servings vegetables with ≥2 servings as raw leafy vegetables per day	• 1/2 cup (125 mL) fresh, frozen, canned vegetables • 1 medium vegetable • 1 cup (250 mL) raw or leafy vegetables	total 1.0 (0.4–1.7) leafy 0.0 (0.0–0.5)	total 1.9 (1.0–3.0) leafy 0.5 (0–1.0)	0 (0)	1 (3)
• ≥3 servings fruit and unsweetened fruit juice per day	• 1/2 cup (125 mL) fresh, frozen, canned fruit • 1 medium fruit • 1/2 cup (125 mL) unsweetened fruit juice	1.8 (1.3–3.3)	1.4 (0.9–2.6)	9 (27)	7 (21)
• <2 servings of red meat, hamburger, or processed meat such as ham, sausage, etc. per day	• 85 g (3 oz) meat • 1/2 cup (125 mL)	1.7 (1.0–2.0)	0.7 (0.3–1.5)	23 (70)	28 (82)
• <1 serving of butter, hydrogenated margarine or cream per day	• 1 Tbsp (15 mL)	n/a	n/a	27 (82)	27 (79)
• <1 sugar sweetened beverage per day	• Yes, No answer	n/a	n/a	31 (94)	27 (79)
• ≥3 servings beans, peas, lentils per week	• 3/4 cup (175 mL)	0.0 (0.0–0.0)	0.0 (0.0–0.2)	3 (9)	3 (9)
• ≥3 servings fish and/or shellfish per week	• CFG = 85 g (3 oz.) • 100 g (3.5 oz) fish • 200 g (7.0 oz) shellfish	fish 0.0 (0.0–0.0) seafood 0.0 (0.0–0.0)	fish 0.0 (0.0–3.1) seafood 0.0 (0.0–0.0)	7 (21)	11 (32)
• Eat <3 times a week baked goods, sweets, pastries or candy	• Yes, No answer	n/a	n/a	19 (58)	19 (56)
• ≥3 servings nuts per week	• 1/4 cup nuts or whole large seeds (30 g) • 2 Tbsp (30 mL) nut and seed butters or small/ground seeds	0.0 (0.0–5.4)	0.4 (0.0–2.6)	12 (36)	8 (24)
• Choose chicken, turkey or rabbit more often than veal, pork, hamburger or sausage	• Yes, No answer	n/a	n/a	12 (36)	18 (53)
• Consume sofrito sauce ≥2 times per week	• Yes, No answer	n/a	n/a	4 (12)	11 (32)
Total mean MDS Score (possible score out of 13)				4.5 (1.1)	4.7 (1.8)

Abbreviations: interquartile range (IQR); No significant differences in P-MDS criteria were evident using chi-square tests between males and females for categorical variables and independent sample t-tests for mean MDS score ($p < 0.05$).

4. Discussion

The present study is a description of the dietary patterns and food intake at one time point at a single center, in adult patients in remission with CD. To our knowledge, this was the first study to report on P-MDS in an adult cohort of patients with CD, and to examine the population data and gender differences in nutrient intakes. Major study findings identified significantly different (a) micronutrient intakes between CD patients and a representative sample of individuals; (b) micronutrient intakes between male and female CD patients; and (c) dietary patterns compared to the P-MDS recommendations.

Few published studies have identified dietary predictors of relapse. One such study in 103 CD and ulcerative colitis (UC) patients used a cross-sectional design to evaluate the association between food intake and course of disease; half with active disease [19]. Intake of legumes and potato were inversely associated with the risk of active disease, defined as fecal calprotectin >150, with close to 80% of the highest quartile consumers of legumes at a lower risk of active disease (adjusted Odds Ratio (OR) 0.21, 95% CI 0.57–0.81). Similarly, patients consuming the highest intake of meat coincided with a higher risk of active disease (unadjusted OR 3.6). In the Tasson study [19], significant effects for fruits and vegetables on disease relapse were not identified. The duration of active inflammation before data collection prevented the authors from inferring the causality of diet determinants of relapse. It is compelling to observe that in our current study, only three individuals consumed three or more servings of legumes, and 30% of male patients demonstrated meat overconsumption.

Similar to our study, significant micronutrient deficits were observed including suboptimal intakes of vitamins A, E, C, folate, and zinc. Vitamins C and E are antioxidants, and supplementation has previously been shown to result in a reduction of oxidative stress [32]. Zinc plays a pivotal role in wound repair, tissue regeneration, and the immune system; zinc deficiency in IBD has been associated with an increased risk of hospitalizations, surgeries, and disease related complications. Normalization of zinc was associated with improvement of these adverse clinical outcomes [33]. Limited dietary diversity including the avoidance of food groups may offer one possible explanation for the deficiency in micronutrient intake. Optimizing dietary diversity through focused nutrition counseling may lead toward an improvement in micronutrient intake.

Compared to the representative sample, dietary MUFA intake from foods like olive and canola oils, avocado, and nuts were low in patients with CD. One recently published study showed that dietary lipid and overall energy intake in a mixed IBD sample was higher than that of the healthy control subjects, however, no differences were observed in protein and carbohydrate intake [34]. Dietary lipid composition, unfortunately, was not reported in this study, rendering the proportion of MUFA and PUFA unknown. An older study in patients stratified by disease severity using the CD Activity Index threshold of 150, showed the mean energy and macronutrient intakes were close to the recommended levels in both patients with active disease and in remission, and reported MUFA intakes of 12% [35]; the MUFA intakes in our CD patients were significantly lower than this. In rheumatoid arthritis, a high intake of MUFAs, was recently demonstrated to be an independent predictor of remission [36].

Gender differences in micronutrient intakes were observed although there was a large degree of variability in the sample. Females consumed less thiamin compared to males, however, they still met 80% of the DRI. Given the adequacy of intake, the clinical relevance of this finding is likely not significant. Males only consumed half of the recommended potassium intake, and had lower intakes than females. Both males and females had low intakes of biotin compared to DRI recommendations; however, females were significantly lower than males at 25%. The consequence and etiology for these findings are not readily apparent, although likely result from the extremely low intakes of legumes, fruit and vegetables, and nuts and seeds. Although both males and females exceeded the DRI recommendation for sodium, males had a significantly greater intake, possibly a surrogate for a greater intake of processed foods. Both males and females exceeded DRIs for sodium in the representative sample, however, to a lesser extent than our sample of patients with CD. While the dietary intake of sodium is under-reported in IBD, there are signs that show a diet enriched in sodium chloride enhances inflammatory cytokine production and exacerbates colitis in animal models [37].

The dietary composition in our patient sample differed from the P-MDS criteria. Olive oil was seldom used as the primary culinary fat of choice, and few patients in our sample met the P-MDS criteria for intake of vegetables or legumes and fruit including fruit juice, and median intakes were 50% below the recommended three or more fruit servings a day. For fruit and vegetable intake, the P-MDS criteria are similar to the North American dietary recommendations. Thirty percent of males exceeded the recommendations for red or processed meats per P-MDS criteria. Over 80% of patients reported inadequate intake of fish and nuts.

Data evaluating the relationship between Mediterranean diets (MD) and disease characteristics (severity and relapse) in IBD are limited. Drawing from the cardiovascular literature, the incidence of major cardiovascular events was lower among participants assigned to an energy-unrestricted MD, and MD supplemented with extra-virgin olive oil or nuts when compared to those assigned to a reduced-fat diet [23]. A subsequent study identified significant reductions in plasma concentrations of high-sensitivity C-reactive protein, interleukin-6, and tumor necrosis factor in patients following a MD supplemented with extra-virgin olive oil or nuts compared to a low fat diet, identifying anti-inflammatory signals to explain the observed clinical findings [38]. Recently, Arpon et al. identified that specific components of the MD, particularly nuts and extra virgin olive oil, were able to induce methylation changes in several peripheral white blood cells, showing a role for specific fatty acids on epigenetic modulation [39]. To our knowledge, studies assessing the gut microbiome composition in long term MD consumers compared to habitual diet in humans have not yet been completed. However, a very recent study identified significant microbiome differences in non-human primates consuming MD when compared to a Western diet [40].

The results of our study provoke further curiosity into the relationships between dietary patterns, nutrition adequacy, and disease pathogenesis in IBD. Protective mechanistic roles for MD patterns in IBD are plausible, mediated through anti-oxidant effects, microbiome changes, and anti-inflammatory effects. Interventional studies are required to test the efficacy of MD patterns on disease severity. Promising effects on disease activity have been observed with elimination diets such as the specific carbohydrate diet [41] and the autoimmune protocol diet [42], among other test diets in the recent literature, highlighting the growing interest in undertaking intervention studies in this population of patients.

The P-MDS was useful in identifying low intakes of foods rich in the deficient micronutrients like olive oil, legumes, nuts, and fruits and vegetables. In patients with suboptimal intakes of these foods, early referral to effective nutrition intervention programs and/or supplementation should be considered. At the present time, in our center, patients are not routinely referred for dietary assessment and counseling, nor do they receive nutrition risk screening. Gastroenterologists and nurse practitioners providing care to patients with IBD at our site generally refrain from offering diet-focused therapies as a solution for disease management in the absence of overt malnutrition. We recognize that the lack of dietary focus as therapy may differ from other centers. We also recognize that patients with IBD assessed at our center are interested in dietary therapies, although the source for nutrition education is not readily apparent. Patients with IBD had a higher dietary fiber intake compared to the representative sample, and 70% met the serving recommendations to limit butter, sugar sweetened beverages, and processed meat.

There are study limitations that should be noted. This study was conducted at a single Canadian center with a small sample, and therefore, the generalizability of the study findings may be limited. While there are limitations to the use of the 3-day food record to capture dietary intake such as biased estimates of intake due to underreporting or changes in normal dietary patterns, this validated tool has been used extensively to measure food intake in a variety of populations. Deficient dietary intake may not be synonymous with deficient total body stores of micronutrients. The current study design was unable to infer a relationship between intake and body stores. In addition, the representative sample data did not report on several micronutrients, so comparisons between patients with IBD and this population were not possible for all micronutrients. This study was underpowered to detect a medium difference between males and females and produced point estimates with a large degree of variability; therefore, results should be interpreted with caution. In addition, multiple analyses were conducted, increasing the risk of type 1 error; however, due to the exploratory nature of this study and limited sample size, a statistical correction was not made and results should be interpreted with this in mind. Additional studies with larger numbers are recommended to confirm this study's conclusions.

Studies such as this one are necessary to identify the need for dietary intervention and offers potential dietary targets for intervention in patients with CD in an ambulatory care setting. Future directions include a further description of dietary patterns in patients with CD and dietary intervention studies to test the feasibility, acceptability, compliance, and efficacy of a MD pattern on disease related outcomes. Dietary intervention studies may be regarded as complex interventions, and should be developed based on established frameworks that may include a needs assessment of the population, rationale for intervention development, and pilot studies to inform the details of a subsequent robust clinical trial [43].

5. Conclusions

Differences in dietary quality and micronutrient intakes were observed between a representative population and male and female patients with CD. Compared with a MD pattern shown to have anti-inflammatory properties, patients with CD reported food choices that promote a more restricted nutrient intake. These results suggest patients with CD should be screened for nutrient deficiencies and inadequacy of dietary patterns. Using a simple tool such as the P-MDS may be a practical and effective way to identify pro-inflammatory dietary patterns at an individual level. These data may be used to inform future dietary interventions in this population to optimize dietary intake. Further investigation into the efficacy of nutrition interventions to improve MD quality and the effect this has on clinical outcomes and nutrient deficiency is warranted.

Author Contributions: L.T. made substantial contributions to the analyses and interpretation of data, drafted the article, revised the article critically for important intellectual content, and provided final approval of the version to be submitted. A.A. made substantial contributions to the acquisition of data, drafted the article, and provided final approval of the version to be submitted. N.S. made substantial contributions to the acquisition of data, revised the article critically for important intellectual content, and provided final approval of the version to be submitted. R.F. made substantial contributions to the conception and design of the study, revised the article critically for important intellectual content, and provided final approval of the version to be submitted. S.G. made substantial contributions to the conception and design of the study, data interpretation, revised the article critically for important intellectual content, and provided final approval of the version to be submitted. R.A.R. made substantial contributions to the conception and design of the study, revised the article critically for important intellectual content, and provided final approval of the version to be submitted. R.P. made substantial contribution to the analysis and interpretation of data, revised the article critically for important intellectual content, and provided final approval of the version to be submitted. M.R. made substantial contributions to the conception and design of the study, data interpretation, drafted the article, and provided final approval of the version to be submitted.

Acknowledgments: I would like to acknowledge the IBD group at the University of Calgary for referring patients, and Nutrition Services, Calgary Zone for supporting this work through contributing Registered Dietitian expertise. Subrata Ghosh is supported by the NIHR, Biomedical Research Centre, Birmingham.

References

1. Dutta, A.K.; Chacko, A. Influence of environmental factors on the onset and course of inflammatory bowel disease. *World J. Gastroenterol.* **2016**, *22*, 1088–1100. [CrossRef] [PubMed]
2. David, L.A.; Maurice, C.F.; Carmody, R.N.; Gootenberg, D.B.; Button, J.E.; Wolfe, B.E.; Ling, A.V.; Devlin, A.S.; Varma, Y.; Fischbach, M.A.; et al. Diet rapidly and reproducibly alters the human gut microbiome. *Nature* **2014**, *505*, 559–563. [CrossRef] [PubMed]

3. Wu, G.D.; Chen, J.; Hoffmann, C.; Bittinger, K.; Chen, Y.Y.; Keilbaugh, S.A.; Bewtra, M.; Knights, D.; Walters, W.A.; Knight, R.; et al. Linking long-term dietary patterns with gut microbial enterotypes. *Science* **2011**, *334*, 105–108. [CrossRef] [PubMed]

4. Bull, M.J.; Plummer, N.T. Part 1: The human gut microbiome in health and disease. *Integr. Med.* **2014**, *13*, 17–22.

5. Limdi, J.K.; Aggarwal, D.; McLaughlin, J.T. Dietary practices and beliefs in patients with inflammatory bowel disease. *Inflamm. Bowel Dis.* **2016**, *22*, 164–170. [CrossRef] [PubMed]

6. Hartman, C.; Eliakim, R.; Shamir, R. Nutritional status and nutritional therapy in inflammatory bowel diseases. *World J. Gastroenterol.* **2009**, *15*, 2570–2578. [CrossRef] [PubMed]

7. Vadan, R.; Gheorghe, L.S.; Constantinescu, A.; Gheorghe, C. The prevalence of malnutrition and the evolution of nutritional status in patients with moderate to severe forms of Crohn's disease treated with infliximab. *Clin. Nutr.* **2011**, *30*, 86–91. [CrossRef] [PubMed]

8. Lomer, M.C. Dietary and nutritional considerations for inflammatory bowel disease. *Proc. Nutr. Soc.* **2011**, *70*, 329–335. [CrossRef] [PubMed]

9. Benjamin, J.; Makharia, G.K.; Kalaivani, M.; Joshi, Y.K. Nutritional status of patients with Crohn's disease. *Indian J. Gastroenterol.* **2008**, *27*, 195–200. [PubMed]

10. Weisshof, R.; Chermesh, I. Micronutrient deficiencies in inflammatory bowel disease. *Curr. Opin. Clin. Nutr. Metab. Care* **2015**, *18*, 576–581. [CrossRef] [PubMed]

11. Lucendo, A.J.; De Rezende, L.C. Importance of nutrition in inflammatory bowel disease. *World J. Gastroenterol.* **2009**, *15*, 2081–2088. [CrossRef] [PubMed]

12. Fabisiak, N.; Fabisiak, A.; Watala, C.; Fichna, J. Fat-soluble vitamin deficiencies and inflammatory bowel disease: Systematic review and meta-analysis. *J. Clin. Gastroenterol.* **2017**, *51*, 878–889. [CrossRef] [PubMed]

13. Guglielmetti, S.; Fracassetti, D.; Taverniti, V.; Del Bo', C.; Vendrame, S.; Klimis-Zacas, D.; Arioli, S.; Riso, P.; Porrini, M. Differential modulation of human intestinal bifidobacterium populations after consumption of a wild blueberry (Vaccinium angustifolium) drink. *J. Agric. Food Chem.* **2013**, *61*, 8134–8140. [CrossRef] [PubMed]

14. Clifford, M.N. Diet-derived phenols in plasma and tissues and their implications for health. *Planta Med.* **2004**, *70*, 1103–1114. [CrossRef] [PubMed]

15. Rajendran, N.; Kumar, D. Role of diet in the management of inflammatory bowel disease. *World J. Gastroenterol.* **2010**, *16*, 1442–1448. [CrossRef] [PubMed]

16. Riordan, A.M.; Ruxton, C.H.; Hunter, J.O. A review of associations between Crohn's disease and consumption of sugars. *Eur. J. Clin. Nutr.* **1998**, *52*, 229–238. [CrossRef] [PubMed]

17. Li, F.; Liu, X.; Wang, W.; Zhang, D. Consumption of vegetables and fruit and the risk of inflammatory bowel disease: A meta-analysis. *Eur. J. Gastroenterol. Hepatol.* **2015**, *27*, 623–630. [CrossRef] [PubMed]

18. Shivappa, N.; Hebert, J.R.; Rashvand, S.; Rashidkhani, B.; Hekmatdoost, A. Inflammatory potential of diet and risk of ulcerative colitis in a case-control study from Iran. *Nutr. Cancer* **2016**, *68*, 404–409. [CrossRef] [PubMed]

19. Tasson, L.; Canova, C.; Vettorato, M.G.; Savarino, E.; Zanotti, R. Influence of diet on the course of inflammatory bowel disease. *Dig. Dis. Sci.* **2017**, *62*, 2087–2094. [CrossRef] [PubMed]

20. Estruch, R. Anti-inflammatory effects of the Mediterranean diet: The experience of the PREDIMED study. *Proc. Nutr. Soc.* **2010**, *69*, 333–340. [CrossRef] [PubMed]

21. Steck, S.; Shivappa, N.; Tabung, F.; Harmon, B.E.; Wirth, M.D.; Hurley, T.G.; Hebert, J.R. The dietary inflammatory index: A new tool for assessing diet quality based on inflammatory potential. *Digest* **2014**, *49*, 1–9.

22. Giugliano, D.; Ceriello, A.; Esposito, K. The effects of diet on inflammation: Emphasis on the metabolic syndrome. *J. Am. Coll. Cardiol.* **2006**, *48*, 677–685. [CrossRef] [PubMed]

23. Estruch, R.; Ros, E.; Salas-Salvado, J.; Covas, M.I.; Corella, D.; Aros, F.; Gomez-Gracia, E.; Ruiz-Gutierrez, V.; Fiol, M.; Lapetra, J.; et al. Primary prevention of cardiovascular disease with a mediterranean diet supplemented with extra-virgin olive oil or nuts. *N. Engl. J. Med.* **2018**, *378*, e34. [CrossRef] [PubMed]

24. Leblanc, V.; Begin, C.; Hudon, A.M.; Royer, M.M.; Corneau, L.; Dodin, S.; Lemieux, S. Gender differences in the long-term effects of a nutritional intervention program promoting the Mediterranean diet: Changes in dietary intakes, eating behaviors, anthropometric and metabolic variables. *Nutr. J.* **2014**, *13*, 107. [CrossRef] [PubMed]

25. ESHA Research. *Food Processor Nutrition Analysis Software 11.3 X*; ESHA Research: Salem, Oregon, 2018.
26. Schroder, H.; Fito, M.; Estruch, R.; Martinez-Gonzalez, M.A.; Corella, D.; Salas-Salvado, J.; Lamuela-Raventos, R.M.; Ros, E.; Salaverria, I.; Fiol, M.; et al. A short screener is valid for assessing Mediterranean diet adherence among older spanish men and women. *J. Nutr.* **2011**, *141*, 1140–1145. [CrossRef] [PubMed]
27. Health Canda; Statistics Canada. Canadian Community Health Survey, Cycle 2.2, Nutrition (2004)—Nutrient Intakes from Food, Provincial, Regional and National Summary Data Tables, Volume 1, 2 and 3. Available online: https://www.canada.ca/en/health-canada/services/food-nutrition/food-nutrition-surveillance/health-nutrition-surveys/canadian-community-health-survey-cchs/canadian-community-health-survey-cycle-2-2-nutrition-focus-food-nutrition-surveillance-health-canada.html#p1 (accessed on 3 January 2018).
28. Health Canada, Office of Nutrition Policy and Promotion Health Products and Food Branch. Canadian Community Health Survey 2.2, Nutrition (2004): A Guide to Accessing and Interpreting the Data 2006. Available online: https://www.canada.ca/en/health-canada/services/food-nutrition/food-nutrition-surveillance/health-nutrition-surveys/canadian-community-health-survey-cchs/canadian-community-health-survey-cycle-2-2-nutrition-2004-guide-accessing-interpreting-data-health-canada-2006.html (accessed on 12 November 2018).
29. Food and Nutrition Board: Institute of Medicine. Dietary Reference Intakes for Energy, Carbohydrate, Fiber, Fat, Fatty Acids, Cholesterol, Protein, and Amino Acids. Available online: http://www.nap.edu/openbook.php?record_id=10490 (accessed on 12 November 2018).
30. Academy of Nutrition and Dietetics. Position of the academy of nutrition and dietetics: dietary fatty acids for healthy adults. *J. Acad. Nutr. Dietetics.* **2014**, *114*, 136–153. [CrossRef] [PubMed]
31. Food and Nutrition Board: Institute of Medicine, Health Canada. Dietary Reference Intakes Tables. 2010. Available online: https://www.canada.ca/en/health-canada/services/food-nutrition/healthy-eating/dietary-reference-intakes/tables.html (accessed on 12 November 2018).
32. Aghdassi, E.; Wendland, B.E.; Steinhart, A.H.; Wolman, S.L.; Jeejeebhoy, K.; Allard, J.P. Antioxidant vitamin supplementation in Crohn's disease decreases oxidative stress. A randomized controlled trial. *Am. J. Gastroenterol.* **2003**, *98*, 348–353. [PubMed]
33. Siva, S.; Rubin, D.T.; Gulotta, G.; Wroblewski, K.; Pekow, J. Zinc deficiency is associated with poor clinical outcomes in patients with inflammatory bowel disease. *Inflamm. Bowel Dis.* **2017**, *23*, 152–157. [CrossRef] [PubMed]
34. Principi, M.; Losurdo, G.; Iannone, A.; Contaldo, A.; Deflorio, V.; Ranaldo, N.; Pisani, A.; Ierardi, E.; Di Leo, A.; Barone, M. Differences in dietary habits between patients with inflammatory bowel disease in clinical remission and a healthy population. *Ann. Gastroenterol.* **2018**, *31*, 469–473. [CrossRef] [PubMed]
35. Aghdassi, E.; Wendland, B.E.; Stapleton, M.; Raman, M.; Allard, J.P. Adequacy of nutritional intake in a canadian population of patients with Crohn's disease. *J. Am. Diet. Assoc.* **2007**, *107*, 1575–1580. [CrossRef] [PubMed]
36. Matsumoto, Y.; Sugioka, Y.; Tada, M.; Okano, T.; Mamoto, K.; Inui, K.; Habu, D.; Koike, T. Monounsaturated fatty acids might be key factors in the Mediterranean diet that suppress rheumatoid arthritis disease activity: The TOMORROW study. *Clin. Nutr.* **2018**, *37*, 675–680. [CrossRef] [PubMed]
37. Monteleone, I.; Marafini, I.; Dinallo, V.; Di Fusco, D.; Troncone, E.; Zorzi, F.; Laudisi, F.; Monteleone, G. Sodium chloride-enriched diet enhanced inflammatory cytokine production and exacerbated experimental colitis in mice. *J. Crohn's Colitis* **2017**, *11*, 237–245. [CrossRef] [PubMed]
38. Casas, R.; Sacanella, E.; Urpi-Sarda, M.; Corella, D.; Castaner, O.; Lamuela-Raventos, R.M.; Salas-Salvado, J.; Martinez-Gonzalez, M.A.; Ros, E.; Estruch, R. Long-term immunomodulatory effects of a Mediterranean diet in adults at high risk of cardiovascular disease in the PREvencion con DIeta MEDiterranea (PREDIMED) randomized controlled trial. *J. Nutr.* **2016**, *146*, 1684–1693. [CrossRef] [PubMed]
39. Arpon, A.; Milagro, F.I.; Razquin, C.; Corella, D.; Estruch, R.; Fito, M.; Marti, A.; Martinez-Gonzalez, M.A.; Ros, E.; Salas-Salvado, J.; et al. Impact of consuming extra-virgin olive oil or nuts within a Mediterranean diet on DNA methylation in peripheral white blood cells within the PREDIMED-Navarra randomized controlled trial: A role for dietary lipids. *Nutrients* **2017**, *10*, 15. [CrossRef] [PubMed]
40. Nagpal, R.; Shively, C.A.; Appt, S.A.; Register, T.C.; Michalson, K.T.; Vitolins, M.Z.; Yadav, H. Gut microbiome composition in non-human primates consuming a western or Mediterranean diet. *Front. Nutr.* **2018**, *5*, 28. [CrossRef] [PubMed]

41. Suskind, D.L.; Cohen, S.A.; Brittnacher, M.J.; Wahbeh, G.; Lee, D.; Shaffer, M.L.; Braly, K.; Hayden, H.S.; Klein, J.; Gold, B.; et al. Clinical and fecal microbial changes with diet therapy in active inflammatory bowel disease. *J. Clin. Gastroenterol.* **2018**, *52*, 155–163. [CrossRef] [PubMed]

42. Konijeti, G.G.; Kim, N.; Lewis, J.D.; Groven, S.; Chandrasekaran, A.; Grandhe, S.; Diamant, C.; Singh, E.; Oliveira, G.; Wang, X.; et al. Efficacy of the autoimmune protocol diet for Inflammatory Bowel Disease. *Inflamm. Bowel Dis.* **2017**, *23*, 2054–2060. [CrossRef] [PubMed]

43. Craig, P.; Dieppe, P.; Macintryre, S.; Michie, S.; Nazareth, I.; Petticrew, M. Developing and evaluating complex interventions: The new Medical Research Council guidance. *BMJ* **2008**, *337*, a1655.

Influence of Vitamin D Deficiency on Inflammatory Markers and Clinical Disease Activity in IBD Patients

Pedro López-Muñoz [1][iD], Belén Beltrán [1,2,3,*], Esteban Sáez-González [1,2], Amparo Alba [4], Pilar Nos [1,2,3] and Marisa Iborra [1,2,3]

[1] IBD Unit, Department of Gastroenterology, Hospital Universitari i Politècnic la Fe, 46026 Valencia, Spain; pedro.lopez8928@gmail.com (P.L.-M.); esteban.digestivo@gmail.com (E.S.-G.); nos_pil@gva.es (P.N.); marisaiborra@hotmail.com (M.I.)

[2] IBD Research Group, Medical Research Institute Hospital la Fe (IIS La Fe), 46026 Valencia, Spain

[3] Networked Biomedical Research Center for Hepatic and Digestive Diseases (CIBEREHD), Institute of Health Carlos III, 28029 Madrid, Spain

[4] Department of Clinical Analysis, Hospital Universitari i Politècnic la Fe, 46026 Valencia, Spain; alba_amp@gva.es

* Correspondence: belenbeltranniclos@gmail.com

Abstract: Vitamin D has recently been discovered to be a potential immune modulator. Low serum vitamin D levels have been associated with risk of relapse and exacerbation of clinical outcomes in Crohn's disease (CD) and ulcerative colitis (UC). A retrospective, longitudinal study was conducted to determine the association between vitamin D levels and inflammatory markers and clinical disease activity in inflammatory bowel disease (IBD). In addition, circulating $25(OH)D_3$ progression was evaluated according to vitamin D supplementation. Participants were separated into three groups according to their vitamin D level: severe deficiency (SD), moderate deficiency (MD) and sufficiency (S). Serum $25(OH)D_3$ was inversely correlated with faecal calprotectin (FC) for CD and UC but was only correlated with C-reactive protein (CRP) for UC patients. In the multivariate analysis of FC, CRP and fibrinogen (FBG), we predicted the presence of a patient in the SD group with 80% accuracy. A deficiency of $25(OH)D_3$ was associated with increased hospitalisations, flare-ups, the use of steroids and escalating treatment. Supplemental doses of vitamin D were likely to be insufficient to reach adequate serum levels of $25(OH)D_3$. Vitamin D intervention studies are warranted to determine whether giving higher doses of vitamin D in IBD might reduce intestinal inflammation or disease activity.

Keywords: vitamin D; Crohn's disease; ulcerative colitis; faecal calprotectin; C-reactive protein

1. Introduction

Vitamin D is a lipophilic hormone synthesised in the skin under the influence of ultraviolet (UV) sunlight. Although most foods contain little vitamin D, it can be obtained from the diet to a lesser extent. The most important sources of this vitamin are fatty fish and egg yolk [1,2].

UV type B light exposure causes 7-dehydrocholesterol transformation into cholecalciferol or vitamin D_3. However, this UV-mediated conversion varies with time of the year, latitude and altitude. During approximately six months of the year, UVB radiation intensity is insufficient for vitamin D synthesis at 45° latitude near sea level (e.g., France or Italy). This period of time increases with the distance from the equator and is also known as vitamin D winter [3]. Along these lines, in countries where there is limited skin exposure to sunlight a dietary supply of vitamin D is important. Cholecalciferol is hydroxylated in the liver into 25-hydroxyvitamin D3 (25(OH)D3) and subsequently in the kidney into 1,25-dihydroxyvitamin D3 (1,25(OH)2D3), or calcitriol, the active metabolite [4]

(Figure 1). These two steps are catalysed by the enzymes 25-hydroxylase (CYP2R1) and 1α-hydroxylase (CYP27B1) that belong to the family of cytochrome P450 mixed function oxidases (CYPs). CYP2R1 has only been identified in the microsomal fraction of liver. However, although the kidney is the main source of 1,25(OH)$_2$ D$_3$, several other tissues also express CYP27B1. The regulation of the renal CYP27B1 differs from that of the extrarenal version [5]. In this way, renal CYP27B1 is activated by the parathyroid hormone (PTH) and inhibited by fibroblast growth factor 23 (FGF23) as well as by 1,25(OH)$_2$D$_3$ itself. Elevated calcium suppresses CYP27B1 by means of the suppression of PTH, and elevated phosphate suppresses CYP27B1 by means of FGF23 stimulation, although these ions can have direct effects on renal CYP27B1 on their own [5]. Thus, it is known that CYP27B1 is expressed in numerous tissues where vitamin D$_3$ can act as an intracrine or paracrine signal. In this way, several immune system cell types express both CYP27B1 and the vitamin D receptor, with CYP27B1 production controlled by a number of immune-specific inputs [3].

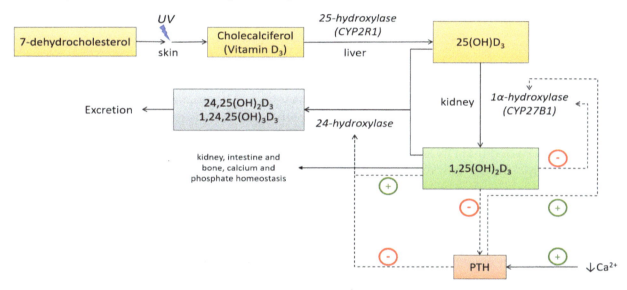

Figure 1. Vitamin D metabolism and functions. Under ultraviolet B light (UVB) exposure, 7-dehydroxycholesterol is converted to vitamin D$_3$ in the skin. First, hydroxylation occurs in the liver where it is converted to 25-hydroxyvitamin D$_3$. 25-hydroxyvitamin D$_3$ is further converted in the kidney to its active metabolite, 1α,25-dihydroxyvitamin D$_3$. In the kidney, 1α-hydroxylase is stimulated by the parathyroid hormone (PTH) and feedback inhibited by 1α,25-dihydroxyvitamin D$_3$. 1α,25-dihydroxyvitamin D$_3$ targets the intestine, kidney and bone to regulate calcium and phosphate homeostasis. Adapted from Lim et al [6].

The half-life of 1,25(OH)$_2$D$_3$ is very short, ranging from 20 to 40 hours [7]; therefore, its serum determination is not clinically relevant. However, the 25(OH)D$_3$ half-life ranges from 12 to 19 days [8], so it appears to be the most reliable source of systemic vitamin D. 1,25(OH)$_2$D$_3$ has its effect on the classic target organs such as bone, intestine and kidney and stimulates calcium transport from these organs to the peripheral blood stream [4].

Calcitriol can influence the expression of targets genes by binding to the vitamin D receptor (VDR), which is present in many cell populations and tissues, such as immune cells. Vitamin D promotes the intestinal absorption of calcium and phosphate and is critical for bone growth and remodelling. Now, however, it is well established that the physiological importance of vitamin D levels extends beyond its classical role in calcium and bone metabolism. Serum vitamin D levels have been associated with inflammatory diseases, such as inflammatory bowel disease (IBD), rheumatoid arthritis, systemic lupus erythematosus, multiple sclerosis, atherosclerosis, and asthma. Regarding inflammation, it has become clear that vitamin D inhibits production of proinflammatory cytokines like IL-6 or TNFα in monocytes via the inhibition of p38 MAP kinase [9], and it can promote anti-inflammatory T-cell pathways to stimulate the antimicrobial effects of macrophages [10].

In terms of gut homeostasis, vitamin D plays a role in protecting the intestinal epithelial barrier, immunity and microbiota, all of which are directly involved in IBD [11].

In-vitro 1,25(OH)2D3 treatment can protect the intestinal epithelial barrier in ulcerative colitis (UC) patients by regulating various pathways involved in tight junction proteins [12]

Similar studies have proposed that lack of VDR leads to hyperfunction of Claudin-2. Claudin-2 is an epithelial protein that forms a water channel to permit the paracellular passage of water through its pores in the epithelium, and its expression is restricted to colonic proliferative cells. An overexpression of Claudin-2 permits intestinal leakage, and is associated with active disease in IBD and reduction of intestinal VDR [13].

Other genetic changes in the VDR gene can contribute to a greater risk for CD. Patients with Crohn's disease (CD) who are homozygous for a certain single nucleotide polymorphism (SNP) in the VDR gene have lower levels of VDR protein expressed in serum monocytes. These individuals have an overactivation of lymphocytic adhesion molecules and a higher risk of developing a penetrating phenotype of CD [14].

Vitamin D has effects on both innate and adaptive immune pathways. 1,25(OH)2D3 modulates the expression of cationic antimicrobial peptides like defensins and cathelicidins. VDR signals through distal enhancers in the NOD2 gene, leading to the expression of defensin beta 2 in macrophages. However, this response was absent in macrophages from patients with CD homozygous for nonfunctional NOD2 variants [15]. It should be noted that NOD2 is also known as IBD1. This gene is located on chromosome 16, in the susceptibility locus for CD, which is responsible for familial aggregation of this disease [16]. It has also been reported that DNA copy number of the beta-defensin gene cluster is highly polymorphic within the healthy population, whereas CD patients appear to present a lower copy number. This results in a diminished beta-defensin expression, predisposing patients to major susceptibility to colonic CD [17]. An induction of human cathelicidin antimicrobial peptide gene was observed under the influence of 1,25(OH)2D3 in colon cancer cells and other tissues [18,19]. Vitamin D is also involved in immune regulation by modulating the role of dendritic cells and macrophages through two methods: firstly, 1,25(OH)2D3 inhibits IL-12, a pivotal interleukin in Th1 development [20]; secondly, it promotes IL-10 to stop maturation from dendritic cells to serum monocytes and leads to apoptosis in mature dendritic cells [21]. Regarding adaptive immunity, 1,25(OH)2D3 affects T-cell polarisation by inhibiting T helper 1(Th) (IFN-gamma production) and promoting Th2 cell development (IL-4, IL-5, and IL-10 production) from naïve T-cells [22]. It has been demonstrated in controlled studies that higher vitamin D levels in UC patients were associated with protective anti-inflammatory serum cytokine profiles [23].

Gut microbiota have become the main research topic in intestinal homeostasis. One recent study demonstrated that individuals with significant intake of vitamin D had different microbiota strains from those without a significant vitamin D intake. These patients had plenty of Bacteroidetes, Prevotella and Megasphera strains, traditionally associated with a noninflammatory status [24]. In another study, administration of vitamin D to CD patients resulted in significant change in the gut microbiota with a high abundance of some strains such as *Alistipes* and *Roseburia* that were not observed in healthy controls [25]. In murine induced colitis, *Alistipes finegoldii* played a protective role [26]. *Roseburia* genii are part of commensal bacteria that produce short-chain fatty acids, especially butyrate, affecting colonic motility, immunity maintenance and anti-inflammatory properties [27]. Therefore, administration of vitamin D might have a positive effect on CD by modulating the intestinal bacterial composition and also by increasing the abundance of potential beneficial bacterial strains [25].

Regarding the epidemiology of vitamin D deficiency in IBD, there is a systematic review and meta-analysis that defined this deficiency as serum 25(OH)D3 below 25 ng/mL. In this study, the prevalence was 38.1% in CD and 31.6% in UC [28].

The latest evidence suggests that low vitamin D levels are involved in changing disease activity and inflammatory markers in IBD. However, these studies sometimes fail to confirm which comes first: are vitamin D levels an independent predictor of clinical activity or it is just a mere bystander of increased inflammation?

Due to chronic malabsorption, IBD patients and particularly those with CD are at greater risk of certain nutritional deficiencies. Micronutrients, including hydro and lipophilic vitamins, iron, calcium and zinc, are the most common problems [29]. Malabsorption, maldigestion and upper protein requirements are directly related to clinical disease activity.

It is unknown why quiescent IBD has a greater prevalence of vitamin D deficiency than other risk groups [30]. Even in patients with IBD in clinical remission, vitamin D malabsorption has been confirmed. This fact led to controversy among researchers about oral intake as standard supplementation. According to several prospective studies, IBD patients with vitamin D deficiency are at greater risk of relapse, hospitalisations and flare-ups [2,31–35]. Schäffler et al. described a correlation between the use of a TNF-alpha inhibitor and higher vitamin D levels in CD patients. This correlation could be explained by a better disease control of these patients [34]. However, they detected a correlation between a higher disease activity and lower vitamin D levels in UC but not in CD. Moreover, the same authors found that in CD located in the small intestine, CD patients after small intestine resections showed significant lower vitamin D levels. Other resections did not lead to changes in the vitamin D levels; therefore, the small intestine plays an important role in vitamin D absorption, particularly in IBD [34]. Despite the immune-modulation role of vitamin D confirmed in translational studies, knowledge about its molecular action in IBD is still scarce. Exhaustive study of vitamin D immune pathways is imperative to identifying new supplementation strategies that correct this deficiency. It is also necessary to establish true sufficiency levels of vitamin D to have a goal for supplementation therapy.

As a result of these findings, our group posed a study to assess outcomes in IBD activity depending on vitamin D status. Thus, the association between vitamin D deficiency and inflammatory markers and clinical disease activity could be evaluated. We also hypothesised that oral supplementation according to practice guidelines was not enough to acquire vitamin D sufficiency.

2. Materials and Methods

2.1. Study Design and Patient Enrolment

We conducted a retrospective, longitudinal and observational study of patients with UC and CD, defined by European Crohn's and Colitis Organization (ECCO) guidelines criteria, which had serial determinations of vitamin D serum samples from the IBD Unit of Hospital Universitari i Politècnic la Fe, a tertiary centre, between 2015 and 2018. Formal consent was collected from all the patients and an ethical committee, according to the declaration of Helsinki, approved the study.

A total of 84 patients divided into three groups according to the 25(OH)D3 (ng/mL) level were enrolled in our study. The first vitamin D serum sample collected was used as a baseline to separate patients into groups and according to core event. A cut-off of <15 ng/mL was considered severe deficiency (SD), >15 and <30 ng/mL moderate deficiency (MD) and >30 ng/mL sufficiency (S). Progression of vitamin D and supplementation from baseline was evaluated. Clinical disease activity (flare-ups, hospitalisations, times to visit IBD clinic, escalating treatment, use of steroids) in the six months before and the six months after the core event was monitored. In addition, inflammatory markers (CRP, FC and fibrinogen (FBG)) were collected to explore the inflammatory status around the vitamin D core event. Two determinations before and two determinations after to the core event were needed for patient inclusion (Figure 2). Two or more consecutive 25(OH)D3 determinations were also required. Other relevant descriptive variables: age, sex, IBD (EC or UC), extraintestinal manifestations, and current therapy (anti-TNF, immunomodulators, etc.) were considered. We sought active supplementation, establishing at least 25,000 IU (international units) of oral, subcutaneous or intramuscular cholecalciferol monthly as adequate supplementation.

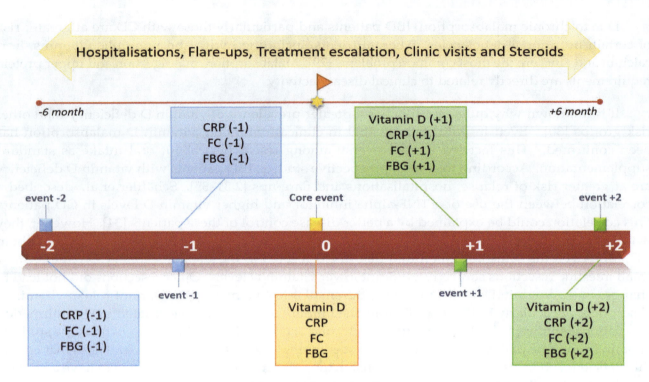

Figure 2. Study timeline.

Patients under 18 years, pregnant patients, those with a previous colectomy in UC, those who had CD surgery in the last three months, those with colorectal cancer or another tumour, those with a severe infection during the time of study and those with malabsorption disease were excluded from enrolment.

Disease activity and laboratory markers were collected from our software OrionClinic (Version 11). Suitable patients to enroll in this study were found by crossing vitamin D measurements from iGestlab software (Cointec iGestlab © 2013. v1.9.9.815, Orihuela, Alicante, Spain) and IBD Unit clinical histories. Patients with several vitamin D samples, inflammatory markers and IBD diagnosis were filtered to assess enrolment.

Serum $25(OH)D_3$ levels (ng/mL) were measured by automated chemiluminescence analyser LIAISON® XL (DiaSorin, Sialuggia, Italy).

A total of 252 patients from IBD Unit and vitamin D measurements were evaluated to enroll. Ultimately, 41 patients with SD, 28 with MD and 16 with sufficient vitamin D levels met the inclusion criteria.

2.2. Statistical Analysis

An ANOVA test on ranks (Kruskal–Wallis test) was performed to compare inflammatory markers with the three different Vitamin D groups (severe deficiency, moderate deficiency and sufficiency). Moreover, a multiple comparison procedure was conducted to quantify the extent of the differences between the groups. The Pearson correlation test was applied to study calprotectin-CRP-fibrinogen correlations with vitamin D. The evolution of vitamin D, FC, CRP and FBG was evaluated by mixed linear regression models. A random effect factor was included to amend the nonindependence of the data (longitudinal study).

Given some patients were supplemented with vitamin D, a comparative study was done with this group and the nonsupplemented ones to analyse the evolution of this parameter. Additionally, the association between vitamin D levels and markers of clinical activity (hospitalisations, flare-ups, escalating treatment, number of times they visited the clinic and the use of steroids) was studied through logistic regression models.

All models included the covariates sex, age and type of disease (CD or UC) as possible confounding factors. R statistic software (3.5.1 version, https://www.r-project.org/), Sigmaplot (SYSTAT, San José, CA, USA) and Minitab (State College, PA, USA) were used in this work. A significance level of 5% was selected. Multivariate discriminant analysis was performed with SIMCA-P (Umetrics, Umeå, Sweden).

3. Results

This study evaluated three concerns: Firstly, the correlation between vitamin D levels, expressed as 25(OH)D3, with both systemic and intestinal inflammation in IBD patients. Secondly, the association between vitamin D deficiency and clinical disease activity markers, collected in a period of time between six months before and after the randomly selected vitamin D core event. During this period, data on admissions, flare-ups, times the patient needed to visit the clinic, the use of steroids and the need for escalating treatment were collected. Thirdly, which patients benefitted from active supplementation was explored.

3.1. Descriptive Statistics

First, a normality study for the continuous quantitative variables (vitamin D, FC, CRP and FBG) was carried out. None of the inflammatory markers (FC, CRP, FBG) followed a normal distribution but their logarithmic transformation leads to data that were normally distributed (Figure 3). However, the vitamin D central values did follow a normal distribution.

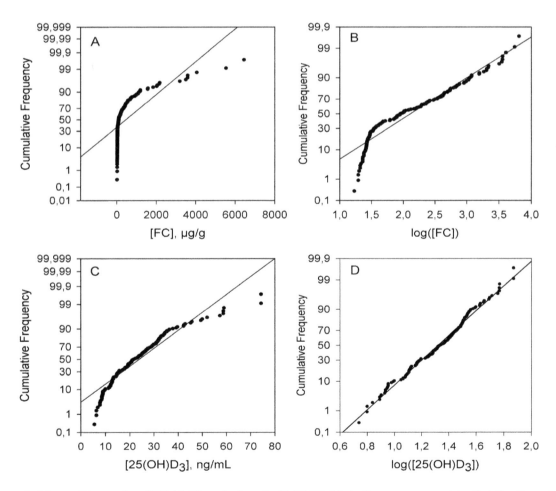

Figure 3. Normality study of FC (**A**,**B**) and vitamin D (**C**,**D**). Note the nonparametric distribution of FC.

Tables 1 and 2 show some of the statistical parameters obtained from the descriptive parametric and nonparametric study. The data have been grouped according to their vitamin D content. The central and dispersion values derived from the parametric and nonparametric treatment of the data are shown. Table 1 shows the parametric descriptive statistics where the deviation of the data with respect to normal behavior is clearly shown. The high values of MSSD (mean of the squared successive differences) clearly indicate a non-random distribution of the results. To obtain a more accurate description of central values and dispersion of inflammatory markers according to their vitamin D content, a robust descriptive statistical study is shown in Table 2. The median of the of inflammatory markers tends to increase when lower vitamin D levels were found. The significant differences found between the groups are noteworthy. The median of all determinations of FC in the group SD was 345.7 µg/g, while in the MD and S groups it was 63.5 and 29.7 µg/g, respectively. The medians of the CRP determinations in the SD, MD and S groups were 5.6, 1.5 and 1.4 mg/dL, respectively.

Table 1. Statistical parameters obtained from vitamin D and inflammatory markers grouped according to vitamin D content.

| Variable | Group | Mean | StDev | CI [a] (95%) | | Skewness | Kurtosis | MSSD |
				CI−	CI+			
Vitamin D	S	40.43	12.7	37.0	43.9	1.34	1.42	78
	MD	24.36	4.7	23.3	25.5	0.32	−0.16	17
	SD	17.83	8.1	16.3	19.3	0.85	0.39	65
CRP	S	2.28	2.37	1.8	2.8	1.82	3.5	1.5
	MD	2.80	3.07	2.3	3.3	1.71	3.01	4.3
	SD	23.6	51.0	16	31	4.48	24.2	1102
FC	S	54	64	39	69	4.09	19.72	2567
	MD	141	164	111	172	1.81	3.00	15,020
	SD	868	1278	665	1070	2.31	5.24	508,909
FBG	S	423	93	401	445	0.35	−0.51	4140
	MD	412	107	392	432	0.57	−0.13	6703
	SD	497	133	475	517	0.08	−0.77	5576

[a] confidence interval; MSSD: mean of the squared successive differences.

Table 2. Robust statistical parameters obtained from vitamin D and inflammatory markers grouped according to vitamin D content.

| Variable | Group | Min | Q1 | Median | Q3 | Max | CI [a] (95%) | |
							CI−	CI+
Vitamin D	S	20.5	32.2	36.2	43.0	74.30	34.1	43.9
	MD	15.3	20.6	24.7	27.4	37.5	22.4	25.5
	SD	4.5	12.2	15.1	22.7	45.7	14.3	19.3
CRP	S	0.20	0.60	1.45	2.97	11.8	0.9	2.0
	MD	0.20	0.60	1.50	3.82	16.5	1.1	2.2
	SD	0.30	1.90	5.60	15.6	364	4.5	7
FC	S	19.6	26.7	29.7	50.7	434	28	37
	MD	17	27.6	63	229	738	43	98
	SD	19	97	346	1065	6450	216	444
FBG	S	262	356	411	491	664	387	446
	MD	201	325	406	475	700	365	432
	SD	151	390	478	602	813	456	502

[a] confidence interval.

3.2. Qualitative Variables Study

Other qualitative variables were also considered and appear in Table 3. The mean age of the patients was 43.7 years, and 39 of the patients were women (46%). Some 60 patients had CD (71%) and 25 presented as UC (29%). Forty-four patients (52%) were supplemented with vitamin D, almost all of them in the SD group. Extraintestinal manifestations were clustered into articular (eight patients) and dermatological manifestations (two patients). Four cases of CD with perianal disease were observed. We collected data on the treatments given during the period of study: biologics (anti-TNFα, vedolizumab, ustekinumab), immunosuppressive agents (azathioprine, methotrexate, 6-mercaptopurine and tacrolimus) and the need for steroids therapy.

Six patients from the SD group required a combination of vedolizumab and steroids during the time of study. None of the individuals in the MD or S groups were on vedolizumab. Some 30 patients from the SD group were on anti-TNFα therapy, 12 of them in combination with azathioprine and eight of them with steroids requirement. However, only 17 patients were on anti-TNFα therapy in MD and S groups altogether. Only three of them required steroids and seven patients were on combination therapy with azathioprine.

Table 3. Baseline clinical characteristics of patients meeting inclusion criteria.

Clinical Characteristic		Number of Participants (Percentage) or Mean ± Standard Deviation
Age, years		43.7 ± 15.9
Female sex		39 (46)
Crohn's disease		60 (71)
Ulcerative colitis		25 (29)
Perianal disease		4 (5)
Extraintestinal manifestations		10 (12)
Vitamin D supplementation		44 (52)
Current therapy	Anti-TNFα	47 (55)
	Vedolizumab	8 (9)
	Ustekinumab	1 (1)
	Steroids	21 (25)
	Azathioprine	31 (36)
	Methotrexate	2 (2)

Clinical disease activity markers collected included flare-ups, hospitalisations, number of times patients visited the clinic, changing or escalating treatment and need for steroid therapy. We found remarkable results between the groups according to vitamin D levels. Among the patients with SD, 16 patients (41%) were hospitalised at least once and 23 patients (58.9%) had at least one flare-up during the time of the study (Figure 4). In the MD group along with the S group, only four flare-ups and one hospitalisation were reported. In the SD group, patients visited the clinic an average of 5.33 times, while in the MD and S groups they visited 3.61 times.

Changes or escalations in current therapy were made for 69.23% of the patients with SD, while only 8.7% in the MD and S groups required such changes. Eighteen patients in the SD group (46.15%) required steroids during the time of study, while only three patients in the SD and S groups did (6.53%).

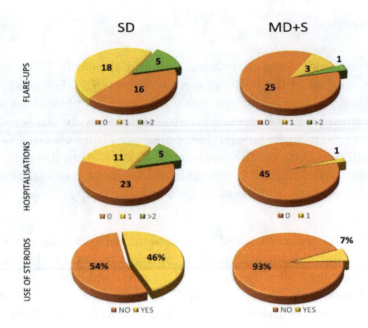

Figure 4. Results of the study of certain qualitative variables depending on vitamin D levels (SD or MD+S).

3.3. Linear Correlation Study of Quantitative Variables

Table 4 shows the median and interquartile range values of inflammatory markers. In nonsupplemented patients, the median and interquartile range of FC increased in cases of severe deficiency. This also occurred when vitamin D was supplemented, but to a lesser extent. A similar behaviour was observed for CRP in terms of the median but not for the interquartile range.

Table 4. Median and interquartile range of FC and CRP grouped by vitamin D levels for patients with and without vitamin D supplementation.

	Group	FC, µg/g Median	Q3–Q1	CRP, mg/dL Median	Q3–Q1
Not supplemented	S	33	25	1.3	1.8
	MD	85	211	1.9	4.2
	SD	524	2230	8.9	3.1
Supplemented	S	29	38	2.3	4.6
	MD	55	328	2.1	4.9
	SD	362	943	6.7	3.1

A nonparametric linear correlation study of vitamin D with FC, CRP and FBG was performed. A Pearson correlation coefficient (R) of −0.533 ($p < 0.001$) was obtained for vitamin D and FC in all patients. When two groups of patients were considered, both CD and UC showed a good correlation (Figure 5). As can be seen, this correlation was almost independent of the disease, given there was no significant differences between both slopes for UC and CD ($p = 0.686$).

For CRP, in patients with UC and CD, a Pearson correlation coefficient of −0.512 and −0.16 ($p = 0.01$ and 0.256), respectively, was obtained (Figure 5). These results demonstrate a strong correlation between CRP and vitamin D exclusively in patients with UC, not in CD. Therefore, there are significant differences between the correlation slopes ($p = 0.02$). No linear correlation was found between FBG values and vitamin D levels (R near 0).

The statistical normality study of FC, CRP and FBG showed a non-normal distribution and, as a consequence, a Kruskal–Wallis test for groups comparison was performed. Significant differences for FC were found between the medians of the SD (345 µg/g), MD (46 µg/g) and S (30 µg/g) groups with a *p*-value < 0.001 (Figure 6). A similar study for CRP also showed significant differences (*p* = 0.01) while no differences were obtained for FBG. Figure 7 shows box and whisker plots of inflammatory markers depending on vitamin D levels. Data were normalised for representation purposes. As can be seen, there were significant differences at 99% (**) in the contents of CRP and FC depending on the vitamin D levels.

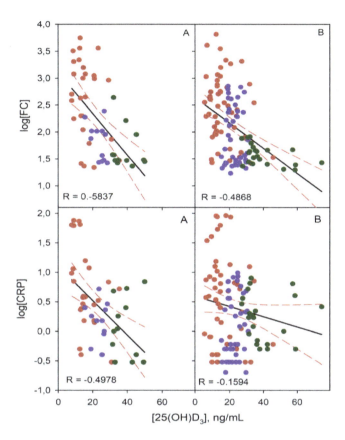

Figure 5. Linear correlation graphs of FC and CRP (log transform) with vitamin D for UC (**A**) and CD (**B**) patients. Red, blue and green points correspond to SD, MD and S vitamin D level, respectively.

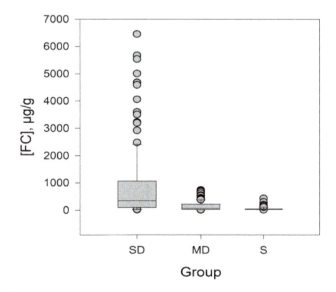

Figure 6. Box and whisker plot to represent the nonparametric variable FC, the values inside the box conform the 25th and 75th percentile, while the horizontal line that crosses the box marks the median. The values outside the whiskers are considered atypical.

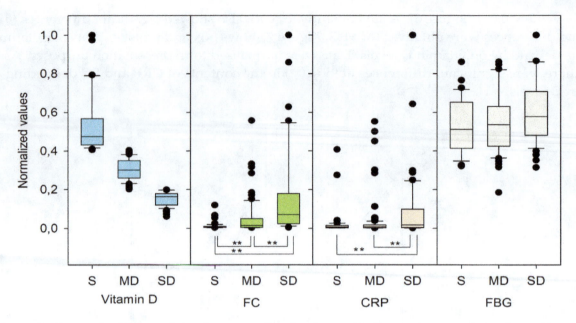

Figure 7. Box and whisker plot using normalised values of inflammatory markers depending on vitamin D levels. (**) correspond to significant differences at 99% (Dun's test for multiple comparisons on the Kruskal–Wallis test).

A multivariate discriminant analysis of FC, CRP and FBG shows a discriminant level of 80%. In this way, 74% of SD patients and 85% of S patients were correctly classified by the model.

3.4. Vitamin D Progression

The progression of vitamin D levels over time was evaluated. Patients were divided according to active supplementation. The mean vitamin D determination in the third event did not reach more than 25 ng/mL of vitamin D despite supposedly adequate supplementation. The Bonferroni test indicated significant differences between situations 0 with 1 and 0 with 2, while showing no differences between situations 1 and 2. This behaviour was the same in the group of patients who were supplemented and not supplemented (Figure 8).

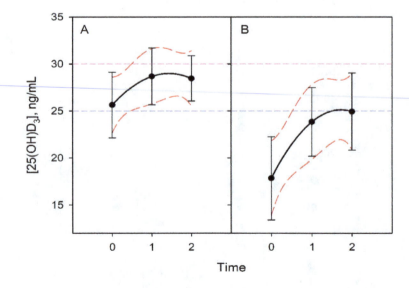

Figure 8. Evolution of vitamin D content in nonsupplemented individuals (**A**). The graph presents the lines of regression of the contents and their slopes. Active supplementation (**B**) did not guarantee levels of sufficiency in these patients.

3.5. Categorical Variables Study

For the categorical variables, a logistic regression analysis was used. Negative binomial regression showed an association between the SD group and a higher probability of having flare-ups, hospitalisations and clinic visit (*p*-value = 0.002). Graphically, it can be seen that for vitamin D levels below 20 ng/mL, the flare-up and hospitalisation rates increased exponentially regardless of the group (Figure 9).

There was a correlation between those patients in the SD group and the probability of receiving treatment with steroids. Another correlation was also observed with the probability of introducing changes or the need for escalating treatment. All these results were statistically significant ($p < 0.001$).

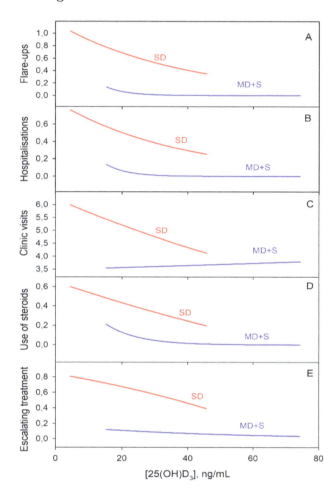

Figure 9. Logistic regression of clinical disease activity markers with vitamin D content. From A to E: Flare-ups, hospitalisations, clinic visits, use of steroids and escalating treatment, respectively.

4. Discussion

In this retrospective longitudinal study, we succeeded in describing an inverse correlation between serum vitamin D levels and both systemic inflammatory markers (CRP) and intestinal inflammatory markers (FC). Our findings confirm that vitamin D levels are also correlated with clinical disease activity, as represented in hospitalisations, flare-ups, number of clinic visits, use of steroids and changes in therapy. Additionally, we evaluated the vitamin D progression under oral supplementation, finding an insufficient absorptive capacity.

Other studies support the association between vitamin D and inflammation. In a cross-sectional study, Meckel et al. [32] demonstrated that serum $25(OH)D_3$ concentrations are inversely correlated with endoscopic and histologic inflammation and disease activity. In addition, they found that $25(OH)D_3$ concentrations correlated with the mucosal expression of VDR as well as epithelial junction proteins. Moreover, in a retrospective cohort of 60 patients, it was reported that vitamin D was inversely correlated with erythrocyte sedimentation rate (ESR), FC and clinical disease activity measured by Harvey–Bradshaw Index > 5 [36].

Supporting the results of our study, Kabbani et al. [37], in one of the largest prospective cohort studies, demonstrated that patients with low vitamin D levels required more hospitalisations, biologic therapy, steroids, surgeries and healthcare utilisation. We have demonstrated a strong correlation between vitamin D and FC as other authors [38] have done in similar studies. We describe an inverse correlation between vitamin D status and systemic inflammation (CRP levels) in UC. In another prospective study, Gubatan et al. [39] demonstrated that those patients with vitamin levels below 35 ng/mL were at greater risk of future clinical relapse.

However, there are some uncertainties not resolved yet concerning vitamin D influence on IBD. Several translational studies are emerging to attempt to understand its hormonal pathophysiology, and there are some interventional studies trying to evaluate its active supplementation. Despite the importance of sunlight exposure in vitamin D levels, only a few studies have considered the season where the sample was collected. Baseline vitamin D levels are not yet established to evaluate deficiency and sufficiency. Thus, it is difficult to assess which patients are at real risk of developing clinical consequences. In our study, we set that limit at <15 ng/mL, but other authors set it at <20 or <35 ng/mL. The extent of the supplementation that should be given to our patients and what leads to sufficiency during IBD clinical activity is also unclear.

In our study, several limitations must be considered. Despite describing a strong association between vitamin D deficiency and higher inflammatory markers and disease activity, we cannot confirm a causal relationship due to the retrospective collection of data. A notable cohort study of patients was included in our study, but the inclusion enrolment was in only one single centre by the main researcher. Thus, methodological flaws are possible, including selection bias. Finally, our study is observational and limited by the inability to account for potential unmeasured confounders. Although we evaluated active vitamin D supplementation, we did not consider baseline dietary vitamin D intake, summer or winter season measurement, body mass index, physical activity and adherence to medical therapy and supplementation. There is a relationship between vitamin D receptor genes (VDR), autophagy and gut microbial assemblage that is essential for maintaining intestinal homeostasis and contributes to the pathophysiology of IBD. However, genetic data regarding VDR polymorphisms has not been considered in this study.

Garg et al. [40] designed an interventional study on vitamin D supplementation where the enrolled IBD patients were given up to 10,000 IU (international units) of oral cholecalciferol. Despite achieving improved symptom-based activity scores and a mean of 41.6 ng/mL of $25(OH)D_3$, no significant reduction in FC levels was observed. It is remarkable that there was no control group in this study. Sharifi et al. [41], on the other hand, in a randomised trial, demonstrated a significant decrease in CRP and ESR levels with a single dose of 30,000 IU intramuscular vitamin D supplement. These results support the findings in our study in terms of insufficient supplementation. Doses recommended by guidelines, although suitable for bone health, appear to be clearly insufficient for IBD patients. Considering chronic oral malabsorption, future studies are warranted to explore significant differences in clinical scores or intestinal inflammation depending on the route of vitamin D administration. A higher target $25(OH)D_3$ concentrations during active supplementation should also be evaluated to clarify beneficial outcomes in IBD patients.

5. Conclusions

Vitamin D deficiency is now recognised as another predictor of clinical disease activity according to recent research. This study demonstrates that low serum circulating $25(OH)D_3$ is associated with intestinal inflammation (FC) in IBD and systemic inflammation (CRP) in UC. Deficiency of $25(OH)D_3$ is associated with more hospitalisations, flare-ups, use of steroids and escalating treatment. Standard vitamin D oral dose of supplementation is probably insufficient to reach normal serum $25(OH)D_3$.

Vitamin D intervention studies are warranted to determine whether raising serum 25(OH)D$_3$ level with higher doses of oral vitamin D in IBD may reduce intestinal inflammation or disease activity.

Author Contributions: P.L.-M.: planning and/or conducting the study, collecting and/or interpreting data, and/or drafting the manuscript. He approved the final draft submitted. B.B.: planning and/or conducting the study, collecting and/or interpreting data, and/or drafting the manuscript. She approved the final draft submitted. E.S.-G.: collecting and/or interpreting data. He approved the final draft submitted. She approved the final draft submitted. A.A.: providing laboratory support in vitamin D measurement, collecting and/or interpreting data. She approved the final draft submitted. P.N.: collecting and/or interpreting data. She approved the final draft submitted. M.I.: planning and/or conducting the study, collecting and/or interpreting data, and/or drafting the manuscript. She approved the final draft submitted.

Acknowledgments: We are very thankful to Victoria Fornes from the Department of Biostatistics of Hospital la Fe.

References

1. Stamp, T.C.; Haddad, J.G.; Twigg, C.A. Comparison of oral 25-hydroxycholecalciferol, vitamin D, and ultraviolet light as determinants of circulating 25-hydroxyvitamin D. *Lancet* **1977**, *1*, 1341–1343. [CrossRef]
2. Alrefai, D.; Jones, J.; El-Matary, W.; Whiting, S.J.; Aljebreen, A.; Mirhosseini, N.; Vatanparast, H. The Association of Vitamin D Status with Disease Activity in a Cohort of Crohn's Disease Patients in Canada. *Nutrients* **2017**, *9*. [CrossRef] [PubMed]
3. White, J.H. Vitamin D metabolism and signaling in the immune system. *Rev. Endocr. Metab. Disord.* **2012**, *13*, 21–29. [CrossRef] [PubMed]
4. Lips, P. Vitamin D physiology. *Prog. Biophys. Mol. Biol.* **2006**, *92*, 4–8. [CrossRef]
5. Bikle, D.D. Vitamin D metabolism, mechanism of action, and clinical applications. *Chem. Biol.* **2014**, *21*, 319–329. [CrossRef]
6. Lim, W.-C.; Hanauer, S.B.; Li, Y.C. Mechanisms of Disease: Vitamin D and inflammatory bowel disease. *Nat. Clin. Pract. Gastroenterol. Hepatol.* **2005**, *2*, 308. [CrossRef] [PubMed]
7. Levine, B.S.; Song, M. Pharmacokinetics and efficacy of pulse oral versus intravenous calcitriol in hemodialysis patients. *J. Am. Soc. Nephrol.* **1996**, *7*, 488–496.
8. Jones, K.S.; Assar, S.; Harnpanich, D.; Bouillon, R.; Lambrechts, D.; Prentice, A.; Schoenmakers, I. 25(OH)D-2 Half-Life Is Shorter Than 25(OH)D-3 Half-Life and Is Influenced by DBP Concentration and Genotype. *J. Clin. Endocrinol. Metab.* **2014**, *99*, 3373–3381. [CrossRef] [PubMed]
9. Wobke, T.K.; Sorg, B.L.; Steinhilber, D. Vitamin D in inflammatory diseases. *Front. Physiol.* **2014**, *5*, 244. [CrossRef] [PubMed]
10. Cantorna, M.T.; Zhu, Y.; Froicu, M.; Wittke, A. Vitamin D status, 1,25-dihydroxyvitamin D3, and the immune system. *Am. J. Clin. Nutr.* **2004**, *80*, 1717s–1720s. [CrossRef]
11. Gubatan, J.; Moss, A.C. Vitamin D in inflammatory bowel disease: More than just a supplement. *Curr. Opin. Gastroenterol.* **2018**, *34*, 217–225. [CrossRef]
12. Stio, M.; Retico, L.; Annese, V.; Bonanomi, A.G. Vitamin D regulates the tight-junction protein expression in active ulcerative colitis. *Scand. J. Gastroenterol.* **2016**, *51*, 1193–1199. [CrossRef] [PubMed]
13. Zhang, Y.G.; Lu, R.; Xia, Y.; Zhou, D.; Petrof, E.; Claud, E.C.; Sun, J. Lack of Vitamin D Receptor Leads to Hyperfunction of Claudin-2 in Intestinal Inflammatory Responses. *Inflamm. Bowel Dis.* **2019**, *25*, 97–110. [CrossRef]
14. Gisbert-Ferrandiz, L.; Salvador, P.; Ortiz-Masia, D.; Macias-Ceja, D.C.; Orden, S.; Esplugues, J.V.; Calatayud, S.; Hinojosa, J.; Barrachina, M.D.; Hernandez, C. A Single Nucleotide Polymorphism in the Vitamin D Receptor Gene Is Associated with Decreased Levels of the Protein and a Penetrating Pattern in Crohn's Disease. *Inflamm. Bowel Dis.* **2018**, *24*, 1462–1470. [CrossRef] [PubMed]
15. Wang, T.T.; Dabbas, B.; Laperriere, D.; Bitton, A.J.; Soualhine, H.; Tavera-Mendoza, L.E.; Dionne, S.; Servant, M.J.; Bitton, A.; Seidman, E.G.; et al. Direct and indirect induction by 1,25-dihydroxyvitamin D3 of the NOD2/CARD15-defensin beta2 innate immune pathway defective in Crohn disease. *J. Biol. Chem.* **2010**, *285*, 2227–2231. [CrossRef]
16. Hugot, J.P.; Chamaillard, M.; Zouali, H.; Lesage, S.; Cezard, J.P.; Belaiche, J.; Almer, S.; Tysk, C.; O'Morain, C.A.; Gassull, M.; et al. Association of NOD2 leucine-rich repeat variants with susceptibility to Crohn's disease. *Nature* **2001**, *411*, 599–603. [CrossRef] [PubMed]

17. Fellermann, K.; Stange, D.E.; Schaeffeler, E.; Schmalzl, H.; Wehkamp, J.; Bevins, C.L.; Reinisch, W.; Teml, A.; Schwab, M.; Lichter, P.; et al. A chromosome 8 gene-cluster polymorphism with low human beta-defensin 2 gene copy number predisposes to Crohn disease of the colon. *Am. J. Hum. Genet.* **2006**, *79*, 439–448. [CrossRef]

18. Gombart, A.F.; Borregaard, N.; Koeffler, H.P. Human cathelicidin antimicrobial peptide (CAMP) gene is a direct target of the vitamin D receptor and is strongly up-regulated in myeloid cells by 1,25-dihydroxyvitamin D3. *FASEB J.* **2005**, *19*, 1067–1077. [CrossRef]

19. Wang, T.T.; Nestel, F.P.; Bourdeau, V.; Nagai, Y.; Wang, Q.; Liao, J.; Tavera-Mendoza, L.; Lin, R.; Hanrahan, J.W.; Mader, S.; et al. Cutting edge: 1,25-dihydroxyvitamin D3 is a direct inducer of antimicrobial peptide gene expression. *J. Immunol.* **2004**, *173*, 2909–2912. [CrossRef]

20. D'Ambrosio, D.; Cippitelli, M.; Cocciolo, M.G.; Mazzeo, D.; Di Lucia, P.; Lang, R.; Sinigaglia, F.; Panina-Bordignon, P. Inhibition of IL-12 production by 1,25-dihydroxyvitamin D3. Involvement of NF-kappaB downregulation in transcriptional repression of the p40 gene. *J. Clin. Investig.* **1998**, *101*, 252–262. [CrossRef]

21. Penna, G.; Adorini, L. 1 Alpha,25-dihydroxyvitamin D3 inhibits differentiation, maturation, activation, and survival of dendritic cells leading to impaired alloreactive T cell activation. *J. Immunol.* **2000**, *164*, 2405–2411. [CrossRef] [PubMed]

22. Boonstra, A.; Barrat, F.J.; Crain, C.; Heath, V.L.; Savelkoul, H.F.; O'Garra, A. 1alpha,25-Dihydroxyvitamin d3 has a direct effect on naive CD4(+) T cells to enhance the development of Th2 cells. *J. Immunol.* **2001**, *167*, 4974–4980. [CrossRef] [PubMed]

23. Gubatan, J.; Mitsuhashi, S.; Longhi, M.S.; Zenlea, T.; Rosenberg, L.; Robson, S.; Moss, A.C. Higher serum vitamin D levels are associated with protective serum cytokine profiles in patients with ulcerative colitis. *Cytokine* **2018**, *103*, 38–45. [CrossRef]

24. Luthold, R.V.; Fernandes, G.R.; Franco-de-Moraes, A.C.; Folchetti, L.G.; Ferreira, S.R. Gut microbiota interactions with the immunomodulatory role of vitamin D in normal individuals. *Metabolism* **2017**, *69*, 76–86. [CrossRef] [PubMed]

25. Schaffler, H.; Herlemann, D.P.R.; Klinitzke, P.; Berlin, P.; Kreikemeyer, B.; Jaster, R.; Lamprecht, G. Vitamin D administration leads to a shift of the intestinal bacterial composition in Crohn's disease patients, but not in healthy controls. *J. Dig. Dis.* **2018**, *19*, 225–234. [CrossRef]

26. Dziarski, R.; Park, S.Y.; Kashyap, D.R.; Dowd, S.E.; Gupta, D. Pglyrp-Regulated Gut Microflora Prevotella falsenii, Parabacteroides distasonis and Bacteroides eggerthii Enhance and Alistipes finegoldii Attenuates Colitis in Mice. *PLoS ONE* **2016**, *11*. [CrossRef] [PubMed]

27. Tamanai-Shacoori, Z.; Smida, I.; Bousarghin, L.; Loreal, O.; Meuric, V.; Fong, S.B.; Bonnaure-Mallet, M.; Jolivet-Gougeon, A. Roseburia spp.: A marker of health? *Future Microbiol.* **2017**, *12*, 157–170. [CrossRef] [PubMed]

28. Del Pinto, R.; Pietropaoli, D.; Chandar, A.K.; Ferri, C.; Cominelli, F. Association Between Inflammatory Bowel Disease and Vitamin D Deficiency: A Systematic Review and Meta-analysis. *Inflamm. Bowel Dis.* **2015**, *21*, 2708–2717. [CrossRef]

29. Filippi, J.; Al-Jaouni, R.; Wiroth, J.B.; Hebuterne, X.; Schneider, S.M. Nutritional deficiencies in patients with Crohn's disease in remission. *Inflamm. Bowel Dis.* **2006**, *12*, 185–191. [CrossRef] [PubMed]

30. Raftery, T.; Merrick, M.; Healy, M.; Mahmud, N.; O'Morain, C.; Smith, S.; McNamara, D.; O'Sullivan, M. Vitamin D Status Is Associated with Intestinal Inflammation as Measured by Fecal Calprotectin in Crohn's Disease in Clinical Remission. *Dig. Dis. Sci.* **2015**, *60*, 2427–2435. [CrossRef]

31. Frigstad, S.O.; Hoivik, M.; Jahnsen, J.; Dahl, S.R.; Cvancarova, M.; Grimstad, T.; Berset, I.P.; Huppertz-Hauss, G.; Hovde, O.; Torp, R.; et al. Vitamin D deficiency in inflammatory bowel disease: Prevalence and predictors in a Norwegian outpatient population. *Scand. J. Gastroenterol.* **2017**, *52*, 100–106. [CrossRef] [PubMed]

32. Meckel, K.; Li, Y.C.; Lim, J.; Kocherginsky, M.; Weber, C.; Almoghrabi, A.; Chen, X.; Kaboff, A.; Sadiq, F.; Hanauer, S.B.; et al. Serum 25-hydroxyvitamin D concentration is inversely associated with mucosal inflammation in patients with ulcerative colitis. *Am. J. Clin. Nutr.* **2016**, *104*, 113–120. [CrossRef]

33. Santos-Antunes, J.; Nunes, A.C.; Lopes, S.; Macedo, G. The Relevance of Vitamin D and Antinuclear Antibodies in Patients with Inflammatory Bowel Disease Under Anti-TNF Treatment: A Prospective Study. *Inflamm. Bowel Dis.* **2016**, *22*, 1101–1106. [CrossRef] [PubMed]

34. Schaffler, H.; Schmidt, M.; Huth, A.; Reiner, J.; Glass, A.; Lamprecht, G. Clinical factors are associated with vitamin D levels in IBD patients: A retrospective analysis. *J. Dig. Dis.* **2018**, *19*, 24–32. [CrossRef] [PubMed]

35. Venkata, K.V.R.; Arora, S.S.; Xie, F.L.; Malik, T.A. Impact of vitamin D on the hospitalization rate of Crohn's disease patients seen at a tertiary care center. *World J. Gastroenterol.* **2017**, *23*, 2539–2544. [CrossRef]

36. Scolaro, B.L.; Barretta, C.; Matos, C.H.; Malluta, E.F.; Almeida, I.B.T.d.; Braggio, L.D.; Bobato, S.; Specht, C.M. Deficiency of vitamin D and its relation with clinical and laboratory activity of inflammatory bowel diseases. *JCOL* **2018**, *38*, 99–104. [CrossRef]

37. Kabbani, T.A.; Koutroubakis, I.E.; Schoen, R.E.; Ramos-Rivers, C.; Shah, N.; Swoger, J.; Regueiro, M.; Barrie, A.; Schwartz, M.; Hashash, J.G.; et al. Association of Vitamin D Level with Clinical Status in Inflammatory Bowel Disease: A 5-Year Longitudinal Study. *Am. J. Gastroenterol.* **2016**, *111*, 712–719. [CrossRef]

38. Garg, M.; Rosella, O.; Lubel, J.S.; Gibson, P.R. Association of circulating vitamin D concentrations with intestinal but not systemic inflammation in inflammatory bowel disease. *Inflamm. Bowel Dis.* **2013**, *19*, 2634–2643. [CrossRef]

39. Gubatan, J.; Mitsuhashi, S.; Zenlea, T.; Rosenberg, L.; Robson, S.; Moss, A.C. Low Serum Vitamin D During Remission Increases Risk of Clinical Relapse in Patients with Ulcerative Colitis. *Clin. Gastroenterol. Hepatol.* **2017**, *15*, 240–246. [CrossRef]

40. Garg, M.; Rosella, O.; Rosella, G.; Wu, Y.; Lubel, J.S.; Gibson, P.R. Evaluation of a 12-week targeted vitamin D supplementation regimen in patients with active inflammatory bowel disease. *Clin. Nutr.* **2018**, *37*, 1375–1382. [CrossRef]

41. Sharifi, A.; Hosseinzadeh-Attar, M.J.; Vahedi, H.; Nedjat, S. A randomized controlled trial on the effect of vitamin D3 on inflammation and cathelicidin gene expression in ulcerative colitis patients. *Saudi J. Gastroenterol.* **2016**, *22*, 316–323. [CrossRef] [PubMed]

10

Dietary Protein Intake Level Modulates Mucosal Healing and Mucosa-Adherent Microbiota in Mouse Model of Colitis

Sandra Vidal-Lletjós [1], Mireille Andriamihaja [1], Anne Blais [1], Marta Grauso [1], Patricia Lepage [2], Anne-Marie Davila [1], Roselyne Viel [3], Claire Gaudichon [1], Marion Leclerc [2], François Blachier [1] and Annaïg Lan [1,*]

[1] UMR PNCA, AgroParisTech, INRA, Université Paris-Saclay, 75005 Paris, France; sandravidalll@gmail.com (S.V.-L.); mireille.andriamihaja@agroparistech.fr (M.A.); anne.blais@agroparistech.fr (A.B.); marta.grausoculetto@agroparistech.fr (M.G.); anne-marie.davila-gay@agroparistech.fr (A.-M.D.); claire.gaudichon@agroparistech.fr (C.G.); francois.blachier@agroparistech.fr (F.B.)

[2] UMR MICALIS, AgroParisTech, INRA, Université Paris-Saclay, 78350 Jouy-en-Josas, France; patricia.lepage@inra.fr (P.L.); marion.leclerc@inra.fr (M.L.)

[3] H2P2, Biosit-Biogenouest, Université de Rennes 1, 35005 Rennes, France; roselyne.viel@univ-rennes1.fr

[*] Correspondence: annaig.lan@agroparistech.fr

Abstract: Mucosal healing after an inflammatory flare is associated with lasting clinical remission. The aim of the present work was to evaluate the impact of the amount of dietary protein on epithelial repair after an acute inflammatory episode. C57BL/6 DSS-treated mice received isocaloric diets with different levels of dietary protein: 14% (P14), 30% (P30) and 53% (P53) for 3 (*day 10*), 6 (*day 13*) and 21 (*day 28*) days after the time of colitis maximal intensity. While the P53 diet worsened the DSS- induced inflammation both in intensity and duration, the P30 diet, when compared to the P14 diet, showed a beneficial effect during the epithelial repair process by accelerating inflammation resolution, reducing colonic permeability and increasing epithelial repair together with epithelial hyperproliferation. Dietary protein intake also impacted mucosa-adherent microbiota composition after inflammation since P30 fed mice showed increased colonization of butyrate-producing genera throughout the resolution phase. This study revealed that in our colitis model, the amount of protein in the diet modulated mucosal healing, with beneficial effects of a moderately high-protein diet, while very high-protein diet displayed deleterious effects on this process.

Keywords: dietary protein level; colitis; epithelial repair; mucosa-adherent microbiota

1. Introduction

In recent years, mucosal healing (MH) has become a therapeutic goal for the prevention of the complications of inflammatory bowel diseases (IBD) [1–4]. MH relies on concomitant cellular events that provide epithelial repair to restore the tissue integrity and the physiological functions of the colon such as barrier function and water absorption [4,5], these events being presumably protein and energy consuming processes. In addition, the nutritional status is known to be impaired during and after an intestinal inflammatory episode due in particular to the catabolic action of the pro-inflammatory cytokines [6]. Although there is some evidence that the daily protein needs of IBD patients may differ from those of healthy controls, further experimental and clinical data are required to fully validate this concept. The European Society for Clinical Nutrition and Metabolism recommends to increase the protein intake in active IBD to 1.2–1.5 g/kg body weight/day in adults and to maintain a similar level as it is recommended for the general population during remission (about 1 g/kg body weight/day) [7]. However, the beneficial effects of increasing dietary protein level have been barely studied. Notwithstanding, majoring dietary protein intake may impact the colonic mucosa in the healthy gut as recently reviewed [8] by altering colonocyte biology [9,10] and colonic luminal environment [11–14]. Furthermore, we showed that a high protein (HP, 53% of total energy provided by protein) intake exacerbated acute colonic inflammation when simultaneously given with colitis induction [15]. Interestingly, the same study showed that this protein level in the diet was rather beneficial after the acute episode of colitis as it enhanced colonic epithelium restoration in surviving animals, thus indicating a potential effect of the dietary protein level on colonic crypt repair after acute inflammation [15]. Actually, supplementation with some AA, alone or in combination, improved parameters related to mucosal healing in colitis model such as epithelial regeneration and colonic barrier function (for review, see Reference [16]). Moreover, published data suggest that the availability of some amino acids, such as threonine or cysteine, is limiting under conditions of colonic inflammation [17,18] and that dietary supplementation of protein or amino acids is needed to promote favorably epithelial repair. However, AA supplementation may also exert deleterious impact as it has been recently shown with threonine during colitis [19]. To date, the positive effect of any AA supplementation on colitis has never been demonstrated in clinical studies.

We then hypothesized that increasing dietary protein intake might influence colon epithelial repair by a direct effect of additional AA blood supply or via microbiota-derived effects. The present study thus aims to evaluate the impact of different level of dietary proteins (normoproteic (14% of the total energy provided by protein, P14)), moderately HP diet (30%, P30) and an elevated HP diet (53%, P53) on some relevant barrier function parameters after the acute inflammatory episode in the DSS-mouse model of colitis.

2. Materials and Methods

2.1. Animals and Diets

Seven-week-old C57BL/6 male mice were obtained from ENVIGO, France (144, weight 18–23 g). Animals were housed in a 12:12-h light-dark circle at 23 °C and controlled humidity (55 $\pm$ 10%) and acclimated for one week with free access to standard mouse chow and tap water. Each mouse was maintained in an individual cage with a grid and was allowed to acclimate to the P14 diet after three days of a standard mouse chow/fresh P14 diet (Table 1). The study was performed according to the European directive for the use and care of laboratory animals (2010/63/UE) and received the agreement of the local animal ethics committee and of the ministerial committee for animal experimentation (registration number: APAFIS#3987-2016012214388658).

Table 1. Composition of the experimental diets.

	P14	P30	P53
Weight content (g/kg)			
Acid casein (Armor Protéines®, ref. #139860)	112	232	424
Whey protein (Armor Protéines®, Protarmor 80, ref. #139805)	28	58	96
Corn starch	622.4	493.2	287
Sucrose	100.3	79.5	45.7
Cellulose	50	50	50
Soybean oil	40	40	40
Mineral Mixture (AIN 93-M)	35	35	35
Vitamin Mixture (AIN 93-V)	10	10	10
Choline	2.3	2.3	2.3
Energy content (%)			
Protein	14	30	55
Carbohydrate	76	60	35
Fat	10	10	10
Energy density (kJ/g)	14.5	14.5	14.5

2.2. Experimental Design

Three types of experimental isocaloric diets (14.5 kJ/g) were used in this study: a normoproteic diet (P14, 140 g/kg milk protein), a moderately HP diet (P30, 300 g/kg of milk protein) and an elevated HP diet (P53, 530 g/kg of milk protein) isocellulose diet with similar energy content (Table 1). Healthy controls (non-treated mice at *day 0*, n = 12) received fresh tap water. DSS-treated mice (n = 132) were given 3.5% (wt/vol) DSS (36,000–50,000 MW, MP Biomedicals Illkirch-Graffenstaden, France) in the drinking water for 5 days, from *day 1* to *day 5* (fresh DSS solution being prepared every two days) to induce an acute colitis episode (Figure 1). At *day 7*, corresponding to the maximal intensity of colon inflammation, mice were divided into three groups with the same mean body weight (BW) and were fed either the P14, the P30 or the P53 diet during 3, 6 or 21 days. Food and drink were given ad libitum and measured daily. Disease activity was scored based on stool consistency, rectal bleeding and percentage of body weight loss, as previously described [15]. For each parameter, a score of 0 to 3 was attributed: loss of weight (0, none; 1, 0%–10%; 2, 10%–20%; 3, >20%), stool consistency (0, normal pellets; 1, slightly loose feces; 2, loose feces; 3, watery diarrhea) and visible fecal blood (0, negative; 1, slightly bloody; 2, bloody; 3, blood in the whole colon). Mice were euthanized to evaluate the impact of diet on epithelial repair kinetics at *days 10* (n = 12), *13* (n = 12) and *28* (n = 16) per diet group (Figure 1). Body fat and lean body mass of mice belonging to *day 28* group, were measured every nine days with dual-energy x-ray absorptiometry (DEXA) using a PIXImus imager (GE Lunar PIXImus, GE Healthcare, Fitchburg, WI, USA). Mice were euthanized if they lost more than 20% BW, as per approved animal protocol guidelines, to meet the end point criteria.

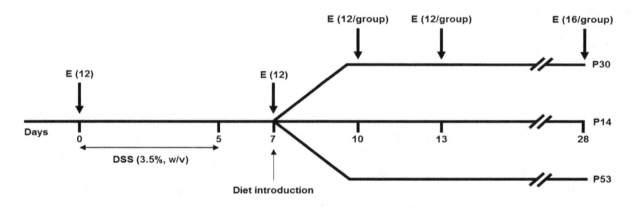

Figure 1. Schematic representation of the experimental design. Mice received either P14 (14% of proteins), P30 (30% of proteins) or P53 (53% of proteins) diet from D7 to D28. Mice were euthanized (E) at *day 0, 7*, and during the resolution phase at *days 10, 13* and *28*.

2.3. Intestinal Permeability Assessment

Firstly, epithelial barrier integrity was assessed in vivo with the 4 kDa paracellular marker fluorescein isothiocyanate (FITC)-labeled dextran (FD4, Sigma-Aldrich, St Quentin Fallavier, France) at *days 9, 12* and *18*. Food was withdrawn for 4h before gavage (600 mg/kg BW of FD4) and plasma was collected from the tail 4 h later (n = 8/diet group). Fluorescence intensity of each sample was later used to calculate permeability using standard curves generated by serial dilution of FD4. Secondly, at euthanasia, the proximal colon section was mounted in EasyMount Ussing chambers (Physiologic Instrument Inc, San Diego, CA, USA), within 15 min from dissection as previously described [13]. Paracellular permeability was assessed by measuring the mucosal-to-serosal flux of FD4 at a final concentration of 0.25 mg/mL, and fluorescence units (FU) were measured 90 min later with the Infinite® 200 Pro spectrofluorimeter (TECAN, Männedorf, Switzerland). Tissue viability was assessed at the end of each recording by adding the cholinergic drug carbachol (10^{-4} M) on the serosal side.

2.4. Tissue Collection

Mice were euthanized by an intracardiac puncture after sedation by isoflurane. Plasma was frozen and kept at $-80\,°C$ for later measurement of cytokines and lipopolysaccharide binding protein (LBP) concentrations. Colon was resected, measured, weighted and the proximal colon section mounted in Ussing chamber. Proximal colon mucosa was scraped for latter mucosa-adherent bacterial DNA extraction procedure. Colon samples were harvested for RNA analysis, myeloperoxidase (MPO) activity and protein expression assays, immediately frozen in liquid nitrogen and stored at $-80\,°C$ after resection. Histological analysis was performed with distal colon fixed in 4% buffered formaldehyde.

2.4.1. Determination of Local and Systemic Inflammatory Markers

Colon inflammation was assayed with MPO assay measurement as described in Reference [20] and colonic IL-1β and IL-6 concentrations were measured by Luminex technology in total colon protein lysate by using Bio-Plex kits (Bio-Rad, Marnes-La- Coquette, France). Plasma concentration of LBP was determined with a commercial solid-phase sandwich ELISA (PikoKine ELISA Kit Mouse, Set EK1274; Boechout, Belgium).

2.4.2. Histological Analysis

Histological and re-epithelization scores on hematoxylin-and-eosin (HE) stained colonic sections were calculated as previously described (Vidal-Lletjós, et al., submitted) after blind microscopic assessment performed by the histological platform Histalim (Montpellier, France). Quantitative evaluation of well-oriented crypts and cell numeration in periodic acid-schiff (PAS) stained 4-μm transversal colon sections was determined using the image analysis software Pannoramic Viewer v. 1.15.4 (3DHISTECH, Budapest, Hungary). Paraffin-embedded distal colon samples were cut into 4 μm-thick sections, mounted on positively charged slides and dried. Immunohistochemical stainings of Ki67 and Caspase 3 were performed on the Discovery XT Automated IHC stainer using either Ventana DAB MAP detection kit (Ventana Medical Systems, Tucson, AZ, USA) or the Ventana CHROMO MAP detection kit (Ventana Medical Systems, Tucson, AZ, USA). Following deparaffination with Discovery wash solution (Ventana), antigen retrieval was performed using a Tris-based buffer solution. Later, endogen peroxidase was blocked and slides rinsed before incubation with primary antibodies either rabbit anti-ki67 (NB600-1252 Novusbio, Centennial, CO, USA) diluted at 1/100 or rabbit anti-Casp3 (9661, Cell Signaling, Danvers, MA, USA) diluted at 1/250. For Ki67 staining, signal enhancement was performed using Goat anti-Rabbit biotinylated secondary antibody (Vector laboratory, Burlingame, CA, USA) and DAB MAP detection kit. An anti-rabbit HRP (Ventana Medical Systems, Tucson, AZ, USA) secondary antibody and the CHROMO MAP detection kit (Ventana Medical Systems, Tucson, AZ, USA) was used for the caspase 3 staining. Slides were then counterstained with hematoxylin and rinsed. Slides were manually dehydrated and coverslipped. Ki67 labelling index was calculated as the percentage of Ki67 positive cells relative to the total number of cells within the same crypts.

2.4.3. RNA Isolation and Quantitative Real-Time PCR

Total RNA was extracted after tissue homogenization in TRIzol® Reagent (Invitrogen, Cergy Pontoise, France). Purification was performed with the RNeasy Mini Kit (Qiagen, Courtaboeuf, France) and a DNase step (Qiagen, Courtaboeuf, France). After cDNA synthesis from mRNA using a High Capacity cDNA Reverse Transcription Kit (Applied Biosystems, Fisher Scientific, Illkirch, France), quantitative real-time polymerase chain reaction (qRT-PCR) was performed (primer sequences available on demand) with the Fast SYBR Green MasterMix (Applied Biosystems, Fisher Scientific, Illkirch, France) and StepOne Real-Time PCR system (Applied Biosystems, Fisher Scientific, Illkirch, France). Gene expression level was normalized relative to the normalizing gene HPRT and normalized to *day 7* group with $2^{-\Delta\Delta Ct}$ calculation.

2.4.4. Western-Blot Analysis

Frozen colonic tissue was homogenized in a lysis buffer [15], and 25 µg of total protein lysates were loaded onto 4%–12% Criterion XT gel (Bio-Rad, Marnes-La-Coquette, France) before electrophoresis in MOPS buffer (Bio-Rad, Marnes-La-Coquette, France). After transfer onto nitrocellulose membrane and incubation in blocking solution (TBS pH 7.5, 0.05% Tween 20, and 5% (wt/vol) non-fat dry milk), membranes were incubated overnight (4 °C) with rabbit ZO-1 antibody (1/250, 617300, Invitrogen, Cergy Pontoise, France) or with mouse claudin-1 antibody (1/250, 374900, Thermo-Fisher Scientific, Bedford, MA, USA) diluted in blocking solution. After three washes, blots were incubated for 2 h at room temperature with an anti-rabbit or anti-mouse HRP-linked secondary antibody. Revealing was performed using enhanced chemiluminescence (ECL system, Pierce Biotechnology, Courtabœuf, France), and bands were quantified by densitometry using the FluorChem FC2 device and the AlphaView software (Cell Biosciences, Santa Clara, CA, USA). GAPDH expression (Ab9484, mouse monoclonal antibody, Abcam, Cambridge, UK) was used to ensure consistent protein loading and transferring.

2.4.5. Evaluation of Adherent Mucosal Microbiota Composition

From the scrapped adherent-mucosa, bacterial DNA extracts were obtained by using the PowerFecal DNA Isolation kit (MoBio Laboratories, Carlsbad, CA, USA) according to the manufacturer's protocol. Specific regions of the bacterial 16S rDNA gene were amplified using real-time qPCR. Eubacteria were quantified by real-time qPCR using specific primers (HAD-1: 5′-TGGCTCAGGACGAACGCTGGCGGC-3′ and HAD-2: 5′-CCTACTGCTGCCTCCCGTAGGAGT-3′), annealing at 59 °C for total bacteria. In addition, the V3-V4 region amplification of the 16S rDNA gene was performed and sent to the GenoToul platform (Castanet-Tolosan, France) for MiSeq Illumina sequencing using the MiSeq kit V2 2 × 250 bp. Data quality check and analysis were performed using the INRA-Migale server, as previously published [21]. In parallel, sulphate-reducing bacteria group were quantified by real-time qPCR using specific primers targeting Dissimilatory Sulfite Reductase A (DSR-1F: 5′-ACSCACTGGAAGCACGGCGG-3′ and DSR-R: 5′-GTGGMRCCGTGCAKRTTGG-3′), Fast SYBR Green MasterMix (Applied Biosystems, Fisher Scientific, Illkirch, France) and StepOne Real-Time PCR system (Applied Biosystems, Fisher Scientific, Illkirch, France).

2.5. Statistical Analysis

All statistical analysis were performed with R software version 1.0.143 (Boston, MA, USA). For follow-up data, a mixed-model was used with mice as random effect while diet and time repeated factor were used as fixed effects. From *day 7*, the mean of values for each diet were compared using Bonferonni post-hoc tests. For parameters measured at euthanasia, Anova with diet as a fixed effect was used and the means were compared using Bonferonni post-hoc tests. For all statistical tests, the level of significance was set to $p < 0.05$. Principal component analysis (PCA) was performed on family-level taxonomy to assess the influence of diet on the mucosa-adherent microbiota composition at *days 10, 13* and *28* as well as all times combined. The analysis of similarity (Anosim) test was used to assess the correlation between the ecological distance (based on family composition) and diet groups where an R-value of 0 indicates the highest dissimilarity possible and 1 indicates the highest similarity possible.

3. Results

3.1. Dietary Protein Level Influences Colon Inflammation and Body Weight Recovery

High protein diets, which were introduced the day of the maximal inflammatory score (at *day 7*), did not influence mortality, which was similar between the three groups (12.5% per diet) from *day 3* to *day 14*. After an average of 14% BW loss, mild to severe diarrhoea and rectal bleeding, disease activity index (DAI) started to decline after *day 8* for P14 and P30 diets (Figure 2A), while a two-day delay was observed for P53 mice. In this latter group of animals, the DAI was systematically two-point higher from *day 9* to *day 19* when compared to the other two diets (Figure 2A) due mainly to higher stool consistency score. This was confirmed by the area under the curve (AUC) values, even though P14 and P30 were not different between them (P14: 72.6 and P30: 71.03 AUC of DAI measured between 0 and 28 days, NS), both were statistically different from P53 (45.8 AUC of DAI for 28 days, vs P14 and P30, $p < 0.01$). In addition, P30 mice recovered their fat mass more rapidly than with the two other diets (P14: 33.9, P30: 49.2 and P53: 23.0 AUC of fat percentage evolution between *days 7* and *26*, $p < 0.001$) (Figure 2B). These differences were not related to the global energy intake level, since diet intake per day was similar whatever the diet (data not shown). P14 and P30 fed-mice presented a similar level of inflammation based on colon MPO activity (Figure 2C) and IL-6 and IL-1β concentrations (Figure 2D) but these inflammatory biomarkers were higher in P53-fed mice. Colonic MPO activity was indeed significantly increased at *day 28* for P53 mice compared to P30 (Figure 2C), as well as the pro-inflammatory cytokines at *day 10* and at *day 28* for IL-1β (Figure 2D). However, the overall histological score (based on crypt damage, ulceration and erosion, goblet cell depletion and cell infiltration) which showed high inter-individual variability, was not different between groups whatever the time (Figure 3A). Although the histological score was significantly reduced for all the groups when compared to *day 7* (9.3 ± 1.4, $p < 0.05$), some histological abnormalities persisted for all dietary groups at *day 28*.

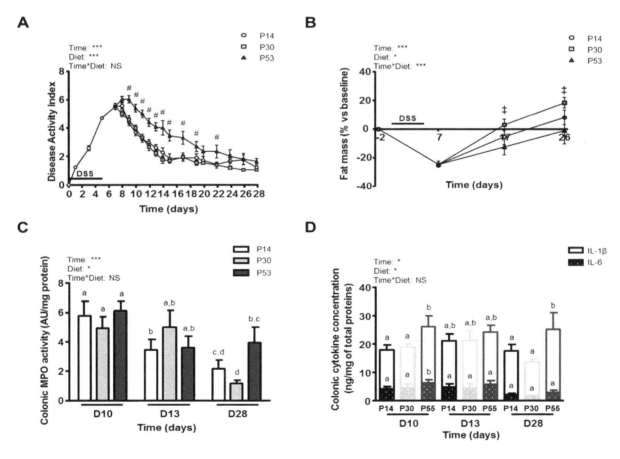

Figure 2. Effects of dietary protein intake level on inflammatory parameters at after 3 (D10), 6 (D13) or 21 days (D28) of dietary intervention with P14, P30 or P53 diet. (**A**): Disease activity index scoring evolution during time. #: $p < 0.05$ DSS P53 vs P14 and P30 at the same time point. (**B**): Evolution of fat mass (percentage vs baseline). ‡: $p < 0.05$ DSS P53 vs P30 at the same time point. (**C**): Colonic MPO activity. (**D**): Colonic concentrations of the pro-inflammatory cytokines IL-6 and IL-1β. Values are means ± SEM ($n = 9$–12). Means that are significantly different ($p < 0.05$) according to the post-hoc test have different letters (a or b or c or d). *: $p < 0.05$; ***: $p < 0.001$; NS: non-significant difference.

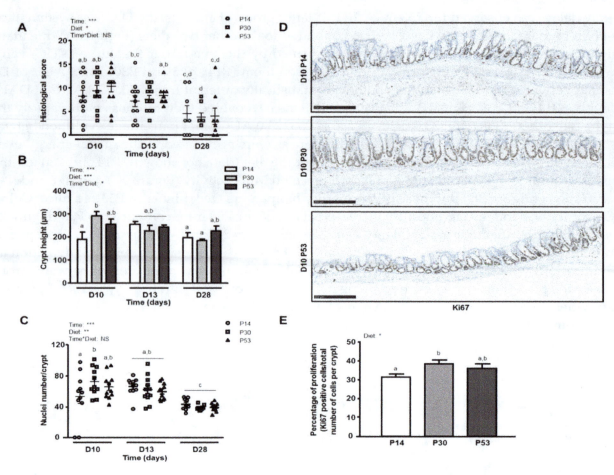

Figure 3. Effects of dietary protein intake on colon histomorphology after 3 (D10), 6 (D13) or 21 days (D28) of dietary intervention with P14, P30 or P53 diet. (**A**): Histological score. (**B**): Colon crypt length. (**C**): Cell numeration. (**D**). Representative illustrations of longitudinal colonic sections immunostained with an anti-Ki67 antibody. (**E**): Percentage of proliferation (Ki67-positive cells/total number of cells per crypt) at *day 10*. Values are means ± SEM (*n* = 9–12). Means that are significantly different (*p* < 0.05) according to the post-hoc test have different letters (a or b or c or d). *: $p < 0.05$; **: $p < 0.01$; ***: $p < 0.001$; NS: non-significant difference.

3.2. P30 Diet Enhances Epithelial Repair Features

P30 mice showed a significant thickening of the colonic wall at *day 10* (colon weight/length ratio: 0.037 ± 0.002) when compared to *day 7* (P30: 0.025 ± 0.002, *p* = 0.0059) and to P14 diet (P14: 0.030 ± 0.002, *p* = 0.0142). P30-fed mice were indeed the only group which recovered initial colonic length at *day 28* (*day 0*: 6.50 ± 0.17 cm vs *day 28* P30: 5.98 ± 0.16 cm, NS) contrastingly to other dietary protein groups (5.70 ± 0.20 cm). This increase in colon weight and length corresponded to a higher crypt height and a higher number of nuclei per crypt in P30 mice than in the P14 group at *day 10* (Figure 3B,C). The percentage of Ki67 positive cells was greater in the colonic tissue of P30 mice (vs P14, *p* = 0.0467), as illustrated in Figure 3D although 30% of the mucosa surface on average was devoid of crypts in all groups at *day 10*, and the number of caspase 3 positive cells was significantly reduced in P30 mice when compared to the other two diets (P30: 0.21 ± 0.07 vs P14: 0.70 ± 0.26 and P53: 0.98 ± 0.26 positive cells per crypt, *p* < 0.05). These epithelial morphometric changes coincided with increased gene expression of the epithelial repair factor *Tgf-β1* in P30-fed mice (Table 2). Interestingly, the gene encoding Gpx2, which protects intestinal tissue against oxidative damage, displayed an increased expression in P30 mice at *day 10* (P30: 1.21 ± 0.21 vs P14: 0.78 ± 0.06 and P53: 0.51 ± 0.12, *p* < 0.05). In addition, the genes encoding *Tff3*, colonic *Saa* (Serum Amyloid A) and *Il-15* were also higher compared to P14 at *day 13* (Table 2).

Table 2. Effects of dietary protein intake level on colonic gene expression. Relative expression level of mRNA expressed as was means ± SEM normalized to *day 7* group (n = 10–12). *: $p < 0.05$; **: $p < 0.01$; ***: $p < 0.001$; NS: non-significant difference. a: vs P14, $p < 0.05$ at the same time, b: vs P53, $p < 0.05$ at the same time.

	Day 10			Day 13			Day 28			Statistical Effect		
	P14	P30	P53	P14	P30	P53	P14	P30	P53	Time	Diet	Interaction
						Epithelial Repair						
Saa	1.05 ± 0.16	0.92 ± 0.21	1.33 ± 0.28	3.40 ± 0.40	4.61 ± 0.55 a	4.01 ± 0.68	3.18 ± 0.30	2.97 ± 0.36	2.45 ± 0.38	***	***	NS
Il-13	0.82 ± 0.08	1.15 ± 0.20	0.98 ± 0.16	0.78 ± 0.10	0.97 ± 0.13	0.91 ± 0.11	2.53 ± 0.39	4.42 ± 0.77 a	4.31 ± 0.84 a	***	*	NS
Il-15	1.67 ± 0.18	2.23 ± 0.42	3.70 ± 0.83	3.61 ± 0.91	6.78 ± 2.06 a	4.59 ± 1.28	4.73 ± 0.86	3.89 ± 0.67	2.37 ± 0.19	**	NS	*
Il-22	0.36 ± 0.08	0.61 ± 0.24	0.38 ± 0.08	0.47 ± 0.14	0.51 ± 0.15	0.57 ± 0.11	0.18 ± 0.04	0.20 ± 0.04	0.19 ± 0.04	***	NS	NS
Il-33	0.60 ± 0.11	0.75 ± 0.10	0.44 ± 0.11	0.43 ± 0.05	0.37 ± 0.07	0.30 ± 0.05	0.26 ± 0.06	0.18 ± 0.04	0.27 ± 0.07	***	NS	NS
Tgf-1ß	0.72 ± 0.07	1.01 ± 0.10 ab	0.60 ± 0.07	0.51 ± 0.07	0.64 ± 0.07 b	0.46 ± 0.05	0.43 ± 0.04	0.44 ± 0.05	0.47 ± 0.07	***	*	NS
Tgf-ß3	0.72 ± 0.10	0.72 ± 0.11	0.67 ± 0.09	0.93 ± 0.12	0.73 ± 0.06	0.85 ± 0.09	1.16 ± 0.16	1.04 ± 0.12	1.08 ± 0.17	**	NS	NS
Tff3	1.05 ± 0.12	1.63 ± 0.36	1.14 ± 0.17	1.62 ± 0.20	2.34 ± 0.35 a	1.70 ± 0.11	1.87 ± 0.13	2.40 ± 0.44	1.63 ± 0.23	*	**	NS
						Mucin genes						
Muc1	0.58 ± 0.09	0.67 ± 0.21	0.70 ± 0.11	1.03 ± 0.14	1.41 ± 0.10	1.34 ± 0.10	0.90 ± 0.11	1.34 ± 0.17	0.75 ± 0.13	***	NS	NS
Muc2	1.72 ± 0.22	2.03 ± 0.21	2.37 ± 0.25	3.03 ± 0.18	3.80 ± 0.44	4.34 ± 0.37 a	3.38 ± 0.21	4.72 ± 0.43 a	5.27 ± 0.50 a	***	***	NS
Muc3	1.25 ± 0.11	1.53 ± 0.14	1.70 ± 0.15	1.73 ± 0.10	2.62 ± 0.44 a	2.65 ± 0.27 a	2.07 ± 0.27	1.94 ± 0.11	1.61 ± 0.08	***	*	*
Muc4	1.66 ± 0.15	2.06 ± 0.33	1.79 ± 0.18	2.32 ± 0.17	2.73 ± 0.34	3.10 ± 0.28	3.43 ± 0.41	3.36 ± 0.36	3.02 ± 0.32	**	NS	NS
						Tight-Junction Proteins						
Cldn1	0.64 ± 0.10	0.84 ± 0.12 b	0.53 ± 0.06	0.39 ± 0.04	0.85 ± 0.17 ab	0.50 ± 0.11	0.38 ± 0.02	0.49 ± 0.07	0.45 ± 0.04	***	*	NS
Cldn2	2.77 ± 0.15	2.69 ± 0.26	3.14 ± 0.25	2.45 ± 0.33	2.34 ± 0.17	2.71 ± 0.23	2.42 ± 0.26	2.13 ± 0.21	2.69 ± 0.13	***	NS	NS
Tjp1	1.17 ± 0.10	1.34 ± 0.08	1.10 ± 0.07	1.30 ± 0.06	1.30 ± 0.05	1.28 ± 0.07	1.29 ± 0.06	1.09 ± 0.08	1.18 ± 0.11	**	NS	NS
Ocln	1.36 ± 0.11	1.52 ± 0.15	1.78 ± 0.44	1.96 ± 0.18	2.61 ± 0.25 b	1.89 ± 0.32	2.21 ± 0.30	2.70 ± 0.32 b	1.54 ± 0.12	***	*	NS

3.3. P30 Diet Improves Dss-Induced Barrier Function Alterations

Interestingly, FD4 challenge showed an intestinal permeability reduction for animals receiving a P30 diet at *days 9* and *12* compared to the P14 group (Figure 4A) and this was confirmed at the colon level where FD4 flux measured in a Ussing chamber was decreased in P30 mice (7119 ± 507 FU) when compared to P14 (9945 ± 303 FU) at *day 10* ($p = 0.014$). This reduction of DSS-induced colon permeability was associated with lower LBP plasmatic concentrations at *days 13* and *28* compared to P14 and P53 groups (Figure 4B). In addition, the gene expression of the tight-junction proteins *Cldn1* and *Ocln* was differentially modulated by dietary protein intake. Indeed, *Cldn1* gene expression was increased by P30 at *days 10* and *13* while *Ocln* increased at *days 13* and *28* (Table 2). This result of *Cldn1* expression has been confirmed by western blotting (Figure 4A), where Claudin-1 protein level was higher in P30 colon at *day 13*. Moreover, ZO-1 was more expressed at *day 13* in P30 mice, when compared to the other two groups, although no significant difference at the gene expression level was detected (*Tjp1*, Table 2) and inter-individual variability was seen (Figure 4C). In addition, the level of dietary protein intake modulated colonic gene expression of several mucins. Indeed, both HP diets increased mRNA expression of the transmembrane mucin *Muc3* at day 13 and the main gel-forming mucin *Muc2* at *day 28* (which was also increased at *day 13* by the P53 diet only). In contrast, neither *Muc1* nor *Muc4* were affected by the diet (Table 2).

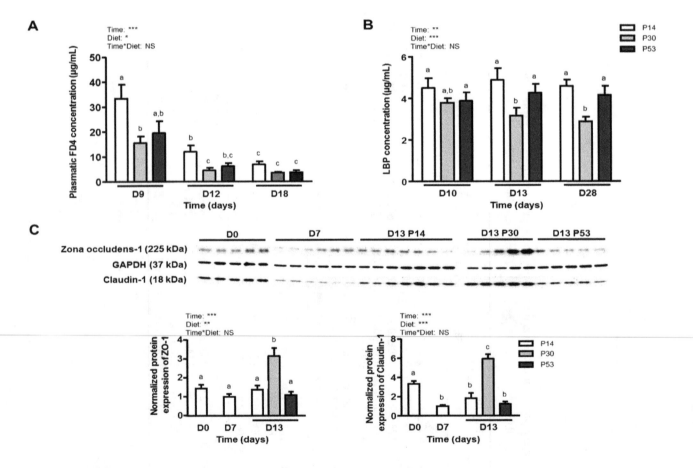

Figure 4. Effects of dietary protein intake level on barrier function after dietary intervention with P14, P30 or P53 diet. (**A**): Evolution of plasmatic FD4 concentration. (**B**): Plasmatic concentration of LPS-binding protein (LBP). (**C**): Western-blot analysis of the tight junction proteins Zona Occludens-1 and Claudin-1, was performed in colonic homogenates of *day 13* mice. GAPDH was used as loading control. Images are representative of four Western blots. Means that are significantly different ($p < 0.05$) according to the *post-hoc* test have different letters (a or b or c). Values are means ± SEM ($n = 10$–12). *: $p < 0.05$; **: $p < 0.01$; ***: $p < 0.001$; NS: non-significant difference.

3.4. DSS-Induced Dysbiosis is not Alleviated by Diet, but P30 Diet Increases the Proportions of Butyrate-Producing Bacteria

DSS-induced dysbiosis was not resolved within 28 days, whatever the diet (Table 3). Diversity and richness were still lower than at *day 0* (6.46 ± 0.07 and 794 ± 55.2 for Shannon and Chao indexes, respectively) and similar to *day 7* (4.75 ± 0.32 and 633 ± 43.7, for Shannon and Chao, respectively). Only the Simpson index was significantly less decreased in P30 group at *day 10* when compared to the two other diets. In addition, the number of observed OTUs at *day 13* was significantly decreased in P53 mice compared to P30 (Table 3).

The overall microbiota composition at the phylum level for each dietary group is shown in Figure 5A and the data describing microbial composition similarities based on family were compared between the diet groups with PCA with the three diet groups as classifying variables (Figure 5B–D). At *day 10*, mucosa-adherent microbial samples clustered by diet groups, as evidenced by their significant ecological distance (R = 0.32, $p < 0.001$) (Figure 5B). P53 group was mostly explained by *Clostridiales* (Firmicutes), *Enterobacteriaceae* (Proteobacteria), *Rikenellaceae* and *Porphyromonaceae* (Bacteroidetes) versus *Eubacteriaceae* (Firmicutes) and *Bifidobacteriaceae* (Actinobacteria) for P30 group (Figure 5B). *Haemophilus* (Proteobacteria) and *Alloprevotella* (Bacteroidetes) proportions were statistically increased in P53 mice at *day 10* while *Desulfovibrio* (Proteobacteria), an H_2S producer, showed a higher abundance at *day 10* for P30 and P14 diets (vs P53, $p < 0.05$) (Table 3). However, the quantification of total sulphato-reducing bacteria did not indicate differences at any time for any diet (data not shown). Interestingly, the Bacteroides genus relative percentage was reduced in the P30 group (vs P14 and P53, $p < 0.001$) while caecal SCFA concentrations were higher (Table 3).

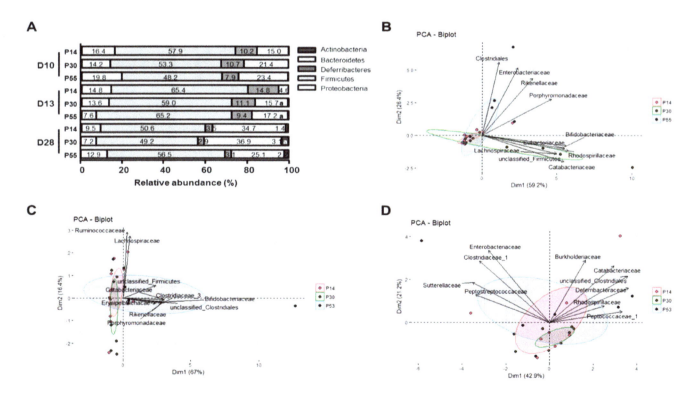

Figure 5. Effects of dietary protein intake on mucosa-associated microbiota composition after 3 (D10), 6 (D13) or 21 days (D28) of dietary intervention with P14, P30 or P53 diet. (**A**). Relative abundance percentages of bacterial phyla in mucosa-adherent microbiota a: vs P14, $p < 0.05$ at the same time. Due to low relative proportions, Tenericutes is not visible in the figure. (**B–D**): Principal coordinate analysis on family relative abundances of mucosa-adherent microbiota at *day 10* (**B**), *day 13* (**C**) and *day 28* (**D**).

Table 3. Effects of dietary protein intake level on characteristics of mucosal-adherent microbiota. Values are means $\pm$ SEM ($n = 10$–12). *: $p < 0.05$; **: $p < 0.01$; ***: $p < 0.001$; NS: non-significant difference. a: vs P14, $p < 0.05$ at the same time, b: vs P53, $p < 0.05$ at the same time.

	Day 10			Day 13			Day 28			Statistical Effect		
	P14	P30	P53	P14	P30	P53	P14	P30	P53	Time	Diet	Interaction
Diversity and richness features												
Shannon Index	4.56 ± 0.28	5.28 ± 0.33	4.53 ± 0.36	4.44 ± 0.26	4.23 ± 0.40	4.96 ± 0.29	5.02 ± 0.29	5.21 ± 0.19	5.31 ± 0.26	*	NS	NS
Simpson Index	0.89 ± 0.02	0.94 ± 0.01 ab	0.88 ± 0.03	0.88 ± 0.03	0.85 ± 0.04	0.92 ± 0.01	0.92 ± 0.02	0.93 ± 0.01	0.94 ± 0.01	***	*	NS
Chao1 Index	593 ± 31.1	678 ± 26.0	673 ± 41.1	635 ± 34.4	566 ± 25.5	642 ± 57.7	606 ± 51.7	648 ± 55.0	605 ± 39.7	**	NS	NS
Observed OTUs	286 ± 36.9	350 ± 30.1	306 ± 32.7	293 ± 24.6	335 ± 29.1 b	261 ± 34.8	285 ± 21.6	342 ± 30.6	305 ± 22.5	***	*	NS
Relative genera composition (%)												
Alloprevotella	0.008 ± 0.006	0.000 ± 0.000 b	0.079 ± 0.014 a	0.013 ± 0.006	0.000 ± 0.000	0.025 ± 0.025	0.003 ± 0.003	0.002 ± 0.002	0.000 ± 0.000	*	*	NS
Bacteroides	11.55 ± 2.771	7.391 ± 1.788 a	15.83 ± 4.937 b	3.082 ± 1.079	14.04 ± 4.541 a	11.92 ± 4.152	20.11 ± 4.979	21.92 ± 4.357 b	7.166 ± 1.920 a	*	*	**
Clostridium_XIVa	5.555 ± 2.733	2.861 ± 0.517	2.950 ± 0.763	8.545 ± 2.801	10.61 ± 3.758 b	3.653 ± 1.709	4.008 ± 1.635	4.212 ± 1.211	5.191 ± 1.197	*	*	NS
Desulfovibrio	3.062 ± 0.643	4.376 ± 0.870 b	1.402 ± 0.272 a	3.643 ± 0.946	3.892 ± 1.142 b	1.565 ± 0.406	1.298 ± 0.306	1.699 ± 0.581	0.939 ± 0.207	**	**	NS
Enterobacter	0.021 ± 0.010	0.013 ± 0.008	0.025 ± 0.019	0.049 ± 0.020	0.023 ± 0.019	0.025 ± 0.013	0.031 ± 0.015	0.012 ± 0.005	0.015 ± 0.008	NS	NS	NS
Enterorhabdus	0.010 ± 0.005	0.009 ± 0.004	0.006 ± 0.003	0.004 ± 0.003	0.028 ± 0.016	0.034 ± 0.012 a	0.030 ± 0.014	0.023 ± 0.008	0.014 ± 0.008	*	*	NS
Ethanoligenens	0.000 ± 0.000	0.000 ± 0.000	0.000 ± 0.000	0.000 ± 0.000	0.000 ± 0.000	0.000 ± 0.000	0.000 ± 0.000	0.000 ± 0.000 b	0.013 ± 0.013 a	**	*	NS
Faecalibacterium	0.000 ± 0.000	0.002 ± 0.002	0.000 ± 0.000	0.004 ± 0.004	0.007 ± 0.002 b	0.001 ± 0.001	0.014 ± 0.014	0.048 ± 0.008 b	0.000 ± 0.000	**	*	NS
Haemophilus	0.000 ± 0.000	0.004 ± 0.004 b	0.017 ± 0.003 a	0.000 ± 0.000	0.013 ± 0.007	0.025 ± 0.012 a	0.002 ± 0.002	0.004 ± 0.004 b	0.043 ± 0.029 a	NS	*	NS
Klebsiella	0.004 ± 0.005	0.000 ± 0.000 b	0.005 ± 0.001	0.000 ± 0.000	0.000 ± 0.000	0.000 ± 0.000	0.002 ± 0.002	0.000 ± 0.000 b	0.005 ± 0.001	*	*	NS
Porphyromonas	0.000 ± 0.000	0.000 ± 0.000	0.000 ± 0.000	0.000 ± 0.000	0.000 ± 0.000	0.000 ± 0.000	0.000 ± 0.000	0.000 ± 0.000 b	0.012 ± 0.012 a	**	**	NS
Roseburia	0.005 ± 0.005	0.009 ± 0.004	0.010 ± 0.005	0.011 ± 0.006	0.006 ± 0.003	0.011 ± 0.008	0.009 ± 0.006	0.029 ± 0.004 ab	0.011 ± 0.001	***	***	NS
Caecal SCFA (μmol/g)												
Total	0.06 ± 0.04	2.05 ± 1.56 a	0.38 ± 0.27	0.14 ± 0.07	1.32 ± 0.44 a	0.99 ± 0.46	4.88 ± 1.08	6.85 ± 1.65 b	12.32 ± 3.65 a	***	*	NS
Acetate	0.04 ± 0.04	1.40 ± 1.04 a	0.28 ± 0.18	0.14 ± 0.07	1.20 ± 0.43 a	1.00 ± 0.38	3.40 ± 0.71	4.66 ± 1.13	8.38 ± 2.42	***	*	NS
Propionate	0.00 ± 0.00	0.44 ± 0.36 a	0.07 ± 0.07	0.00 ± 0.00	0.00 ± 0.00	0.13 ± 0.13	0.90 ± 0.26	1.31 ± 0.35	2.55 ± 0.65	***	*	NS
Butyrate	0.01 ± 0.01	0.21 ± 0.16 a	0.03 ± 0.03	0.00 ± 0.00	0.12 ± 0.05	0.10 ± 0.07	0.59 ± 0.13	0.88 ± 0.26	1.40 ± 0.39	***	*	NS

Although Firmicutes phylum proportions remained stable and similar to *day 0* (Figure 5) whatever the time and the diet, *Clostridium_XIVa* and *Faecalibacterium* proportions were higher in P30 group than in P53 at *day 13* ($p = 0.005$) (Table 3). In contrast to *day 10*, Bacteroidetes relative abundance was higher with both P30 and P53 diets owing to increased proportions of *Bacteroides* genus. Moreover, *Haemophilus* had increased proportions in the P53 group when compared to the P14 group at *day 13*, as well as *Enterorhabdus* (Actinobacteria) (Table 3).

At *day 28*, the impact of dietary protein intake on mucosal-adherent composition was less marked between groups (Figure 5D) especially between P14 and P30 groups (Table 3). However, Actinobacteria, which proportions stayed low before *day 28* (*day 0–day 13*: 0.1%) (Figure 5A), were two-fold higher in P30 (P30: 3.1% vs P14: 1.4%, $p = 0.014$) and in the P53 group, the proportion of *Bifidobacteriaceae* being increased in that latter group ($p = 0.021$, P14: $0.60 \pm 0.28\%$, P30: $1.70 \pm 0.83\%$ and P53: $0.93 \pm 0.36\%$). In addition, the protein intake modulated microbiota activities since total caecal SCFA concentrations increased in both HP groups at *day 28*. Although Deferribacteres proportion was reduced for the three diets when compared to *days 10* and *13*, reaching *day 0* level ($3.7 \pm 1.0\%$, NS vs *day 28* whatever the diet), no other major differences at the phylum level were recorded. Interestingly, *Lachnospiraceae* family (Firmicutes) relative proportion at *day 28* was greater than the one at *day 7* (*day 7*: $13.48 \pm 2.91\%$ vs *day 28*: $24.22 \pm 1.82\%$, $p = 0.0184$). Moreover, higher proportions of *Faecalibacterium* (*Clostridiaceae*) (vs P53) and *Roseburia* (vs P53 and P14) in P30 group were observed at *day 28* (Table 3). Contrastingly, P53 microbiota composition showed again noticeable taxonomic differences compared to P14 and P30 mice, with increased abundance of the genera *Porphyromonas*, *Ethanoligenens* and *Haemophilus* contrasting with a decreased abundance of *Bacteroides* (Table 3).

4. Discussion

The present study showed that the level of dietary protein intake differentially modulated mucosal healing after an acute colon inflammatory episode. While the P53 diet worsened both the intensity and duration of the inflammation induced by DSS treatment, the P30 diet, when compared to P14 diet, accelerated epithelial repair by favoring the restoration of colon barrier architecture and function.

P30 diet indeed induced crypt hyperproliferation associated with increased gene expression of the repairing factors *Tgf-ß1* and *Tff3*, both factors being known to contribute to the integrity of mucosal surface continuity but in an independent manner [22]. In addition, *Saa*, which was over-expressed in P30 mice compared to the two other diets, was recently described as a protective factor against colon epithelium acute injury [23]. Altogether, the increased expression of genes encoding these promoting repair factors as well as tight-junction proteins (Claudin-1 and Zona-Occludens 1), likely contributed to the restoration of colon barrier integrity, as evidenced by lower permeability and bacterial translocation-related marker (LBP) in the systemic flow. Additionally, an increased mRNA level of *Gpx2*, which upregulation is associated with inflammation resolution [24], suggests a lower inflammation-induced oxidative stress in P30 animals. Furthermore, the P30-mediated positive effects on epithelial repair might be related to a modulation of the mucosa-adherent microbiota composition and activities within the first days of colitis resolution. Indeed, the higher relative abundance of bacteria belonging to *Lachnospiraceae*, *Eubacteriaceae* and *Bifidobacteriaceae* families, together with higher concentrations of SCFAs, the major end products of microbiota metabolic activity, may partly explain the beneficial impact of P30 diet on colon mucosa. Interestingly, the P30 diet also longitudinally increased the proportion of *Faecalibacterium*, a commensal butyrate producer, detected in healthy subjects, whose abundance is reduced in IBD patients and is positively correlated with the maintenance of clinical remission [25,26]. Butyrate is well known to be a major fuel for colonic epithelial cells, to exert pluripotent effects on the colon such as the regulation of cell growth and differentiation [27], and to present anti-inflammatory properties [28]. Butyrate deficiency in its concentrations and/or in its transport and metabolism has been indeed observed in the inflamed mucosa [29].

Although minor differences in mucosa-adherent bacterial composition were noticed between the animals fed with P14 or P30 diets in the week following the acute colitis episode (with the notable exception regarding the *Bacteroides* proportion), bacterial populations were severely modulated in P53 mice compared to the two other diets. Indeed, P53 diet consumption in DSS-treated mice decreased the proportions of butyrate-producing bacteria from *Clostridium XIVa*, *Faecalibacterium* and *Roseburia* genera in the mucosa-adherent microbiota. P53 diet-fed mice were also characterized by an increased representation of families and genera previously reported in IBD patients during flares [30,31] such as *Alloprevotella*, *Ethanoligenens*, *Klebsiella*, *Porphyromonas* and *Haemophilus*. In parallel, *Desulfovibrio*, an H_2S producer, was reduced in P53 diet-fed mice as recently reported in the faecal microbiota recovered from UC patients [31], whereas the quantification of sulphato-reducing bacteria was not different between diets. This latter result is somewhat unexpected since an increased protein content in the diet is associated with a higher faecal H_2S concentration [32]. However, substrate availability, microbiote composition and metabolic activity are major parameters for fixing the production of bacterial metabolites [13], and other AA-derived bacterial metabolites that are known to exert deleterious effects on intestinal epithelial cells when present in excess, such as ammonium, p-cresol or hydrogen sulphide [9,33–35], that might have been over-produced in P53-fed mice. Our study is in accordance with Llewellyn et al. study that shows that the level of dietary proteins has an impact on colitis severity that is associated with changes in microbiota composition [36]. In this study, the authors have shown that a high-protein diet (41%) enhanced disease progression when compared to a low-protein diet (6%). However, comparison between this study and ours should take into account the important experimental designs differences, which were the quantity and quality of proteins in the diets. Indeed, we used a mix of milk proteins containing both whey and caseins (20:80) to mimic cow milk composition, while Llewellyn et al. used casein as the only protein source. Furthermore, diets were provided one week prior to the DSS administration, whereas we started to give our different diets after colitis induction at *day 7*. Other studies, outside the scope of the present work, are necessary for determining more precisely the changes in the luminal environment in each experimental conditions. Such changes may partly explain that P53-fed mice showed a higher inflammation state but a level of epithelial crypt repair similar to P30-fed mice. Consequently, in addition to the quantity, the source of dietary proteins may modulate the IBD course [37,38] although association between protein intake and IBD risk has not been found in all studies [39,40], highlighting the urgent need for human studies to decipher the role of quantity and source of dietary proteins in IBD.

Furthermore, the reduction of carbohydrate supply in the diet may also influence colon healing. Indeed, P30 diet proportions might be more suitable to cover the requirements of macronutrients (both carbohydrates and proteins) to sustain the metabolic activity of cells [41] and synthesis of macromolecules involved in epithelial repair and restoration of barrier integrity. Additional experiments, such as the measurement of colon mucosal cell bioenergetics and protein synthesis during acute inflammation and following mucosal healing, would help to decipher these points.

5. Conclusions

Our results fit with the view that an optimized epithelium repair after an acute inflammatory episode can be obtained through the supply of an appropriate amount of dietary protein. It indeed depends upon a balance between the AA originating from dietary and endogenous proteins, which are available from the blood supply for mucosal healing, and the gut microbial activity towards undigested protein that enters the colon. Our study showed that a moderately high dietary protein intake during a post-inflammatory phase appears beneficial to speed up the restoration of the intestinal mucosa integrity when compared to a normoproteic diet, by affecting several key parameters associated with inflammation and healing during and after the inflammatory flare in the DSS model of colitis. In contrast, a further increase in the dietary protein amount appears counter-productive for such a process. As such, our experimental study is in accordance with the need for an increased protein intake during active IBD [7] but suggests that a threshold protein intake value should be not exceeded to avoid deleterious effects on the patients' inflamed mucosa.

Author Contributions: S.V.-L., M.A., A.B., M.G., and A.L. performed experiments. S.V.-L., P.L., A.-M.D., R.V. and A.L. analyzed the data. A.L., M.L., C.G. and F.B. conceived and supervised the study. S.V.-L. and A.L. drafted the manuscript. All of the authors read and approved the final manuscript as submitted and agree to be accountable for all aspects of the work.

Acknowledgments: The authors greatly acknowledge R. Onifarasoaniaina and M. Favier from the Cochin HistIM Facility, Morgane Dufay who helped to take care of the animals, Maxime Evrard and Julie Bonnereau for their involvement in the experiment. Also, they want to thank Armor Protéines (Saint-Brice-en-Cogles, France) for providing the dietary proteins used to prepare diets.

References

1. Danese, S.; Fiocchi, C. Ulcerative colitis. *N. Engl. J. Med.* **2011**, *365*, 1713–1725. [CrossRef] [PubMed]
2. Neurath, M.F.; Travis, S.P.L. Mucosal healing in inflammatory bowel diseases: A systematic review. *Gut* **2012**, *61*, 1619–1635. [CrossRef] [PubMed]
3. Papi, C.; Fascì-Spurio, F.; Rogai, F.; Settesoldi, A.; Margagnoni, G.; Annese, V. Mucosal healing in inflammatory bowel disease: Treatment efficacy and predictive factors. *Dig. Liver Dis.* **2013**, *45*, 978–985. [CrossRef] [PubMed]
4. Neurath, M.F. New targets for mucosal healing and therapy in inflammatory bowel diseases. *Mucosal Immunol.* **2014**, *7*, 6–19. [CrossRef] [PubMed]
5. Sturm, A.; Dignass, A.U. Epithelial restitution and wound healing in inflammatory bowel disease. *World J. Gastroenterol.* **2008**, *14*, 348–353. [CrossRef] [PubMed]
6. Forbes, A.; Goldesgeyme, E.; Paulon, E. Nutrition in inflammatory bowel disease. *JPEN. J. Parenter. Enteral Nutr.* **2011**, *35*, 571–580. [CrossRef]
7. Forbes, A.; Escher, J.; Hébuterne, X.; Kłęk, S.; Krznaric, Z.; Schneider, S.; Shamir, R.; Stardelova, K.; Wierdsma, N.; Wiskin, A.E.; et al. ESPEN guideline: Clinical nutrition in inflammatory bowel disease. *Clin. Nutr.* **2017**, *36*, 321–347. [CrossRef] [PubMed]
8. Vidal-Lletjós, S.; Beaumont, M.; Tomé, D.; Benamouzig, R.; Blachier, F.; Lan, A. Dietary Protein and Amino Acid Supplementation in Inflammatory Bowel Disease Course: What Impact on the Colonic Mucosa? *Nutrients* **2017**, *9*, 310. [CrossRef] [PubMed]
9. Andriamihaja, M.; Davila, A.-M.; Eklou-Lawson, M.; Petit, N.; Delpal, S.; Allek, F.; Blais, A.; Delteil, C.; Tomé, D.; Blachier, F. Colon luminal content and epithelial cell morphology are markedly modified in rats fed with a high-protein diet. *Am. J. Physiol. Gastrointest. Liver Physiol.* **2010**, *299*, G1030–G1037. [CrossRef] [PubMed]
10. Blachier, F.; Beaumont, M.; Andriamihaja, M.; Davila, A.-M.; Lan, A.; Grauso, M.; Armand, L.; Benamouzig, R.; Tomé, D. Changes in the luminal environment of the colonic epithelial cells and physiopathological consequences. *Am. J. Pathol.* **2017**, *187*, 476–486. [CrossRef] [PubMed]
11. Geypens, B.; Claus, D.; Evenepoel, P.; Hiele, M.; Maes, B.; Peeters, M.; Rutgeerts, P.; Ghoos, Y. Influence of dietary protein supplements on the formation of bacterial metabolites in the colon. *Gut* **1997**, *41*, 70–76. [CrossRef] [PubMed]
12. Liu, X.; Blouin, J.-M.; Santacruz, A.; Lan, A.; Andriamihaja, M.; Wilkanowicz, S.; Benetti, P.-H.; Tomé, D.; Sanz, Y.; Blachier, F.; et al. High-protein diet modifies colonic microbiota and luminal environment but not colonocyte metabolism in the rat model: The increased luminal bulk connection. *Am. J. Physiol. Gastrointest. Liver Physiol.* **2014**, *307*, G459–G470. [CrossRef] [PubMed]
13. Beaumont, M.; Portune, K.J.; Steuer, N.; Lan, A.; Cerrudo, V.; Audebert, M.; Dumont, F.; Mancano, G.; Khodorova, N.; Andriamihaja, M.; et al. Quantity and source of dietary protein influence metabolite production by gut microbiota and rectal mucosa gene expression: A randomized, parallel, double-blind trial in overweight humans. *Am. J. Clin. Nutr.* **2017**, *106*, 1005–1019. [CrossRef] [PubMed]
14. Blachier, F.; Beaumont, M.; Portune, K.J.; Steuer, N.; Lan, A.; Audebert, M.; Khodorova, N.; Andriamihaja, M.; Airinei, G.; Benamouzig, R.; et al. High-protein diets for weight management: Interactions with the intestinal microbiota and consequences for gut health. A position paper by the my new gut study group. *Clin. Nutr.* **2018**. [CrossRef] [PubMed]
15. Lan, A.; Blais, A.; Coelho, D.; Capron, J.; Maarouf, M.; Benamouzig, R.; Lancha, A.H.; Walker, F.; Tomé, D.; Blachier, F. Dual effects of a high-protein diet on DSS-treated mice during colitis resolution phase. *Am. J. Physiol. Gastrointest. Liver Physiol.* **2016**, *311*, G624–G633. [CrossRef] [PubMed]

16. Liu, Y.; Wang, X.; Hu, C.-A. Therapeutic Potential of Amino Acids in Inflammatory Bowel Disease. *Nutrients* **2017**, *9*, 920. [CrossRef] [PubMed]

17. Sprong, R.C.; Schonewille, A.J.; van der Meer, R. Dietary cheese whey protein protects rats against mild dextran sulfate sodium-induced colitis: Role of mucin and microbiota. *J. Dairy Sci.* **2010**, *93*, 1364–1371. [CrossRef] [PubMed]

18. Faure, M.; Moënnoz, D.; Montigon, F.; Mettraux, C.; Breuillé, D.; Ballèvre, O. Dietary threonine restriction specifically reduces intestinal mucin synthesis in rats. *J. Nutr.* **2005**, *135*, 486–491. [CrossRef] [PubMed]

19. Gaifem, J.; Gonçalves, L.G.; Dinis-Oliveira, R.J.; Cunha, C.; Carvalho, A.; Torrado, E.; Rodrigues, F.; Saraiva, M.; Castro, A.G.; Silvestre, R. L-Threonine Supplementation During Colitis Onset Delays Disease Recovery. *Front. Physiol.* **2018**, *9*, 1247. [CrossRef] [PubMed]

20. Lan, A.; Blachier, F.; Benamouzig, R.; Beaumont, M.; Barrat, C.; Coelho, D.; Lancha, A.; Kong, X.; Yin, Y.; Marie, J.-C.; et al. Mucosal healing in inflammatory bowel diseases: Is there a place for nutritional supplementation? *Inflamm. Bowel Dis.* **2015**, *21*, 198–207. [CrossRef] [PubMed]

21. Chemouny, J.M.; Gleeson, P.J.; Abbad, L.; Lauriero, G.; Boedec, E.; Le Roux, K.; Monot, C.; Bredel, M.; Bex-Coudrat, J.; Sannier, A.; et al. Modulation of the microbiota by oral antibiotics treats immunoglobulin A nephropathy in humanized mice. *Nephrol. Dial. Transplant.* **2018**, 1–10. [CrossRef] [PubMed]

22. Dignass, A.; Lynch-devaney, K.; Kindon, H.; Thim, L.; Podolsky, D.K. Trefoil peptides promote epithelial migration through a transforming growth factor beta-independent pathway. *J. Clin. Investig.* **1994**, *94*, 376–383. [CrossRef] [PubMed]

23. Zhang, G.; Liu, J.; Wu, L.; Fan, Y.; Sun, L.; Qian, F.; Chen, D.; Ye, R.D. Elevated Expression of Serum Amyloid a 3 Protects Colon Epithelium against Acute Injury Through TLR2-Dependent Induction of Neutrophil IL-22 Expression in a Mouse Model of Colitis. *Front. Immunol.* **2018**, *9*, 1503. [CrossRef] [PubMed]

24. Hiller, F.; Besselt, K.; Deubel, S.; Brigelius-Flohé, R.; Kipp, A.P. GPx2 induction is mediated through STAT transcription factors during acute colitis. *Inflamm. Bowel Dis.* **2015**, *21*, 2078–2089. [CrossRef] [PubMed]

25. Sokol, H.; Seksik, P.; Furet, J.P.; Firmesse, O.; Nion-Larmurier, I.; Beaugerie, L.; Cosnes, J.; Corthier, G.; Marteau, P.; Doraé, J. Low counts of faecalibacterium prausnitzii in colitis microbiota. *Inflamm. Bowel Dis.* **2009**, *15*, 1183–1189. [CrossRef] [PubMed]

26. Machiels, K.; Joossens, M.; Sabino, J.; De Preter, V.; Arijs, I.; Eeckhaut, V.; Ballet, V.; Claes, K.; Van Immerseel, F.; Verbeke, K.; et al. A decrease of the butyrate-producing species Roseburia hominis and Faecalibacterium prausnitzii defines dysbiosis in patients with ulcerative colitis. *Gut* **2014**, *63*, 1275–1283. [CrossRef] [PubMed]

27. Macfarlane, G.T.; Macfarlane, S. Bacteria, colonic fermentation, and gastrointestinal health. *J. AOAC Int.* **2012**, *95*, 50–60. [CrossRef] [PubMed]

28. Chang, P.V.; Hao, L.; Offermanns, S.; Medzhitov, R. The microbial metabolite butyrate regulates intestinal macrophage function via histone deacetylase inhibition. *Proc. Natl. Acad. Sci. USA* **2014**, *111*, 2247–2252. [CrossRef] [PubMed]

29. Thibault, R.; Blachier, F.; Darcy-Vrillon, B.; de Coppet, P.; Bourreille, A.; Segain, J.-P.P. Butyrate utilization by the colonic mucosa in inflammatory bowel diseases: A transport deficiency. *Inflamm. Bowel Dis.* **2010**, *16*, 684–695. [CrossRef] [PubMed]

30. Lucke, K.; Miehlke, S.; Jacobs, E.; Schuppler, M. Prevalence of Bacteroides and *Prevotella* spp. in ulcerative colitis. *J. Med. Microbiol.* **2006**, *55*, 617–624. [CrossRef] [PubMed]

31. Ma, H.-Q.; Yu, T.-T.; Zhao, X.-J.; Zhang, Y.; Zhang, H.-J. Fecal microbial dysbiosis in Chinese patients with inflammatory bowel disease. *World J. Gastroenterol.* **2018**, *24*, 1464–1477. [CrossRef] [PubMed]

32. Magee, E.A.; Richardson, C.J.; Hughes, R.; Cummings, J.H. Contribution of dietary protein to sulfide production in the large intestine: An in vitro and a controlled feeding study in humans. *Am. J. Clin. Nutr.* **2000**, *72*, 1488–1494. [CrossRef] [PubMed]

33. Andriamihaja, M.; Lan, A.; Beaumont, M.; Audebert, M.; Wong, X.; Yamada, K.; Yin, Y.; Tomé, D.; Carrasco-Pozo, C.; Gotteland, M.; et al. The deleterious metabolic and genotoxic effects of the bacterial metabolite p-cresol on colonic epithelial cells. *Free Radic. Biol. Med.* **2015**, *85*, 219–227. [CrossRef] [PubMed]

34. Beaumont, M.; Andriamihaja, M.; Lan, A.; Khodorova, N.; Audebert, M.; Blouin, J.M.; Grauso, M.; Lancha, L.; Benetti, P.H.; Benamouzig, R.; et al. Detrimental effects for colonocytes of an increased exposure to luminal hydrogen sulfide: The adaptive response. *Free Radic. Biol. Med.* **2016**, *93*, 155–164. [CrossRef] [PubMed]

35. Portune, K.J.; Beaumont, M.; Davila, A.-M.; Tomé, D.; Blachier, F. Gut microbiota role in dietary protein metabolism and health-related outcomes: The two sides of the coin. *Trends Food Sci. Technol.* **2016**, *57*, 213–232. [CrossRef]

36. Llewellyn, S.R.; Britton, G.J.; Contijoch, E.J.; Vennaro, O.H.; Mortha, A.; Colombel, J.F.; Grinspan, A.; Clemente, J.C.; Merad, M.; Faith, J.J. Interactions Between Diet and the Intestinal Microbiota Alter Intestinal Permeability and Colitis Severity in Mice. *Gastroenterology* **2018**, *154*, 1037–1046.e2. [CrossRef] [PubMed]

37. Jantchou, P.; Morois, S.; Clavel-Chapelon, F.; Boutron-Ruault, M.-C.; Carbonnel, F. Animal protein intake and risk of inflammatory bowel disease: The E3N prospective study. *Am. J. Gastroenterol.* **2010**, *105*, 2195–2201. [CrossRef] [PubMed]

38. Jowett, S.L.; Seal, C.J.; Pearce, M.S.; Phillips, E.; Gregory, W.; Barton, J.R.; Welfare, M.R. Influence of dietary factors on the clinical course of ulcerative colitis: A prospective cohort study. *Gut* **2004**, *53*, 1479–1484. [CrossRef] [PubMed]

39. Spooren, C.E.G.M.; Pierik, M.J.; Zeegers, M.P.; Feskens, E.J.M.; Masclee, A.A.M.; Jonkers, D.M.A.E. Review article: The association of diet with onset and relapse in patients with inflammatory bowel disease. *Aliment. Pharmacol. Ther.* **2013**, *38*, 1172–1187. [CrossRef] [PubMed]

40. Racine, A.; Carbonnel, F.; Chan, S.S.M.; Hart, A.R.; Bas Bueno-De-Mesquita, H.; Oldenburg, B.; Van Schaik, F.D.M.; Tjønneland, A.; Olsen, A.; Dahm, C.C.; et al. Dietary Patterns and Risk of Inflammatory Bowel Disease in Europe: Results from the EPIC Study. *Inflamm. Bowel Dis.* **2016**, *22*, 345–354. [CrossRef] [PubMed]

41. Kominsky, D.J.; Campbell, E.L.; Colgan, S.P. Metabolic shifts in immunity and inflammation. *J. Immunol.* **2010**, *184*, 4062–4068. [CrossRef] [PubMed]

Inflammatory Bowel Diseases and Food Additives: To Add Fuel on the Flames!

Rachel Marion-Letellier [1,2,*], Asma Amamou [1,2], Guillaume Savoye [1,2,3] and Subrata Ghosh [4]

[1] INSERM unit 1073, Normandie University, UNIROUEN, 22 boulevard Gambetta, F-76183 Rouen, France; asma.amamou@etu.univ-rouen.fr (A.A.); guillaume.savoye@chu-rouen.fr (G.S.)

[2] Institute for Research and Innovation in Biomedicine (IRIB), Normandie University, UNIROUEN, F-76183 Rouen, France

[3] Department of Gastroenterology, Rouen University Hospital, 1 rue de Germont, F-76031 Rouen, France

[4] Institute of Translational Medicine, University of Birmingham, Birmingham B15 2TT, UK; sughosh@ymail.com

* Correspondence: rachel.letellier@univ-rouen.fr

Abstract: Inflammatory bowel diseases (IBDs) develop in genetically predisposed individuals in response to environmental factors. IBDs are concomitant conditions of industrialized societies, and diet is a potential culprit. Consumption of ultra-processed food has increased over the last decade in industrialized countries, and epidemiological studies have found associations between ultra-processed food consumption and chronic diseases. Further studies are now required to identify the potential culprit in ultra-processed food, such as a poor nutritional composition or the presence of food additives. In our review, we will focus on food additives, i.e., substances from packaging in contact with food, and compounds formed during production, processing, and storage. A literature search using PubMed from inception to January 2019 was performed to identify relevant studies on diet and/or food additive and their role in IBDs. Manuscripts published in English from basic science, epidemiological studies, or clinical trials were selected and reviewed. We found numerous experimental studies highlighting the key role of food additives in IBD exacerbation but epidemiological studies on food additives on IBD risk are still limited. As diet is a modifiable environmental risk factor, this may offer a scientific rationale for providing dietary advice for IBD patients.

Keywords: colitis; food additive; diet; emulsifiers; high salt diet; inflammatory bowel diseases

---

1. Introduction

The most common types of inflammatory bowel diseases (IBDs) are Crohn's disease (CD) and ulcerative colitis (UC). IBD etiology is unknown, but IBDs develop in genetically predisposed individuals in response to environmental factors and the result of an exacerbated mucosal immune response to intestinal microbiota. IBDs are concomitant conditions of industrialized societies [1]. Indeed, IBD prevalence has continued to increase in Western countries, and newly industrialized countries in Asia, the Middle East, Africa, and South America have exhibited a rapid increase of IBD prevalence [1].

Environmental factors are supposed to play a decisive role in the pathogenesis of IBDs. Diet is considered to be a potential culprit and we previously reviewed the potential effect of specific nutrients in IBDs [2]. With this study, we aimed to focus on another potential dietary culprit: food additives.

Consumption of ultra-processed food (UPF) has increased over the last decade, in particular in industrialized societies [3–5], and studies from the French web-based NutriNet-Santé cohort have found an association between UPF consumption and chronic diseases, such as a higher cancer risk [6]. UPF now represent an important part of the diet of French individuals: UPF accounted for 16% of food consumed by weight, corresponding to 33% of total energy intake [7]. In addition, the authors also reported an association between these dietary patterns and a higher irritable bowel syndrome risk (OR Q4 vs. Q1 [95% CI]: 1.25 [1.12–1.39], p-trend < 0.0001) [7]. Similar associations between UPF consumption and chronic diseases are globally observed, such as metabolic syndrome in the US [4] or depression in Spain [5]. Further studies are now required to identify the potential culprit in UPF, such as a poor nutritional composition or the presence of food additives. In our review, we will focus on food additives, i.e., substances from packaging in contact with food, and compounds formed during production, processing, and storage.

2. IBD Patients and Dietary Beliefs

Diet is a crucial point for IBD patients [8–10] and exclusion diets are commonly reported. In a French study, the dietary beliefs of 244 IBD patients were studied using a questionnaire of 14 items [8]. The majority of IBD patients (58%) believed that food can play a role in causing a relapse and this strongly affects quality of life because IBD patients may refuse outdoor dining for fear of causing IBD symptoms [8]. In a study conducted in the UK, 400 IBD patients received a dietary questionnaire and data from this study were in accordance with the French study. In this study, deteriorating symptoms were associated with certain foods from 60% of IBD patients [10]. Similar results were found in a Dutch study conducted in 294 IBD patients through an online questionnaire [9]. Interestingly, 81% of IBD patients from the Dutch study reported that their main nutritional knowledge came from their own experience, while 71% reported that they received professional dietary advice mainly from dieticians [9]. In a Spanish study, the majority of IBD patients (86%) refrained from eating some foods to avoid a worsening of flare-ups [11]. In pediatric IBD populations, food avoidance is also commonly reported for 53% of patients [12].

3. A Pinch of Salt

Processed food is a high provider of dietary sodium chloride (NaCl). Few recent studies have evaluated the potential impact of dietary salt in colitis models [13–15] (Figure 1). Tubbs et al. calculated the NaCl content of a series of available foods in grocery and fast food restaurants using the SELF Nutrition database, and they reported that these foods contained approximately 4% w/w NaCl [13]. Increased concentration of NaCl from 10 to 80 mM induced inflammatory cytokine production, such as the IL (interleukin)-23/IL-17 pathway in normal intestinal lamina propria mononuclear cells [14]. High-salt diet (HSD) exacerbated chemically induced colitis, while pharmacological inhibition of p38/MAPK abrogated its effect in both models [14]. Tubbs et al. demonstrated the deleterious effect of HSD in numerous colitis models, such IL-10$^{-/-}$ or infectious colitis [13]. Interestingly, Aguiar et al. reported that dietary salt exacerbated colitis but by itself can trigger gut inflammation by increasing intestinal permeability and inflammatory histological score [15]. More recently, HSD also has been shown to have a deleterious impact on intestinal microbiota by decreasing *Lactobaccilus* levels and short-chain fatty acid production [16].

These studies raised the potential role of dietary salt as an environmental trigger for IBD development by creating a deleterious environment that is more vulnerable to inflammatory insults.

Dietary phosphate has been less studied than dietary salt. Nevertheless, dietary inorganic phosphate is abundant in processed food as a food additive, in particular in fast foods and processed meats. Phosphate intake is two or three times higher [17]: 1655 mg/day for men and 1190 mg/day for women in the US compared to dietary reference intake at 700 mg/day in industrialized countries. Its deleterious effect on intestinal inflammation has also been demonstrated. Sugihara et al. fed Sprague–Dawley rats with a diet containing 0.5% to 1.5% phosphate for 7 days before colitis induction [18]. As standard animal diet contains approximatively 5000 mg/kg of phosphate, i.e., 0.5%, the range of phosphate from 0.5% to 1.5% used in the study mimics the human exposure range from 1- to 3-fold of the recommended dietary intake. Dietary phosphate exacerbates colitis by accentuating body weight loss by increasing disease activity index and by activating NF (Nuclear factor)-κB [18]. The authors of the study also found an in vitro increased inflammatory response by 2 mM phosphate in liposaccharide (LPS)-treated RAW264 cells [18].

To our knowledge, only one study has reported clinical data concerning salt consumption and IBDs [19]. In a US cohort from 194,711 women, the authors of this study reported that dietary intake of potassium ($P_{trend} = 0.005$) but not sodium ($P_{trend} = 0.440$) was inversely associated with risk of CD [19]. The authors did not observe any significant association between both dietary potassium and sodium and UC risk [19].

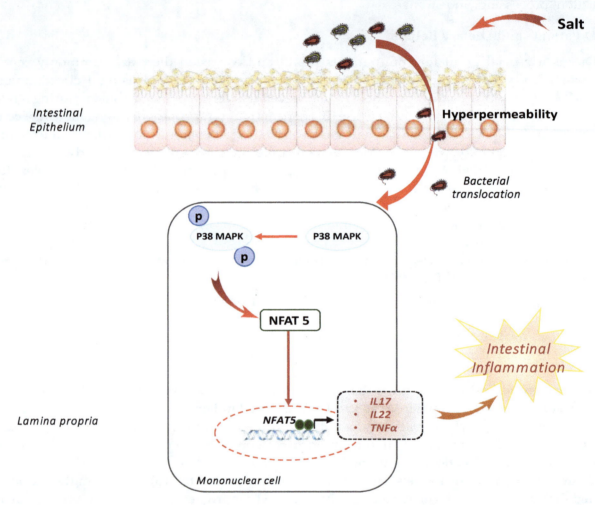

Figure 1. High-salt diet promotes intestinal inflammation. High-salt diet exposure led to higher intestinal permeability and dysbiosis. High-salt diet induced p38 MAPK phosphorylation and NFAT5 in lamina propria mononuclear cells activation with a subsequent expression of inflammatory cytokines expression such as IL17, IL22, and TNFα.

4. Take the Bitter with the Sweet

Carbohydrates are obviously part of a normal diet but their excessive consumption is a feature of the Westernized diet. In addition, industrialized food contains hidden sugars, such as lactose as a texturing agent in sausages. There is currently no evidence of an association between carbohydrate intake and IBD risk in epidemiological studies [20]. Results from the prospective EPIC (European Prospective Investigation into Cancer and Nutrition) study, when excluding cases occurring within the first 2 years after dietary assessment, found a positive association between a "high sugar and soft drinks" pattern and UC risk (1.68 [1.00–2.82]; $P_{trend} < 0.05$). When the authors considered the foods most associated with the pattern, high consumers of sugar and soft drinks were at higher UC risk only if they had low intakes of vegetables [21], but the amount of consumed sugar was not mentioned.

Those with pediatric IBDs had a lower intake of carbohydrates compared to the general population, in particular a decreased intake of food types high in sugar [12].

Polysaccharides are commonly added in UPF as emulsifiers, coating agents, stabilizers, or bulking agents. These ingredients enable a better palatability and a longer shelf like of these products. Some of these ingredients have been studied in experimental models of IBDs [22–25].

Nickerson et al. focused their studies on the effect of the dietary polysaccharide maltodextrin to bacterial-induced intestinal inflammation [22–24]. Maltodextrin is commonly found in processed food and medications. Nickerson et al. demonstrated that maltodextrin can promote *Salmonella* survival in multiple cell types [24]. They also studied the effect of maltodextrin on CD-associated adherent-invasive *Escherichia coli* (AIEC) and found that the presence of maltodextrin enhanced AIEC adhesion by a better biofilm formation [22]. Maltodextrin consumption may promote intestinal dysbiosis and contribute to disease susceptibility. In a recent study, maltodextrin in drinking water exacerbated intestinal inflammation in an indomethacin-induced enteropathy model or in DSS (Dextran sodium sulfate)-colitis. The mechanisms behind maltodextrin's deleterious effects involved endoplasmic reticulum stress and led to mucin-2 depletion [25].

The consumption of sweeteners is becoming more and more frequent in the US general population. A recent study on 16,942 participants reported that 25% of children and 41% of adults in the US consumed foods and beverages containing low-calorie sweeteners [26]. Two large Swedish prospective cohort studies consisting of 83,042 participants did not find any association between sweetened beverages consumption and risk of later-onset CD or UC [27]. In South Korea, food additive consumption (such as sucralose) cannot explain the increased incidence of IBDs [28]. Increased IBD incidence started before the 1980s in South Korea, while sucralose was only approved in 2000 [28]. A recent study demonstrated the deleterious impact of an artificial sweetener called Splenda in experimental IBDs [29]. Splenda contains 1% sucralose and 99% maltodextrin. The authors of this study investigated the impact of 6 weeks of supplementation with Splenda in SAMP1/YitFc mice that spontaneously developed ileitis. Splenda supplementation induced ileal myeloperoxidase activity and promoted dysbiosis, in particular an expansion of proteobacteria [29].

Carrageenan is a polysaccharide commonly used as a food additive. In experimental models, it is also commonly used to induce an inflammatory response in vitro or in vivo [30,31]. The daily consumption of carrageenan in the US diet is approximatively 250 mg per adult. Recently, a small clinical trial was conducted to evaluate the potential benefit of a carrageenan-free diet in UC patients [32]. Patients were instructed to follow a carrageenan-free diet by avoiding carrageenan-containing-food and received either 100 to 200 mg of carrageenan capsules or placebo capsules. Carrageenan-supplemented patients had some higher inflammatory parameters, such as a higher clinical disease index and higher IL-6 and fecal calprotectin [32]. Carrageenan also has an impact on intestinal microbiota [33]. Colitis induction by carrageenan at 20 mg/L in drinking water decreased the level of an anti-inflammatory bacteria *Akkermansia muciniphila* [30].

Chassaing et al. did a remarkable study on two emulsifiers, carboxymethylcellulose (CMC) and polysorbate-80 (P80), on gut barrier [34–36]. They added emulsifiers in the mouse drinking water at a relative low level for 12 weeks in wild-type or IL-10-deficient mice [35]. Dietary emulsifiers altered gut microbiota composition and induced hyperpermeability [35]. Emulsifiers promote colitis in IL-10[-/-] mice by increasing inflammatory markers such as fecal lipocalin-2 or myeloperoxidase activity [35]. They demonstrated microbiota involvement in mediating the emulsifier effect by transferring intestinal microbiota from emulsifier-treated mice into unexposed germ-free mice; upon doing so, they observed that colonized germ-free mice had the same response [35]. They confirmed in a second study the direct impact of the emulsifiers on the microbiota using a mucosal simulator of the human intestinal microbial ecosystem; they observed that emulsifiers-promoted flagellin levels [36]. In another study, Chassaing et al. investigated whether emulsifiers can impact colon carcinogenesis [34]. They exposed mice with colitis-associated cancer to the same emulsifiers for 13 weeks and they observed that emulsifiers promote carcinogenesis through intestinal microbiota alteration, the establishment of a pro-inflammatory environment, and increased proliferation marker Ki67 [34]. Interestingly, they demonstrated in a recent study that emulsifiers also had a significant impact on anxiety [37], and psychological co-morbidities are commonly observed in IBD patients and IBD experimental models [38].

One-third of IBD patient underwent irritable bowel syndrome-like symptoms [39] and a recent meta-analysis confirmed that dietary restriction of fermentable oligosaccharide, disaccharide, monosaccharide, and polyol (FODMAP) reduced functional gastrointestinal symptoms such as bloating [40]. In heathy volunteers, mechanisms behind low-FODMAP diet involved decreased *Bifidobacterium* and reduced breath hydrogen [41].

5. Put the Pedal to the Metal

Aluminum is an abundant element commonly used in our environment. It is used in processed foods and cooking materials such as food packaging or foils. Cosmetic products and drugs are also a source of aluminum. The European Food Safety Authority set the tolerable weekly intake of 1 mg aluminum/kg body weight. Pineton de Chambrun et al. investigated the dietary effect of aluminum in colitis models. The strength of this study from Lille University is that the aluminum dose of 1.5 mg/kg/day that they used was relevant to human exposure [42]. Four weeks of oral administration of aluminum has been shown to worsen chemically-induced colitis models. Indeed, macroscopic and histologic scores and myeloperoxidase activity were higher in colitis mice exposed to aluminum. They also found a similar effect in IL-10$^{-/-}$ mice. Exposure of epithelial cells lines with aluminum phosphate increased constitutive or LPS-induced cytokines mRNA level. Interestingly, aluminum exposure also delays mucosal repair capacity by inhibiting proliferating processes [43]. IBD patients often suffer from visceral pain even in remission periods [39], and a recent study from the same team has shown that dietary exposure of aluminum also induced visceral hypersensitivity in rodents [44]. This effect persisted over time after treatment cessation and involved mast cell activation [44].

6. To Add or Not to Add

Titanium dioxide (TiO$_2$) is a food pigment which increases opacity and confers a white color [45]. Dietary sources of TiO$_2$ are numerous, from sweets to toothpaste, and it is often used to provide a natural whiteness and opacity to foods, such as icing on cakes. TiO$_2$ has an optimal particle diameter of 200–300 nm, but a nano-sized fraction can be found because of manufacturing processes. These TiO$_2$ nanoparticles, in Europe listed as E171, are commonly used as a food additive. We previously investigated the effects of microparticles on macrophages from CD patients, and we observed that microparticles alone did not induce an immune response [46]. By contrast, microparticles act as adjuvants to induce potent cytokine responses in the presence of bacterial antigens such as LPS [46]. In addition, macrophage function has been shown to be impaired in the presence of high concentrations of microparticles [46]. Houdeau et al. investigated the specific effect of E171 on gut barrier [47] at a relevant range for human exposure, because modeling of human exposure to TiO$_2$ estimates an exposure of 2–3 mg/kg/day for children under the age of ten [48]. After one week of dietary exposure to TiO$_2$ at 10 mg/kg, titanium can be detected in Peyer's patches in rats [47] and it is associated with an unfavorable immune cell balance: an increased CD11b/c$^+$ CD103$^+$ MHC-II$^+$ dendritic cell proportion and a decreased proportion of regulatory T cells [47]. This TiO$_2$ effect is not transient because it lasts after 100 days of TiO$_2$ treatment [47]. In addition, long-term exposition for 100 days is associated with low-grade colon inflammation and induced aberrant crypt foci in a chemically induced carcinogenesis model [47]. The effect of dietary exposure to titanium dioxide at 50 to 500 mg/kg on colitis development has been investigated [49]. Dietary titanium dioxide exacerbates acute DSS colitis by inducing a shortening of the colon and increasing infiltration and histological inflammatory scores [49]. The same experiment was performed in inflammasome Nlrp3-/- mice, and the results showed that dietary TiO$_2$ at 500 mg.kg^{-1} did not reproduce colitis exacerbation in Nlrp3/- compared to the response of the wild type mice. The mechanisms behind the dietary effect of TiO$_2$ on colitis involved NLRP3. In vitro works demonstrated the accumulation of TiO_2 in human intestinal epithelial and macrophage cell lines in a dose-dependent manner [49]. In addition, TiO_2 at 20 to 100 µg/mL stimulates oxidative stress and increased intestinal permeability in human intestinal epithelial cell lines. Rogler et al. found that patients with active UC exhibited increased blood levels of titanium [49]. In extra-intestinal organs, dietary exposure at 2.5 to 10 mg/kg to TiO_2 for 6 months upregulated renal TGFβ and SMAD, signaling pathways involved in fibrosis [50]. We speculate that dietary TiO_2 may also promote IBD-induced intestinal fibrosis, but this effect has not been yet documented. Two recent studies have proposed a dietary intervention to counteract TiO_2-induced inflammation in mice. The administration of both flavonoids naringenin or quercetin inhibits TiO_2-induced arthritis by decreasing cytokine production and oxidative stress [51,52].

Oral bisphenol A is a chemical used in food packages. Oral bisphenol A at a dose lower to the tolerable daily intake was able to induce intestinal hyperpermeability in rats, and this effect occurs in a dose-dependent manner [53]. In trinitrobenzene sulfonic acid (TNBS)-induced colitis, perinatal exposure of dietary bisphenol A increased myeloperoxidase activity in female rats but not in male rats [53].

Dietary bisphenol A induced visceral hypersensitivity in response to colorectal distension [53]. A recent study highlighted the effect of bisphenol A in chemically induced colitis in ovariectomized female mice, and the authors demonstrated that bisphenol A exposure led to a worsened colitis through intestinal microbiota metabolites, such as a decreased level of tryptophan [54].

Food heat treatment leads to neoformed compounds such as Maillard reaction products. Exposure to these Maillard reaction products alleviated inflammatory response [55] and dysbiosis in colitis models [56].

7. Exclusion Diets

Exclusion diets are commonly followed by IBD patients [57]. These exclusion diets have poor or no scientific rationale but expose IBD patients to nutritional deficiencies. The last European Society for Clinical Nutrition and Metabolism (ESPEN) guidelines about clinical nutrition in IBD patients declared that there is no IBD diet in active disease (strong consensus—96% agreement) [58]. We will limit our section to a few exclusion diets that may explain some benefits to limit food additive exposure.

Exclusive enteral nutrition (EEN) is recommended as first intention treatment to induce remission in children or teenagers with CD [58], although EEN is not recommended in adult patients. The mechanisms behind EEN are not fully understood, but it may involve dysbiosis correction or gut barrier maintenance [59]. EEN mechanisms may also involve the absence of specific deleterious food components, such as food additive exposure.

There is also concern about the presence of pesticides in the food chain, although there is still no evidence connecting pesticides to IBDs [60]. A recent study from the NutriNet French cohort found that more frequent organic food consumption decreased cancer risk [61].

We previously mentioned the effect of nanoparticles in gut barrier dysfunction in preclinical models, and two clinical trials have investigated the impact of low or microparticle-free diet in IBD patients. The first one was a very small trial in 20 CD patients that showed a beneficial effect of low or microparticle-free diet in ileal CD patients, such as decreased corticosteroids intake [62].

The second study included 84 active CD patients for 16 weeks [63] and the authors did not find any benefit of the microparticle exclusion on inflammatory disease activity index, fecal calprotectin, or intestinal permeability [63]. We previously reported the effects of carrageenan on gut barrier in preclinical models. A small pilot study investigated the effect of carrageenan-free diet in 12 UC patients [32]. Three out of ten UC patients who followed the carrageenan-free diet for 12 months relapsed compared to three out of five patients in the control group (RR (Relative risk) 0.50, 95% CI 0.15 to 1.64), but it may be difficult to conclude that there are potentially beneficial effects because of the very small size of the study.

Lactose-free diets are common in IBD patients. In a small recent study on 78 IBD patients from Iceland, 60% (47 patients) reported limiting their dairy consumption or even excluding it, but only eight of them used calcium supplements [64]. Acquired lactase deficiency is commonly reported in CD patients, in particular in proximal CD. In a clinical trial in 77 UC patients published in 1965, milk-free diets had only a benefit for one out of five patients [65] and did not justify dairy-restricted diets in all IBD patients. In 29 pediatric UC patients, exclusion of cow milk proteins had no influence on induction and/or maintenance of remission [66].

Paleolithic diet is another exclusion diet without scientific rationale. Its principles are that our gastrointestinal system did not evolve alongside our modernized diet and may explain numerous inflammatory diseases. This diet excludes a lot of foodstuffs, such as ultra-processed foods or cereals, and is limited to wild meats and a non-cereal, plant-based diet. To our knowledge, the only published data about paleo diet and IBDs is a Hungarian case report about a teen CD patient's refractory to treatments. This CD patient had a clinical remission after 2 weeks on a paleo diet and was still in remission 15 months later [67]. Extrapolation from a unique case control study is not permitted, and exclusion of so many foodstuffs may be associated with numerous nutritional deficiencies.

One-third of IBD patients underwent IBS-like symptoms, and partial exclusion of some fermentable components may be associated with benefits to functional symptoms. For example, in a small study with 16 CD patients in remission, a strict exclusion diet of wheat and dairy products for 2 weeks significantly decreased function symptoms such as abdominal pain [68]. In a prospective study with 89 IBD patients in remission, a low-FODMAP diet for 6 weeks reduced IBS-like symptoms while it increased quality of life in patients [69].

Exclusion diets are not recommended and may expose patients to numerous nutritional deficiencies. In addition, cofounding factors are often observed, leading to unjustified dietary exclusion. Recently, a double-blind clinical trial identified that fructan composition, instead of gluten, induced functional symptoms in patients with self-reported non-celiac gluten sensitivity [69]. Similar results were previously reported concerning lactose intolerance [70]. Avoiding some foods has been identified as a risk factor for malnutrition in IBD patients in a Spanish cohort [71]. Of note, malnutrition increased further complications, such as higher surgery and hospitalization rates, and malnutrition is associated with altered quality of life in IBD patients [11,72]. In addition, exclusion diets may limit socializing and dining because many IBD patients reportedly refused dining out because doing so would not conform with their exclusion diet [11]. Exclusion of dairy products such as in a lactose-free diet or paleo diet may increase osteoporosis risk in IBD patients, while gluten-free diets are associated with decreased microbiota diversity.

8. Conclusions

Diet is a modifiable environmental risk factor and food additives may act as potentiators of disease. Diet is a crucial point for IBD patients and exclusion diets appear to offer an alternative allowing for relative control of disease development. Nevertheless, the last ESPEN guidelines did not recommend any exclusion diet for induction or maintenance of remission in IBD patients but advised IBD patients to undergo counselling by a dietitian to avoid malnutrition. In addition, it has been recently reported that IBD patients in remission have an unbalanced dietary profile for essential nutrients [73]. Rather than exclusion diets, home-made food may be prioritized to decrease food additive amounts and enable patients to control their exposure to many hidden ingredients, such as added salt or sugars. Home-made food is already recommended in the last nutritional guidelines in France and, contrary to exclusion diets, cooking can represent a form of a convivial time, allowing a better quality of life with increased socialization. In addition, obesity is more and more frequent in IBD patients [74] and food preparation from scratch may be associated with a decreased risk of obesity [75] or decreased amount of dietary energy from ultra-processed food [76].

Abbreviations

AIEC	Adherent-invasive *Escherichia coli*
CD	Crohn's disease
CMC	carboxymethylcellulose
EEN	exclusive enteral nutrition
ESPEN	European Society for Clinical Nutrition and Metabolism
FODMAP	fermentable oligosaccharide, disaccharide monosaccharide, and polyol
HSD	High-salt diet
IBD	inflammatory bowel diseases
LPS	liposaccharide
NFAT5	nuclear factor of activated T cells 5
NLRP	NOD-like receptor pyrin
P80	polysorbate-80
SCFA	short-chain fatty acid
SMAD	small mothers against decapentaplegic
TNBS	trinitrobenzene sulfonic acid
TiO2	titanium dioxide
UC	ulcerative colitis
UPF	ultra-processed food

References

1. Kaplan, G.G.; Ng, S.C. Understanding and preventing the global increase of inflammatory bowel disease. *Gastroenterology* **2017**, *152*, 313–321. [CrossRef]
2. Marion-Letellier, R.; Savoye, G.; Ghosh, S. IBD: In food we trust. *J. Crohn's Colitis* **2016**, *10*, 1351–1361. [CrossRef]
3. Marron-Ponce, J.A.; Tolentino-Mayo, L.; Hernandez, F.M.; Batis, C. Trends in ultra-processed food purchases from 1984 to 2016 in Mexican households. *Nutrients* **2018**, *11*, 45. [CrossRef]
4. Steele, E.M.; Juul, F.; Neri, D.; Rauber, F.; Monteiro, C.A. Dietary share of ultra-processed foods and metabolic syndrome in the US adult population. *Prev. Med.* **2019**. [CrossRef]
5. Gomez-Donoso, C.; Sanchez-Villegas, A.; Martinez-Gonzalez, M.A.; Gea, A.; Mendonca, R.D.; Lahortiga-Ramos, F.; Bes-Rastrollo, M. Ultra-processed food consumption and the incidence of depression in a Mediterranean cohort: The SUN Project. *Eur. J. Nutr.* **2019**, 1–11. [CrossRef]
6. Fiolet, T.; Srour, B.; Sellem, L.; Kesse-Guyot, E.; Alles, B.; Mejean, C.; Deschasaux, M.; Fassier, P.; Latino-Martel, P.; Beslay, M.; et al. Consumption of ultra-processed foods and cancer risk: Results from NutriNet-Sante prospective cohort. *BMJ* **2018**, *360*, k322. [CrossRef]
7. Schnabel, L.; Buscail, C.; Sabate, J.M.; Bouchoucha, M.; Kesse-Guyot, E.; Alles, B.; Touvier, M.; Monteiro, C.A.; Hercberg, S.; Benamouzig, R.; et al. Association between ultra-processed food consumption and functional gastrointestinal disorders: Results from the french nutrinet-sante cohort. *Am. J. Gastroenterol.* **2018**, *113*, 1217–1228. [CrossRef] [PubMed]
8. Zallot, C.; Quilliot, D.; Chevaux, J.B.; Peyrin-Biroulet, C.; Gueant-Rodriguez, R.M.; Freling, E.; Collet-Fenetrier, B.; Williet, N.; Ziegler, O.; Bigard, M.A.; et al. Dietary beliefs and behavior among inflammatory bowel disease patients. *Inflamm. Bowel Dis.* **2013**, *19*, 66–72. [CrossRef] [PubMed]
9. de Vries, J.H.M.; Dijkhuizen, M.; Tap, P.; Witteman, B.J.M. Patient's dietary beliefs and behaviours in inflammatory bowel disease. *Dig. Dis. (Basel Switz.)* **2019**, *37*, 131–139. [CrossRef]
10. Limdi, J.K.; Aggarwal, D.; McLaughlin, J.T. Dietary practices and beliefs in patients with inflammatory bowel disease. *Inflamm. Bowel Dis.* **2016**, *22*, 164–170. [CrossRef] [PubMed]
11. Casanova, M.J.; Chaparro, M.; Molina, B.; Merino, O.; Batanero, R.; Duenas-Sadornil, C.; Robledo, P.; Garcia-Albert, A.M.; Gomez-Sanchez, M.B.; Calvet, X.; et al. Prevalence of malnutrition and nutritional characteristics of patients with inflammatory bowel disease. *J. Crohn's Colitis* **2017**, *11*, 1430–1439. [CrossRef]

12. Diederen, K.; Krom, H.; Koole, J.C.D.; Benninga, M.A.; Kindermann, A. Diet and anthropometrics of children with inflammatory bowel disease: A comparison with the general population. *Inflamm. Bowel Dis.* **2018**, *24*, 1632–1640. [CrossRef]

13. Tubbs, A.L.; Liu, B.; Rogers, T.D.; Sartor, R.B.; Miao, E.A. Dietary salt exacerbates experimental colitis. *J. Immunol.* **2017**, *199*, 1051–1059. [CrossRef]

14. Monteleone, I.; Marafini, I.; Dinallo, V.; Di Fusco, D.; Troncone, E.; Zorzi, F.; Laudisi, F.; Monteleone, G. Sodium chloride-enriched diet enhanced inflammatory cytokine production and exacerbated experimental colitis in mice. *J. Crohn's Colitis* **2017**, *11*, 237–245. [CrossRef] [PubMed]

15. Aguiar, S.L.F.; Miranda, M.C.G.; Guimaraes, M.A.F.; Santiago, H.C.; Queiroz, C.P.; Cunha, P.D.S.; Cara, D.C.; Foureaux, G.; Ferreira, A.J.; Cardoso, V.N.; et al. High-salt diet induces IL-17-Dependent gut inflammation and exacerbates colitis in mice. *Front. Immunol.* **2017**, *8*, 1969. [CrossRef] [PubMed]

16. Miranda, P.M.; De Palma, G.; Serkis, V.; Lu, J.; Louis-Auguste, M.P.; McCarville, J.L.; Verdu, E.F.; Collins, S.M.; Bercik, P. High salt diet exacerbates colitis in mice by decreasing Lactobacillus levels and butyrate production. *Microbiome* **2018**, *6*, 57. [CrossRef]

17. Calvo, M.S.; Moshfegh, A.J.; Tucker, K.L. Assessing the health impact of phosphorus in the food supply: Issues and considerations. *Adv. Nutr.* **2014**, *5*, 104–113. [CrossRef]

18. Sugihara, K.; Masuda, M.; Nakao, M.; Abuduli, M.; Imi, Y.; Oda, N.; Okahisa, T.; Yamamoto, H.; Takeda, E.; Taketani, Y. Dietary phosphate exacerbates intestinal inflammation in experimental colitis. *J. Clin. Biochem. Nutr.* **2017**, *61*, 91–99. [CrossRef]

19. Khalili, H.; Malik, S.; Ananthakrishnan, A.N.; Garber, J.J.; Higuchi, L.M.; Joshi, A.; Peloquin, J.; Richter, J.M.; Stewart, K.O.; Curhan, G.C.; et al. Identification and characterization of a novel association between dietary potassium and risk of Crohn's disease and ulcerative colitis. *Front. Immunol.* **2016**, *7*, 554. [CrossRef]

20. Chan, S.S.; Luben, R.; van Schaik, F.; Oldenburg, B.; Bueno-de-Mesquita, H.B.; Hallmans, G.; Karling, P.; Lindgren, S.; Grip, O.; Key, T.; et al. Carbohydrate intake in the etiology of Crohn's disease and ulcerative colitis. *Inflamm. Bowel Dis.* **2014**, *20*, 2013–2021. [CrossRef]

21. Racine, A.; Carbonnel, F.; Chan, S.S.; Hart, A.R.; Bueno-de-Mesquita, H.B.; Oldenburg, B.; van Schaik, F.D.; Tjonneland, A.; Olsen, A.; Dahm, C.C.; et al. Dietary patterns and risk of inflammatory bowel disease in Europe: Results from the EPIC study. *Inflamm. Bowel Dis.* **2016**, *22*, 345–354. [CrossRef]

22. Nickerson, K.P.; McDonald, C. Crohn's disease-associated adherent-invasive Escherichia coli adhesion is enhanced by exposure to the ubiquitous dietary polysaccharide maltodextrin. *PLoS ONE* **2012**, *7*, e52132. [CrossRef]

23. Nickerson, K.P.; Homer, C.R.; Kessler, S.P.; Dixon, L.J.; Kabi, A.; Gordon, I.O.; Johnson, E.E.; de la Motte, C.A.; McDonald, C. The dietary polysaccharide maltodextrin promotes Salmonella survival and mucosal colonization in mice. *PLoS ONE* **2014**, *9*, e101789. [CrossRef]

24. Nickerson, K.P.; Chanin, R.; McDonald, C. Deregulation of intestinal anti-microbial defense by the dietary additive, maltodextrin. *Gut Microbes* **2015**, *6*, 78–83. [CrossRef]

25. Laudisi, F.; Di Fusco, D.; Dinallo, V.; Stolfi, C.; Di Grazia, A.; Marafini, I.; Colantoni, A.; Ortenzi, A.; Alteri, C.; Guerrieri, F.; et al. The food additive maltodextrin promotes endoplasmic reticulum stress-driven mucus depletion and exacerbates intestinal inflammation. *Cell. Mol. Gastroenterol. Hepatol.* **2019**, *7*, 457–473. [CrossRef]

26. Sylvetsky, A.C.; Jin, Y.; Clark, E.J.; Welsh, J.A.; Rother, K.I.; Talegawkar, S.A. Consumption of low-calorie sweeteners among children and adults in the United States. *J. Acad. Nutr. Diet.* **2017**, *117*, 441–448. [CrossRef]

27. Khalili, H.; Hakansson, N.; Chan, S.S.; Ludvigsson, J.F.; Olen, O.; Chan, A.T.; Hart, A.R.; Wolk, A. No association between consumption of sweetened beverages and risk of later-onset Crohn's disease or ulcerative colitis. *Clin. Gastroenterol. Hepatol. Off. Clin. Pract. J. Am. Gastroenterol. Assoc.* **2019**, *17*, 123–129. [CrossRef]

28. Ahn, H.S. Increased incidence of inflammatory bowel disease in Korea may not be explained by food additives. *Inflamm. Bowel Dis.* **2015**, *21*, E17. [CrossRef]

29. Rodriguez-Palacios, A.; Harding, A.; Menghini, P.; Himmelman, C.; Retuerto, M.; Nickerson, K.P.; Lam, M.; Croniger, C.M.; McLean, M.H.; Durum, S.K.; et al. The artificial sweetener splenda promotes gut proteobacteria, dysbiosis, and myeloperoxidase reactivity in Crohn's disease-like ileitis. *Inflamm. Bowel Dis.* **2018**, *24*, 1005–1020. [CrossRef]

30. Shang, Q.; Sun, W.; Shan, X.; Jiang, H.; Cai, C.; Hao, J.; Li, G.; Yu, G. Carrageenan-induced colitis is associated with decreased population of anti-inflammatory bacterium, Akkermansia muciniphila, in the gut microbiota of C57BL/6J mice. *Toxicol. Lett.* **2017**, *279*, 87–95. [CrossRef]

31. Fahoum, L.; Moscovici, A.; David, S.; Shaoul, R.; Rozen, G.; Meyron-Holtz, E.G.; Lesmes, U. Digestive fate of dietary carrageenan: Evidence of interference with digestive proteolysis and disruption of gut epithelial function. *Mol. Nutr. Food Res.* **2017**, *61*. [CrossRef] [PubMed]

32. Bhattacharyya, S.; Shumard, T.; Xie, H.; Dodda, A.; Varady, K.A.; Feferman, L.; Halline, A.G.; Goldstein, J.L.; Hanauer, S.B.; Tobacman, J.K. A randomized trial of the effects of the no-carrageenan diet on ulcerative colitis disease activity. *Nutr. Healthy Aging* **2017**, *4*, 181–192. [CrossRef] [PubMed]

33. Munyaka, P.M.; Sepehri, S.; Ghia, J.-E.; Khafipour, E. Carrageenan gum and adherent invasive escherichia coli in a piglet model of inflammatory bowel disease: Impact on Intestinal mucosa-associated microbiota. *Front. Microbiol.* **2016**, *7*, 462. [CrossRef]

34. Viennois, E.; Merlin, D.; Gewirtz, A.T.; Chassaing, B. Dietary emulsifier-induced low-grade inflammation promotes colon carcinogenesis. *Cancer Res.* **2017**, *77*, 27–40. [CrossRef]

35. Chassaing, B.; Koren, O.; Goodrich, J.K.; Poole, A.C.; Srinivasan, S.; Ley, R.E.; Gewirtz, A.T. Dietary emulsifiers impact the mouse gut microbiota promoting colitis and metabolic syndrome. *Nature* **2015**, *519*, 92–96. [CrossRef]

36. Chassaing, B.; Van de Wiele, T.; De Bodt, J.; Marzorati, M.; Gewirtz, A.T. Dietary emulsifiers directly alter human microbiota composition and gene expression ex vivo potentiating intestinal inflammation. *Gut* **2017**, *66*, 1414–1427. [CrossRef] [PubMed]

37. Holder, M.K.; Peters, N.V.; Whylings, J.; Fields, C.T.; Gewirtz, A.T.; Chassaing, B.; de Vries, G.J. Dietary emulsifiers consumption alters anxiety-like and social-related behaviors in mice in a sex-dependent manner. *Sci. Rep.* **2019**, *9*, 172. [CrossRef]

38. Salameh, E.; Meleine, M.; Gourcerol, G.; do Rego, J.C.; do Rego, J.L.; Legrand, R.; Breton, J.; Aziz, M.; Guerin, C.; Coeffier, M.; et al. Chronic colitis-induced visceral pain is associated with increased anxiety during quiescent phase. *Am. J. Physiol. Gastrointest. Liver Physiol.* **2019**. [CrossRef]

39. Vivinus-Nebot, M.; Frin-Mathy, G.; Bzioueche, H.; Dainese, R.; Bernard, G.; Anty, R.; Filippi, J.; Saint-Paul, M.C.; Tulic, M.K.; Verhasselt, V.; et al. Functional bowel symptoms in quiescent inflammatory bowel diseases: Role of epithelial barrier disruption and low-grade inflammation. *Gut* **2014**, *63*, 744–752. [CrossRef]

40. Zhan, Y.L.; Zhan, Y.A.; Dai, S.X. Is a low FODMAP diet beneficial for patients with inflammatory bowel disease? A meta-analysis and systematic review. *Clin. Nutr. (Edinb. Scotl.)* **2018**, *37*, 123–129. [CrossRef]

41. Sloan, T.J.; Jalanka, J.; Major, G.A.D.; Krishnasamy, S.; Pritchard, S.; Abdelrazig, S.; Korpela, K.; Singh, G.; Mulvenna, C.; Hoad, C.L.; et al. A low FODMAP diet is associated with changes in the microbiota and reduction in breath hydrogen but not colonic volume in healthy subjects. *PLoS ONE* **2018**, *13*, e0201410. [CrossRef]

42. Greger, J.L.; Sutherland, J.E. Aluminum exposure and metabolism. *Crit. Rev. Clin. Lab. Sci.* **1997**, *34*, 439–474. [CrossRef] [PubMed]

43. de Chambrun, G.P.; Body-Malapel, M.; Frey-Wagner, I.; Djouina, M.; Deknuydt, F.; Atrott, K.; Esquerre, N.; Altare, F.; Neut, C.; Arrieta, M.C.; et al. Aluminum enhances inflammation and decreases mucosal healing in experimental colitis in mice. *Mucosal Immunol.* **2014**, *7*, 589–601. [CrossRef]

44. Esquerre, N.; Basso, L.; Dubuquoy, C.; Djouina, M.; Chappard, D.; Blanpied, C.; Desreumaux, P.; Vergnolle, N.; Vignal, C.; Body-Malapel, M. Aluminum ingestion promotes colorectal hypersensitivity in rodents. *Cell. Mol. Gastroenterol. Hepatol.* **2018**, *7*, 185–196. [CrossRef] [PubMed]

45. Winkler, H.C.; Notter, T.; Meyer, U.; Naegeli, H. Critical review of the safety assessment of titanium dioxide additives in food. *J. Nanobiotechn.* **2018**, *16*, 51. [CrossRef] [PubMed]

46. Butler, M.; Boyle, J.J.; Powell, J.J.; Playford, R.J.; Ghosh, S. Dietary microparticles implicated in Crohn's disease can impair macrophage phagocytic activity and act as adjuvants in the presence of bacterial stimuli. *Inflamm. Res. Off. J. Eur. Histamine Res. Soc.* **2007**, *56*, 353–361. [CrossRef] [PubMed]

47. Bettini, S.; Boutet-Robinet, E.; Cartier, C.; Comera, C.; Gaultier, E.; Dupuy, J.; Naud, N.; Tache, S.; Grysan, P.; Reguer, S.; et al. Food-grade TiO2 impairs intestinal and systemic immune homeostasis, initiates preneoplastic lesions and promotes aberrant crypt development in the rat colon. *Sci. Rep.* **2017**, *7*, 40373. [CrossRef] [PubMed]

48. Weir, A.; Westerhoff, P.; Fabricius, L.; Hristovski, K.; von Goetz, N. Titanium dioxide nanoparticles in food and personal care products. *Environ. Sci. Technol.* **2012**, *46*, 2242–2250. [CrossRef]

49. Ruiz, P.A.; Moron, B.; Becker, H.M.; Lang, S.; Atrott, K.; Spalinger, M.R.; Scharl, M.; Wojtal, K.A.; Fischbeck-Terhalle, A.; Frey-Wagner, I.; et al. Titanium dioxide nanoparticles exacerbate DSS-induced colitis: Role of the NLRP3 inflammasome. *Gut* **2017**, *66*, 1216–1224. [CrossRef] [PubMed]

50. Hong, F.; Wu, N.; Ge, Y.; Zhou, Y.; Shen, T.; Qiang, Q.; Zhang, Q.; Chen, M.; Wang, Y.; Wang, L.; et al. Nanosized titanium dioxide resulted in the activation of TGF-beta/Smads/p38MAPK pathway in renal inflammation and fibration of mice. *J. Biomed. Mater. Res. Part A* **2016**, *104*, 1452–1461. [CrossRef]

51. Borghi, S.M.; Mizokami, S.S.; Pinho-Ribeiro, F.A.; Fattori, V.; Crespigio, J.; Clemente-Napimoga, J.T.; Napimoga, M.H.; Pitol, D.L.; Issa, J.P.M.; Fukada, S.Y.; et al. The flavonoid quercetin inhibits titanium dioxide (TiO2)-induced chronic arthritis in mice. *J. Nutr. Biochem.* **2018**, *53*, 81–95. [CrossRef]

52. Manchope, M.F.; Artero, N.A.; Fattori, V.; Mizokami, S.S.; Pitol, D.L.; Issa, J.P.M.; Fukada, S.Y.; Cunha, T.M.; Alves-Filho, J.C.; Cunha, F.Q.; et al. Naringenin mitigates titanium dioxide (TiO2)-induced chronic arthritis in mice: Role of oxidative stress, cytokines, and NFkappaB. *Inflamm. Res. Off. J. Eur. Histamine Res. Soc.* **2018**, *67*, 997–1012. [CrossRef]

53. Braniste, V.; Jouault, A.; Gaultier, E.; Polizzi, A.; Buisson-Brenac, C.; Leveque, M.; Martin, P.G.; Theodorou, V.; Fioramonti, J.; Houdeau, E. Impact of oral bisphenol A at reference doses on intestinal barrier function and sex differences after perinatal exposure in rats. *Proc. Natl. Acad. Sci. USA* **2010**, *107*, 448–453. [CrossRef] [PubMed]

54. DeLuca, J.A.; Allred, K.F.; Menon, R.; Riordan, R.; Weeks, B.R.; Jayaraman, A.; Allred, C.D. Bisphenol-A alters microbiota metabolites derived from aromatic amino acids and worsens disease activity during colitis. *Exp. Biol. Med.* **2018**, *243*, 864–875. [CrossRef]

55. Al Amir, I.; Dubayle, D.; Heron, A.; Delayre-Orthez, C.; Anton, P.M. Maillard reaction products from highly heated food prevent mast cell number increase and inflammation in a mouse model of colitis. *Nutr. Res.* **2017**, *48*, 26–32. [CrossRef] [PubMed]

56. Jahdali, N.A.L.; Gadonna-Widehem, P.; Delayre-Orthez, C.; Marier, D.; Garnier, B.; Carbonero, F.; Anton, P.M. Repeated oral exposure to N (epsilon)-Carboxymethyllysine, a maillard reaction product, alleviates gut microbiota dysbiosis in colitic mice. *Dig. Dis. Sci.* **2017**, *62*, 3370–3384. [CrossRef]

57. Limketkai, B.N.; Iheozor-Ejiofor, Z.; Gjuladin-Hellon, T.; Parian, A.; Matarese, L.E.; Bracewell, K.; MacDonald, J.K.; Gordon, M.; Mullin, G.E. Dietary interventions for induction and maintenance of remission in inflammatory bowel disease. *Cochrane Database Syst. Rev.* **2019**, *2*, CD012839. [CrossRef]

58. Forbes, A.; Escher, J.; Hebuterne, X.; Klek, S.; Krznaric, Z.; Schneider, S.; Shamir, R.; Stardelova, K.; Wierdsma, N.; Wiskin, A.E.; et al. ESPEN guideline: Clinical nutrition in inflammatory bowel disease. *Clin. Nutr. (Edinb. Scotl.)* **2017**, *36*, 321–347. [CrossRef]

59. Altomare, R.; Damiano, G.; Abruzzo, A.; Palumbo, V.D.; Tomasello, G.; Buscemi, S.; Lo Monte, A.I. Enteral nutrition support to treat malnutrition in inflammatory bowel disease. *Nutrients* **2015**, *7*, 2125–2133. [CrossRef]

60. Arcella, D.; Boobis, A.; Cressey, P.; Erdely, H.; Fattori, V.; Leblanc, J.C.; Lipp, M.; Reuss, R.; Scheid, S.; Tritscher, A.; et al. Harmonized methodology to assess chronic dietary exposure to residues from compounds used as pesticide and veterinary drug. *Crit. Rev. Toxicol.* **2019**, 1–10. [CrossRef]

61. Baudry, J.; Assmann, K.E.; Touvier, M.; Alles, B.; Seconda, L.; Latino-Martel, P.; Ezzedine, K.; Galan, P.; Hercberg, S.; Lairon, D.; et al. Association of frequency of organic food consumption with cancer risk: Findings from the nutrinet-sante prospective cohort study. *JAMA Intern. Med.* **2018**, *178*, 1597–1606. [CrossRef] [PubMed]

62. Lomer, M.C.; Harvey, R.S.; Evans, S.M.; Thompson, R.P.; Powell, J.J. Efficacy and tolerability of a low microparticle diet in a double blind, randomized, pilot study in Crohn's disease. *Eur. J. Gastroenterol. Hepatol.* **2001**, *13*, 101–106. [CrossRef]

63. Lomer, M.C.; Grainger, S.L.; Ede, R.; Catterall, A.P.; Greenfield, S.M.; Cowan, R.E.; Vicary, F.R.; Jenkins, A.P.; Fidler, H.; Harvey, R.S.; et al. Lack of efficacy of a reduced microparticle diet in a multi-centred trial of patients with active Crohn's disease. *Eur. J. Gastroenterol. Hepatol.* **2005**, *17*, 377–384. [CrossRef]

64. Vidarsdottir, J.B.; Johannsdottir, S.E.; Thorsdottir, I.; Bjornsson, E.; Ramel, A. A cross-sectional study on nutrient intake and -status in inflammatory bowel disease patients. *Nutr. J.* **2016**, *15*, 61. [CrossRef] [PubMed]

65. Wright, R.; Truelove, S.C. A controlled therapeutic trial of various diets in ulcerative colitis. *Br. Med. J.* **1965**, *2*, 138–141. [CrossRef]
66. Strisciuglio, C.; Giannetti, E.; Martinelli, M.; Sciorio, E.; Staiano, A.; Miele, E. Does cow's milk protein elimination diet have a role on induction and maintenance of remission in children with ulcerative colitis? *Acta Paediatr.* **2013**, *102*, e273–e278. [CrossRef]
67. Tóth, C.; Dabóczi, A.; Howard, M.; Miller, N.J.; Clemens, Z. Crohn's disease successfully treated with the paleolithic ketogenic diet. *Int. J. Case Rep. Images* **2016**, *7*, 570–578. [CrossRef]
68. Komperod, M.J.; Sommer, C.; Mellin-Olsen, T.; Iversen, P.O.; Roseth, A.G.; Valeur, J. Persistent symptoms in patients with Crohn's disease in remission: An exploratory study on the role of diet. *Scand. J. Gastroenterol.* **2018**, *53*, 573–578. [CrossRef] [PubMed]
69. Pedersen, N.; Ankersen, D.V.; Felding, M.; Wachmann, H.; Vegh, Z.; Molzen, L.; Burisch, J.; Andersen, J.R.; Munkholm, P. Low-FODMAP diet reduces irritable bowel symptoms in patients with inflammatory bowel disease. *World J. Gastroenterol.* **2017**, *23*, 3356–3366. [CrossRef]
70. Suarez, F.L.; Savaiano, D.A.; Levitt, M.D. A comparison of symptoms after the consumption of milk or lactose-hydrolyzed milk by people with self-reported severe lactose intolerance. *N. Engl. J. Med.* **1995**, *333*, 1–4. [CrossRef]
71. Lim, H.S.; Kim, S.K.; Hong, S.J. Food elimination diet and nutritional deficiency in patients with inflammatory bowel disease. *Clin. Nutr. Res.* **2018**, *7*, 48–55. [CrossRef] [PubMed]
72. Rocha, R.; Sousa, U.H.; Reis, T.L.M.; Santana, G.O. Nutritional status as a predictor of hospitalization in inflammatory bowel disease: A review. *World J. Gastrointest. Pharmacol. Ther.* **2019**, *10*, 50–56. [CrossRef]
73. Taylor, L.; Almutairdi, A.; Shommu, N.; Fedorak, R.; Ghosh, S.; Reimer, R.A.; Panaccione, R.; Raman, M. Cross-sectional analysis of overall dietary intake and mediterranean dietary pattern in patients with Crohn's disease. *Nutrients* **2018**, *10*, 1761. [CrossRef] [PubMed]
74. Moran, G.W.; Dubeau, M.F.; Kaplan, G.G.; Panaccione, R.; Ghosh, S. The increasing weight of Crohn's disease subjects in clinical trials: A hypothesis-generatings time-trend analysis. *Inflamm. Bowel Dis.* **2013**, *19*, 2949–2956. [CrossRef] [PubMed]
75. Mejean, C.; Lampure, A.; Si Hassen, W.; Gojard, S.; Peneau, S.; Hercberg, S.; Castetbon, K. Influence of food preparation behaviors on 5-year weight change and obesity risk in a French prospective cohort. *Int. J. Behav. Nutr. Phys. Act.* **2018**, *15*, 120. [CrossRef] [PubMed]
76. Lam, M.C.L.; Adams, J. Association between home food preparation skills and behaviour, and consumption of ultra-processed foods: Cross-sectional analysis of the UK National Diet and nutrition survey (2008–2009). *Int. J. Behav. Nutr. Phys. Act.* **2017**, *14*, 68. [CrossRef] [PubMed]

Dietary Support in Elderly Patients with Inflammatory Bowel Disease

Piotr Eder *,†, Alina Niezgódka †, Iwona Krela-Kaźmierczak, Kamila Stawczyk-Eder, Estera Banasik and Agnieszka Dobrowolska

Department of Gastroenterology, Dietetics and Internal Medicine, Poznan University of Medical Sciences, Heliodor Święcicki Hospital, 60-355 Poznań, Poland; niezgodkaalina@gmail.com (A.N.); krela@op.pl (I.K.-K.); kamilastawczyk@wp.pl (K.S.-E.); esta717@gmail.com (E.B.); agdob@ump.edu.pl (A.D.)
* Correspondence: piotr.eder@op.pl
† These two authors contribute equally to this paper.

Abstract: Ageing of the human population has become a big challenge for health care systems worldwide. On the other hand, the number of elderly patients with inflammatory bowel disease (IBD) is also increasing. Considering the unique clinical characteristics of this subpopulation, including many comorbidities and polypharmacy, the current therapeutic guidelines for the management of IBD should be individualized and applied with caution. This is why the role of non-pharmacological treatments is of special significance. Since both IBD and older age are independent risk factors of nutritional deficiencies, appropriate dietary support should be an important part of the therapeutic approach. In this review paper we discuss the interrelations between IBD, older age, and malnutrition. We also present the current knowledge on the utility of different diets in the management of IBD. Considering the limited data on how to support IBD therapy by nutritional intervention, we focus on the Mediterranean and Dietary Approaches to Stop Hypertension diets, which seem to be the most beneficial in this patient group. We also discuss some new findings on their hypothetical anti-inflammatory influence on the course of IBD.

Keywords: inflammatory bowel disease; malnutrition; Mediterranean diet; older age

1. Introduction

The frequency of Crohn's disease (CD) and ulcerative colitis (UC), two forms of inflammatory bowel disease (IBD), is increasing worldwide [1–3]. Simultaneously with the demographic ageing of the human population observed in recent decades, especially in developed countries, the number of elderly IBD patients is also increasing [4–8]. Considering the definition of elderly as aged 60 years and above, it is estimated that 25–35% of CD and UC patients meet this criterion. These data encompass both those who were diagnosed before reaching 60 and those who were diagnosed when over 60 (elderly onset). The latter group, representing 10–15% of all IBD patients, reflects the second peak of CD and UC morbidity [9]. UC is the more frequent IBD subtype in this age range, since one in eight UC patients is older than 60, compared to one in 20 CD cases [9]. A population-based cohort study by Charpentier et al. revealed that, among elderly people suffering from IBD, 65% are between 60 and 70 years old, 25% between 70 and 80 years old, and 10% are older than 80 [10].

There is an increasing body of evidence showing several differences in the clinical course and management of elderly IBD patients, compared with those suffering from UC or CD at a younger age. One of the most important characteristics is a tendency for less aggressive therapeutic regimens [11–13]. On the other hand, the significance of non-pharmacological and non-surgical interventions is higher. Since both IBD and older age are independent risk factors of nutritional deficiencies, appropriate dietary support is needed, especially in the cases of patients older than 60 with UC or CD [12,14,15]. In this review, we discuss the influence of older age on the physiology of the gastrointestinal tract and the mechanisms leading to malnutrition, especially in the context of IBD in the elderly. We summarize the main differences in the clinical course and management of IBD in the elderly with special emphasis on the role of diet. We also present some recommendations for nutritional support for this unique population.

In order to analyze the current literature on dietary support among elderly IBD patients, we searched the PubMed and Web of Science databases using the key words "diet and IBD", "elderly IBD", "diet in elderly people", and "nutrition in elderly IBD patients". We identified mainly review papers, meta-analyses, and guidelines published after 2010. Moreover, we analyzed conference abstracts from the Congresses of the European Crohn's and Colitis Organisation (ECCO) in 2018 and 2019.

1.1. Elderly IBD Patient—Differences in Clinical Course and Management

There are several characteristic features of elderly IBD. The delay in the diagnosis of CD or UC is longer than that in younger patients. This is related to less specific symptoms and to a frequent co-existence of other comorbidities and polypharmacy. Differential diagnosis encompasses many entities like ischemic colitis, infectious diseases, drug adverse reactions (non-steroidal anti-inflammatory drugs, anticoagulation, anti-platelet drugs, chemotherapy, etc.), diverticulitis, radiation colitis, and microscopic colitis. Performing invasive diagnostic investigations (like colonoscopy) can also be challenging, since older age, other comorbidities and drugs used are risk factors for severe complications [5,6,16,17].

The clinical course of elderly IBD seems to be less aggressive [6,8]. In CD, there is a higher frequency of colonic location [16,18]. On the other hand, complications like strictures or perianal involvement and extraintestinal manifestations are less common. As a result, the clinical presentation of elderly CD can be similar to UC, with rectal bleeding as a main symptom. Abdominal pain, weight loss, and diarrhea are less typical [16,18–20]. In the case of elderly UC, the predominant location is E2 or E3 according to the Montreal classification, whereas isolated proctitis is rare [20,21]. The disease is more stable over time and there is a low frequency of proximal disease colonic extension [19,20]. The need for a colectomy is also relatively low. A French population-based registry (EPIMAD) showed that only 16% of elderly onset UC patients underwent a colectomy in a ten-year follow-up period [6,8,22–24].

Despite a milder clinical course in long-term observation, the first IBD episode can be paradoxically more severe than in younger patients [18]. Older age also seems to be related to a more frequent hospitalization rate in IBD [18,20]. A study by Ananthakrishnan et al. revealed that hospitalized IBD patients older than 65 are at a higher risk of significant malnutrition, anaemia, and hypovolemia [25]. The frequency of thromboembolic complications is increased due to hypercoagulability, dehydration, prolonged bed rest, and immobilization. This is why the hospitalization of elderly IBD patients seems to be connected with higher fatality [18,26–29].

Although there are no randomized, controlled trials assessing the therapeutic strategies for IBD in the elderly, medical and surgical management is often different from patients of a younger age [30–34]. The usage of many medications is limited due to their higher toxicity (e.g., corticosteroids), the risk of interactions (e.g., thiopurines with allopurinol, mesalamine with anticoagulants), contraindications (e.g., renal insufficiency in the case of mesalamine, severe congestive heart failure in the case of anti-tumor necrosis factor alpha antibodies), and higher rates of adverse events (e.g., serious infections, diabetes, arterial hypertension, mental disorders in the case of corticosteroids or neoplastic complications in the case of thiopurines) [7,35–53]. The safety of newly registered immunosuppressive molecules and biological agents (tofacitinib, anti-integrins–vedolizumab, or anti-IL-12/23 antibodies–ustekinumab) in elderly IBD patients has not been studied at all [54].

General indications for surgery in IBD patients aged >60 are similar, when compared with the younger subgroup, however, a decision to use surgical intervention should be taken with caution since there is a higher risk of post-operative complications and mortality [5,11]. Nevertheless, in many cases surgery is inevitable, which is why, in order to improve therapeutic outcomes, optimal treatment should be applied preoperatively, with minimization of corticosteroid use and extensive nutritional support [5,11,55–57].

The rules for disease monitoring in elderly IBD patients should be also adjusted for age and concomitant morbidities. Since repeated endoscopic assessment is often impossible, the importance of non-invasive markers of inflammatory activity, like fecal calprotectin or C-reactive protein, is high [58,59]. In terms of cross-sectional imaging methods, repeated computed tomography or magnetic resonance (MR) imaging can be difficult and, in many cases, contraindicated [60]. This is due to the fact that a significant proportion of older patients suffer from renal insufficiency or are at a high risk of this complication, which makes the administration of an intravenous contrast agent impossible. Another limitation for MR imaging is the high frequency of metallic implants (e.g., after a total hip or knee replacement or after the implantation of a cardiac rhythm control device) in elderly people. This is why more common use of an abdominal ultrasound should be advised for the objective assessment of morphological abnormalities in the gastrointestinal tract [60].

1.2. Ageing, IBD, and Malnutrition—What Are the Connections?

As discussed above, there are many limitations for the routine application of classical therapeutic approaches in the case of IBD in elderly patients. Thus, non-pharmacological and non-surgical interventions are of great importance. The role of dietary support is especially high, since ageing by itself increases the risk of malnutrition. Epidemiological analyses show that 5%–20% of European citizens aged 60 and older suffer from malnutrition, while for hospitalized patients or those in long-term care, these numbers are even higher [61]. Thus, obligatory assessment of the nutritional status of all older patients is recommended by both the American Society for Parenteral and Enteral Nutrition (ASPEN) and the European Society for Parenteral and Enteral Nutrition (ESPEN). A Mini Nutritional Assessment (MNA) is believed to be the most appropriate tool for this purpose [62–64].

The etiology of malnutrition in older people is multifactorial. There are multiple medical conditions associated with a high risk of weight loss and nutritional deficiencies, like cancer, pulmonary disorders (chronic obstructive pulmonary disease), diabetes, cerebrovascular and neurological diseases, and gastrointestinal disorders. Many of those conditions are characterized by an increased catabolism, loss of appetite, and dysphagia. Multimorbidity and polypharmacy—typical phenomena among elderly people—are also connected with higher hospitalization rates, and increased probability of significant drug interactions [65]. These factors can independently promote malnutrition [65–67]. Another important problem is poor oral health and dental status leading to chewing difficulties and mouth dryness, which can cause lower food intake [68,69]. Depression, anxiety, dementia, and many other neuropsychological factors can result in unintentional weight loss and nutritional deficiencies [70–72]. There are also many social determinants of malnutrition risk, like poverty, loneliness and isolation, an inability to shop or cook, secondary to cognitive disorders and/or physical disability [73,74]. Interestingly, although ageing per se is not always associated with malnutrition, there are several physiological phenomena increasing the risk of weight loss. Decreasing appetite among elderly and otherwise healthy people can be explained by a reduction in stomach capacity and impairment of gastric relaxation, accompanied by lower gastric emptying. One of the etiological hypotheses for these processes in older people is fluctuation in the production and secretion of several enterohormones. There are data suggesting that higher levels of cholecystokinin and lower concentration of ghrelin can contribute to early satiation after food consumption. Moreover, degenerative processes in the gastrointestinal tract can result in the reduction in the number of taste buds, which can be accompanied by a deterioration in the sense of smell. These phenomena can additionally demotivate the patients to consume regularly [75–77].

Since the mechanisms underlying malnutrition in elderly people are complex, three types of weight loss proposed by Roubenoff can coexist: wasting, cachexia, and sarcopenia [78,79]. Wasting is associated with inadequate dietary intake and results in involuntary weight loss [80]. Cachexia is caused by induced catabolic processes, with pro-inflammatory cytokines like interleukin-1 (IL-1), tumor necrosis factor–alpha (TNF-alpha), IL-6, and others having a predominant role. The main consequence of cachexia is a decrease in fat-free mass and body cell mass [81]. Sarcopenia is defined as a loss of muscle mass [78,79,82]. The etiology of this phenomenon is poorly understood, however, a dominant role is hypothetically played by a lack of physical activity, induction of the pro-inflammatory response, and dysregulation of anabolic hormones, like testosterone or growth hormone [83,84].

IBD is independently associated with an increased risk of malnutrition. Epidemiological data shows that 65%–75% of CD patients and 18%–62% of UC patients have nutritional deficiencies [85]. The discrepancies in these numbers are a consequence of the different definitions of malnutrition. Body mass index (BMI) is among the most frequently used criteria, but it has been widely criticized recently, since it does not take into account several qualitative and quantitative parameters like the relation between fat and muscle mass, the concentration of micro- and macronutrients, recent changes in body mass or disease activity [86]. There are many data showing that low body mass is only one of the dimensions reflecting malnutrition in IBD. Among other parameters, which have been frequently reported, are deficiencies in iron, calcium, selenium, vitamin D and/or vitamin K [85].

The etiology of malnutrition in IBD is complex. It encompasses disease-related and treatment-related factors [85]. In the first group, a decrease in food intake seems to be the most important. This phenomenon can be related to IBD symptoms, like nausea, vomiting, abdominal pain, diarrhea, fever or fatigue. Also, it has been shown that hospitalization is associated with a higher risk of inappropriate food intake due to a frequent need to fast in preparation for different investigations or due to an inadequate hospital diet [85,87]. Moreover, disease activity by itself, with the production of multiple pro-inflammatory cytokines, induces catabolic processes, and promotes increased energy expenditure, contributing to malnutrition. The absorptive functions of the gastrointestinal tract are also impaired due to bowel wall damage with a loss of epithelial integrity, bacterial overgrowth, and increased intestinal motility. The same factors contribute to enhanced nutrient loss [85,88]. Considering the treatment-related causes of malnutrition, there are data on the negative impact of steroids on body composition. Moreover, nitroimidazoles or immunosuppressive drugs (thiopurines, methotrexate) can also alter the appetite, leading to reduced food intake [85]. On the other hand, multiple surgical resections limit the absorptive gastrointestinal surface, in spite of the high compensatory potential of the remaining parts of the intestines [85].

Taking into consideration the complex etiology and high frequency of malnutrition among elderly people and IBD patients analyzed separately, the significance of this phenomenon among CD and UC patients aged 60 and older becomes especially challenging. In order to prevent and/or adequately treat this unique subpopulation, proper dietary support is needed.

1.3. The Role of Diet in IBD and the Elderly

There are no strict dietitian recommendations for patients with IBD, since there are insufficient data for promoting any special diet. The general rule is that patients should cover their energy demand by eating well-balanced meals containing complex carbohydrates, proteins and fats, mainly of plant origin, rich in vegetables and fruits, with the elimination of highly processed foods [89]. Special attention should be paid to appropriate iron and vitamin D consumption. In each case, however, a highly individualized recommendation should be defined in order to adjust the nutritional needs to a concrete, clinical scenario, especially in older people.

According to current knowledge, in the case of physiological ageing special recommendations should be given for protein, vitamin D, and water consumption. In order to maintain muscle mass, the PROT-AGE study group defined the daily protein requirement, which is 1.0–1.2 g protein/kg body weight [90]. Moreover, all individuals should supplement vitamin D3 in a dose of 800–2000 IU per day [91]. Adults should drink 30–35 mL/kg body weight (at least 1500 mL/day or 1–1.5 mL/1 kcal) of water (preferably medium-carbonized and still water). Since there is an increased risk of dehydration among older people, the recommendations for daily water consumption in this subpopulation (similar to the pediatric population) are more precisely defined as 100 mL of water for the first 10 kg, then 50 mL for second 10 kg, and 15–20 mL for each additional kilogram of body weight [92,93]. In addition, older adults are in the groups at risk of vitamin B12 deficiency. The usual dietary sources of vitamin B12 are animal products, including fish, meat, poultry, eggs, milk, and milk products. Vitamin B12 is generally not present in plant foods, but a lot of these products are fortified. The vitamin B12 recommended dietary allowance for older adults is 2.4 μg/day [94,95].

In the case of high IBD activity, especially in patients with severe diarrhea and abdominal pain due to stricturing CD, it is advisable to avoid a high intake of fiber and lactose, in order to prevent bacterial overgrowth and reduce the number of bowel movements [96]. The daily protein requirement is 1.2–1.5 g protein/kg body weight [96]. Resting energy expenditure during a flare is 25–30 kcal/kg standard body weight [96–98]. Moreover, according to the ESPEN recommendations, oral nutrition supplements (ONS) should be considered in addition to a normal diet for the treatment of nutritional deficiencies in the case of IBD exacerbation [96]. ONS contain high amounts of all (complete) or selected (incomplete) macro- and microelements in relatively small volume products. ONS can be also divided into two categories: standard ONS which contain different nutritional compounds in proportions characteristic for a normal oral diet and specific ONS which is composed adequately for some particular patient populations (e.g., Parkinson's disease, Alzheimer's disease, etc.). ONS can be used together with meals; they contain no lactose, gluten, purines or cholesterol and should be considered in each case of increased malnutrition risk or diagnosed malnutrition [96,99].

Recent years, however, have brought plenty of data about the crucial role of impaired microbiota in the pathogenesis of intestinal inflammation. Moreover, there is a growing body of evidence that also ageing is associated with changes in intestinal microbiota composition. In 2007 the ELDERMET consortium was established to investigate this topic [100]. They found (by using the pyrosequencing of 16S rRNA method) that there was an increase in *Bacteroidetes* and a concomitant decrease in *Firmicutes* species among older people, however there was a significant inter-individual variability in the composition of elderly gut microbiota [101]. One of the reasons was the health status of the investigated subjects. The statistical analysis indicated a clear separation between community-dwelling subjects and long-stay home residents [101]. Another observation was that health status and the diversity of the intestinal microbiota in the ELDERMET study correlated with the patients' nutritional habits. It was shown that the diversity index of the fecal microbiota was significantly associated with a low-fat and high-fiber diet [101]. It is, however, still not known whether changes in gut microbiota are a result of dietary intervention or are more related to unhealthy ageing by itself.

Nevertheless, the possibility of shaping the intestinal microbiota by nutritional interventions would be very attractive. The hypothetical promotion of a "healthy" in-vironment (microbiota) by environmental factors (diet) seems to be an interesting concept for therapeutic intervention also in IBD. This is why dietary intervention is currently considered not only in the context of sufficient nutritional support, but also as a potential modulator of intestinal inflammation [102,103]. Our understanding of the link between nutrition, intestinal microbiota, and inflammatory response is still poor, however, due to the development of new technologies such as metabolic profiling and next-generation DNA sequencing, we know that microbiota composition changes after exposure to different modifying factors [104]. For example, there are data showing that a high-fat and low-fiber diet, as well as an animal-based diet, increase the abundance of *Bacteroidetes* and *Prevotella*, which are believed to participate in the development of chronic inflammation in the gastrointestinal tract [105]. On the other hand, dietary fiber can promote short-chain fatty acids synthesis by colonic microbiota, which can lead to the suppression of pro-inflammatory cytokines from dendritic cells and macrophages [104,106,107]. Another hypothetical association between the diet and inflammation is the epigenetic regulation of gene expression by different nutritional components. There is some evidence that the typical Western diet, deficient in micronutrients, like selenium and folate, can influence DNA methylation, which promotes pro-inflammatory phenomena and seems to increase colorectal cancer susceptibility [104]. What is more, in an experimental model of IBD it was shown that selenium supplementation prevented tissue damage through interfering with the expression of the key genes responsible for inflammation [104,108]. Nevertheless, although these concepts of the associations between diet, microbiota, and inflammatory response are very promising, we are still not able to translate this knowledge into clinical practice. We hope that it will be possible in the future to modulate our microbiota by changing the in-vironmental milieu via nutritional intervention, but we still need more data.

Among different diets already studied in the context of IBD, main attention is being paid to the low-fermentable oligosaccharide, disaccharide, monosaccharide, and polyol (FODMAP) and anti-inflammatory diet (IBD-AID), although supporting scientific evidence is relatively poor [104]. Recently, the advantages of the Mediterranean or the Dietary Approach to Stop Hypertension (DASH) diets in the context of chronic inflammation have also been discussed [105,106].

The main rule of the low-FODMAP diet is to exclude highly fermentable and poorly absorbed carbohydrates and polyols. In this diet, consumption of different food types is strongly discouraged, such as many fruits (e.g., apple, blackberry, grapefruit, mango, nectarine, peach, plum, watermelon), vegetables (e.g., artichoke, asparagus, avocado, onion, cabbage, garlic, leek, pea), dairy (e.g., cow, goat, sheep, condensed and evaporated milk), beverages (e.g., green tea, soft drinks, white tea, coconut water) and many nuts, seeds and legumes. Moreover, breaded meat or meat made with high fructose corn syrup should be avoided. This is not a long-term diet and the dietary limitations should last for only 6–8 weeks. Then patients should gradually restart foods high in FODMAPs in order to establish an individual tolerance to specific oligosaccharides, disaccharides, monosaccharides, and polyols. The utility of the low-FODMAP diet has been shown mainly for patients with irritable bowel syndrome (IBS), since there is a hypothesis that high fermentation in the gastrointestinal lumen can lead to increased intestinal permeability and provoke intestinal hypersensitivity in a genetically susceptible host [107,108]. Data on the usefulness of this diet in IBD are limited and mainly come from retrospective cohorts. It is advised that a low-FODMAP diet can be used in selected IBD patients with IBS-like symptoms in addition to conventional therapy, but only under strict dietitian supervision [104–115].

IBD-AID is a multistep and highly individualized dietary intervention, limiting some specific carbohydrates (e.g., refined sugar, gluten-based grains, certain starches). Olendzki et al., who developed IBD-AID, hypothesized that this can decrease the growth of several pro-inflammatory bacteria in the gastrointestinal tract, preventing dysbiosis [116]. In the next step, the patient should ingest prebiotics and probiotics (e.g., leek, onion, fermented food) to promote restoration of the microbiota. Moreover, the consumption of total and saturated fat, and hydrogenated oils should be avoided, together with the individual identification of dietary intolerances and nutritional deficiencies. The rules of IBD-AID were first published in 2017 and until now there were no randomized, controlled trials conducted in order to confirm the initial, promising reports on the use of this diet as an adjunct therapy for the treatment of IBD [104,116].

Lack of sufficient data for the usefulness of the low-FODMAP diet and IBD-AID in IBD result in a high skepticism of clinicians to promote this kind of dietary intervention. In the case of elderly IBD patients, another important limitation for the use of these diets is their complexity. Moreover, there is a high risk of several nutritional deficiencies due to the restriction and avoidance of different foods, especially when the dietary intervention is conducted without professional support. This can have serious negative consequences, considering the general increased risk of malnutrition and the presence of serious comorbidities in older people. This is why it seems to be more reasonable to promote safer diets, with more robust data in the context of elderly patients.

Considering the nutritional requirements and characteristics of elderly patients with IBD discussed above, as well as the most common disorders among older people (arterial hypertension and other cardiovascular diseases, type 2 diabetes, hypercholesterolemia), the DASH or Mediterranean diet could be recommended for this unique population. The main restrictions in the DASH diet concern carbohydrates and fats, in particular by limiting simple carbohydrates (glucose, fructose, saccharose) and reducing the intake of saturated fats. This means a significant reduction in the consumption of sweets, sugar confectionery, sweeteners, fruit preservatives (less than five portions per week), as well as red meat and highly processed food. Vegetables and fruits should be eaten 4–5 times/day, and whole grain products 6–8 times/day. The DASH diet also includes medium-fat dairy products

(2–3 portions/day), however, this needs to be accompanied with regular consumption of vegetable oils (preferably raw, inter alia, to enable the absorption of fat-soluble vitamins). The recommended frequency for eating fatty saltwater fish (herring, salmon, mackerel, halibut, sardine, codfish, flounder) is 2–4 times/week. Different seeds, nuts, legumes are also an important part of the DASH diet, since they contain (similar to vegetable oils—linseed, soybean or rapeseed oil— and fatty saltwater fish) high amounts of omega-3 polyunsaturated fatty acids (PUFA). Another main rule of this type of diet is a significant reduction in salt (sodium) consumption [117].

Although there are no data on the utility of the DASH diet in IBD, its beneficial effect on general health status and cardiovascular risk is well known [118–121]. Moreover, Nilsson et al. showed that adherence to a DASH-style diet was significantly associated with a lower clustered metabolic risk among older women, and it promoted a systemic anti-inflammatory environment, independently of physical activity [122]. The authors concluded that the DASH diet should be considered as a key target for nutritional intervention among elderly people to prevent age-related metabolic abnormalities.

The general recommendations of the Mediterranean diet are very similar to DASH. It emphasizes eating primarily plant-based foods (fruits, vegetables, whole grains, legumes, nuts, seeds, olive oil), which should be consumed several times per day, together with dairy products (mainly different types of cheese, yogurts). Low or moderate alcohol drinking (preferably red wine with a meal) is also advised. Fish, eggs, and poultry can be consumed several times per week. In contrast, consumption of sweets and red meat should be significantly reduced (a few times per month). The details of the Mediterranean diet can vary depending on the region of the Mediterranean Basin; however, the general rule is to eat foods coming from this geographic area [123,124].

In contrast to the DASH diet, there are some data on the usefulness of Mediterranean diet in IBD. Marlow et al. demonstrated that even a short-term (six weeks) nutritional intervention is beneficial for patients with CD, decreasing the concentration of several pro-inflammatory markers with a trend to normalize the composition of intestinal microbiota. Transcriptomics analyses confirmed small changes in many genes, providing a cumulative anti-inflammatory effect of the diet [125]. In another study, Godny and colleagues showed that the Mediterranean diet is associated with decreased fecal calprotectin in patients after pouch surgery in UC, which is accompanied by an improvement in gut microbiota composition [126]. Moreover, Molendijk et al. demonstrated a beneficial effect of long-term nutritional intervention in IBD. In this study, six months of the Mediterranean diet improved the quality of life and reduced CRP levels. The level of improvement was associated with adherence to the rules of this type of diet [127].

The question remains, which hypothetical mechanisms could be related to the anti-inflammatory properties of the Mediterranean diet in IBD. As discussed above, this diet is characterized by a low intake of omega-6 PUFA, high intake of omega-3 PUFA, and dietary fiber, which seems to be important in the context of IBD. In line with that, the most recent epidemiological data indicate that a higher ratio of omega-6/omega-3 PUFA in the diet can be associated with an increased UC incidence [128]. Moreover, Hou et al. noted that a high intake of omega-6 PUFA, saturated fats, and meat is correlated with an increased risk of developing UC and CD [129]. It was also shown in a murine dextran sulfate sodium (DSS)-induced colitis model that omega-6/omega-3 PUFA ratio in the diet can influence the inflammatory processes in the gastrointestinal tract [130]. The authors observed that an α-linolenic acid (ALA)-enriched diet with a decreased uptake of linoleic acid (LA) resulted in less severe colitis in mice, with a markedly alleviated intestinal inflammation [130]. This was supported by Pearl et al. who showed the association between severity of intestinal inflammation and increased content of omega-6 PUFA in inflamed mucosa in UC patients [131]. Furthermore, Uchiyama et al. investigated the influence of a diet therapy involving the use of an "omega-3 PUFA food exchange table". The authors showed that omega-3 PUFA significantly increased the erythrocyte membrane omega-3/omega-6 PUFA ratio in IBD patients, what was associated with clinical remission of the disease [132]. Recently, another experimental study on the protective role of omega-3 PUFA has been published. Charpentier et al. showed that supplementation of omega-3 PUFA significantly decreased colon inducible nitric oxide synthase (iNOS) and cyclooxygenase-2 (COX-2) expression, as well as IL-6 and leukotriene B4 production in 2,4,6-trinitrobenzene sulfonic acid (TNBS)-induced colitis [133].

Dietary fiber is also believed to have a protective effect on the development of inflammation in the gastrointestinal tract. Moreover, the short-chain fatty acids, regarded as one of the major microbial metabolites of dietary fiber, have the potential to improve intestinal mucosal immunity and maintain homeostasis [134]. There are several experimental and clinical data supporting these hypotheses. Liu et al. showed in a murine DSS-induced colitis model that supplementation of β-glucans at a dose of 500 mg/kg per day reduced the severity of clinical activity of the disease. β-glucans-enriched diet resulted in a smaller weight loss, improvement in the number of bowel movements, and amelioration of the inflammatory response assessed microscopically. It has been also shown that β-glucans supplementation inhibited the expression of pro-inflammatory proteins, such as TNF-α, IL-1, IL-6 or NOS [135]. On the other hand, based on the data from the Nurses' Health Study, it was suggested in a prospective study that a long-term intake of dietary fiber was associated with lower risk of CD, but not UC [136]. A meta-analysis, performed by Liu and colleagues, indicated that the intake of dietary fiber was related to a decreased risk of developing IBD [137]. In a recent study by Andersen et al. an inverse association between the consumption of cereal fiber and CD in non-smokers was confirmed [138].

The only theoretical limitation of the DASH or Mediterranean diet in IBD is the high amount of whole grain cereal products, nuts, and seeds of leguminous plants which can stimulate intestinal peristalsis and increase the frequency of bowel movements. This is why it is advised to reduce the consumption of these particular foods during an IBD flare, whereas in patients in remission the individually tolerated amount of these products should be established.

The main rules of DASH and the Mediterranean diet are presented in Tables 1 and 2.

Table 1. The rules of Dietary Approaches to Stop Hypertension (DASH) diet [117].

The DASH Diet (Dietary Approaches to Stop Hypertension)			
Dietary Product	**The Frequency of Consumption**	**Indicated**	**Contraindicated**
Cereal products	6–8/day	whole grain	refined
Vegetables	4–5/day	all	-
Fruits	4–5/day	all	-
Protein	6 or less/day	fatty saltwater fish, lean meat, seeds of leguminous plants	fatty, red meat
Nuts and seeds	4–5/week	all	-
Fats	2–3/day	vegetable oils rich in unsaturated fatty acids	animal fat, coconut oil, palm oil
Dairy products	2–3/day	low-fat or fat-free	full-fat
Drinks	several times a day	unspecified	drinks containing simple carbohydrates
Other			
Sweets, confectionery products	5 or less/week	-	-
Sodium	Max. 2300 mg/day	-	-

Table 2. The rules of the Mediterranean diet [124].

	The Mediterranean Diet		
Dietary Product	The Frequency of Consumption	Indicated	Contraindicated
Cereal products	several times a day	whole grains	refined
Vegetables	several times a day	all	-
Fruits	several times a day	all	-
Fish and seafood	several times a week (at least 2 times a week)	fatty saltwater fish (tuna, salmon, sardines, herring) and mussels, oysters and shrimps	-
Poultry and eggs	several times a week	all	-
Red meat	a few times a month	-	-
Nuts and seeds of leguminous plants	several times a day	all	-
Fats	several times a day	olive oil	animal fats such as lard, butter, fatty beef, fatty pork, poultry with skin
Dairy products	several times a day	all	-
Drinks	several times a day	still water	sugary drinks
Sweets, confectionery products	few times a week	-	-
Red wine	every day; women max. 1, men max. 2 glasses/day	-	-

2. Conclusions

The ageing of the human population has become a big challenge for health care systems worldwide. The increasing proportion of elderly people is a result of significant improvements in medical care, successful prophylaxis of infectious diseases, and declining birth rates in developed countries. On the other hand, the number of elderly IBD patients is also increasing and we have to face the problem of managing this unique population. Since there are several important differences in the clinical characteristics of older IBD patients, appropriate nutritional intervention and counseling should become a crucial element of the therapy. Although there are no data on the definite therapeutic influence of any diet on the course of IBD, it seems to be reasonable, considering data presented in this paper, to actively promote a healthy diet among elderly patients with IBD with special emphasis on the DASH or Mediterranean-style diet. Patients with IBD aged >60 are also at increased risk of cardiovascular diseases, type 2 diabetes, and arterial hypertension. This is why these two similar types of nutrition can cover not only the dietary requirements characteristic of a chronic inflammatory condition, but also due to its anti-inflammatory properties, they can improve the metabolic abnormalities typical in older age. Of course, it seems rational to advocate these types of diets only in parallel with classical treatment of IBD and even regardless of subsequent gastrointestinal disorders or any other disease. Nevertheless, since application of the current, aggressive therapeutic approaches in a significant proportion of elderly IBD patients is limited, the use of the Mediterranean and DASH diets is reasonable, especially in this unique population.

Author Contributions: Conceptualization, P.E. and A.N.; formal analysis, P.E. and I.K.-K.; resources, P.E., A.N., K.S.-E., and E.B.; writing—original draft preparation, P.E. and A.N.; writing—review and editing, I.K.-K., K.S.-E., and E.B.; visualization, P.E. and. A.N.; supervision, P.E. and A.D.; project administration, P.E. and A.N.; funding acquisition, P.E. and. A.D.

References

1. Andersen, V.; Chan, S.; Luben, R.; Khaw, K.T.; Olsen, A.; Tjonneland, A.; Kaaks, R.; Grip, O.; Bergmann, M.M.; Boeing, H.; et al. Fiber intake and the development of inflammatory bowel disease: A European prospective multi-centre cohort study (EPIC-IBD). *J. Crohns Colitis* **2018**, *12*, 129–136. [CrossRef] [PubMed]
2. Nimmons, D.; Limdi, J.K. Elderly patients and inflammatory bowel disease. *World J. Gastrointest. Pharmacol. Ther.* **2016**, *7*, 51–65. [CrossRef] [PubMed]
3. Cosnes, J.; Gower-Rousseau, C.; Seksik, P.; Cortot, A. Epidemiology and natural history of inflammatory bowel diseases. *Gastroenterology* **2011**, *140*, 1785–1794. [CrossRef] [PubMed]
4. Molinié, F.; Gower-Rousseau, C.; Yzet, T.; Merle, V.; Grandbastien, B.; Marti, R.; Lerebours, E.; Dupas, J.L.; Colombel, J.F.; Salomez, J.L.; et al. Opposite evolution in incidence of Crohn's disease and ulcerative colitis in Northern France (1988–1999). *Gut* **2004**, *53*, 843–848. [CrossRef] [PubMed]
5. Molodecky, N.A.; Soon, I.S.; Rabi, D.M.; Ghali, W.A.; Ferris, M.; Chernoff, G.; Benchimol, E.; Panaccione, R.; Ghosh, S.; Barkema, H.W.; et al. Increasing incidence and prevalence of the inflammatory bowel diseases with time, based on systematic review. *Gastroenterology* **2012**, *142*, 46–54. [CrossRef] [PubMed]
6. Sturm, A.; Maaser, C.; Mendall, M.; Karagiannis, D.; Karatzas, P.; Ipenburg, N.; Sebastian, S.; Rizzello, F.; Limdi, J.; Katsanos, K.; et al. European Crohn's and colitis organisation topical review on IBD in the elderly. *J. Crohns Colitis* **2017**, *11*, 263–273. [CrossRef] [PubMed]
7. Katz, S.; Pardi, D.S. Inflammatory bowel disease of the elderly: Frequently asked questions (FAQs). *Am. J. Gastroenterol.* **2011**, *106*, 1889–1897. [CrossRef]
8. Taleban, S.; Colombel, J.F.; Mohler, M.J.; Fain, M.J. Inflammatory bowel disease and the elderly: A review. *J. Crohns Colitis* **2015**, *9*, 507–515. [CrossRef] [PubMed]
9. Del Val, J.H. Old-age inflammatory bowel disease onset: A different problem? *World J. Gastroenterol.* **2011**, *17*, 2734–2739. [CrossRef] [PubMed]
10. Hussain, S.W.; Pardi, D.S. Inflammatory bowel disease in the elderly. *Drugs Aging* **2010**, *27*, 617–624. [CrossRef]
11. Charpentier, C.; Salleron, J.; Savoye, G.; Fumery, M.; Merle, V.; Laberenne, J.E.; Vasseur, F.; Dupas, J.L.; Cortot, A.; Dauchet, L.; et al. Natural history of elderly-onset inflammatory bowel disease: A population based cohort study. *Gut* **2014**, *63*, 423–432. [CrossRef] [PubMed]
12. Arnott, I.; Rogler, G.; Halfvarson, J. The Management of Inflammatory Bowel Disease in Elderly: Current Evidence and Future Perspectives. *Inflamm. Intest. Dis.* **2018**, *2*, 189–199. [CrossRef] [PubMed]
13. Kedia, S.; Limdi, J.K.; Ahuja, V. Management of inflammatory bowel disease in older persons: Evolving paradigms. *Intest. Res.* **2018**, *16*, 194–208. [CrossRef]
14. Lobatón, T.; Ferrante, M.; Rutgeerts, P.; Ballet, V.; Van Assche, G.; Vermeire, S. Efficacy and safety of anti-TNF therapy in elderly patients with inflammatory bowel disease. *Aliment. Pharmacol. Ther.* **2015**, *42*, 441–445. [CrossRef] [PubMed]
15. Ha, C.Y.; Katz, S. Clinical implications of ageing for the management of IBD. *Nat. Rev. Gastroenterol. Hepatol.* **2014**, *11*, 128–138. [CrossRef] [PubMed]
16. Wagtmans, M.J.; Verspaget, H.W.; Lamers, C.B.; van Hogezand, R.A. Crohn's disease in the elderly: A comparison with young adults. *J. Clin. Gastroenterol.* **1998**, *27*, 129–133. [CrossRef] [PubMed]
17. Cohen, S.H.; Gerding, D.N.; Johnson, S.; Kelly, C.P.; Loo, V.G.; McDonald, L.C.; Pepin, J.; Wilcox, M.H. Clinical practice guidelines for Clostridium difficile infection in adults: 2010 update by the Society for Healthcare Epidemiology of America (SHEA) and the Infectious Diseases Society of America (IDSA). *Infect. Control Hosp. Epidemiol.* **2010**, *31*, 431–455. [CrossRef]
18. Harper, P.C.; McAuliffe, T.L.; Beeken, W.L. Crohn's disease in the elderly. A statistical comparison with younger patients matched for sex and duration of disease. *Arch Intern. Med.* **1986**, *146*, 753–755. [CrossRef]
19. Greth, J.; Török, H.P.; Koenig, A.; Folwaczny, C. Comparison of inflammatory bowel disease at younger and older age. *Eur. J. Med. Res.* **2004**, *9*, 552–554.
20. Polito, J.M.; Childs, B.; Mellits, E.D.; Tokayer, A.Z.; Harris, M.L.; Bayless, T.M. Crohn's disease: Influence of age at diagnosis on site and clinical type of disease. *Gastroenterology* **1996**, *111*, 580–586. [CrossRef]
21. Silverberg, M.S.; Satsangi, J.; Ahmad, T.; Arnott, I.D.; Bernstein, C.N.; Brant, S.; Caprilli, R.; Colombel, J.F.; Gasche, C.; Geboes, K.; et al. Toward an integrated clinical, molecular and serological classification

of inflammatory bowel disease: Report of a Working Party of the 2005 Montreal World Congress of Gastroenterology. *Can. J. Gastroenterol. Hepatol.* **2005**, *19*, 5–36. [CrossRef] [PubMed]

22. Han, S.W.; McColl, E.; Barton, J.R.; James, P.; Steen, I.N.; Welfare, M.R. Predictors of quality of life in ulcerative colitis: The importance of symptoms and illness representations. *Inflamm. Bowel Dis.* **2005**, *11*, 24–34. [CrossRef] [PubMed]

23. Lakatos, P.L.; David, G.; Pandur, T.; Erdelyi, Z.; Mester, G.; Balogh, M.; Szipocs, I.; Molnar, C.; Komaromi, E.; Kiss, L.S.; et al. IBD in the elderly population: Results from a population-based study in Western Hungary, 1977–2008. *J. Crohns Colitis* **2011**, *5*, 5–13. [CrossRef] [PubMed]

24. Gower-Rousseau, C.; Vasseur, F.; Fumery, M.; Savoye, G.; Salleron, J.; Dauchet, L.; Turck, D.; Cortot, A.; Peyrin-Biroulet, L.; Colombel, J.F. Epidemiology of inflammatory bowel diseases: New insights from a French population-based registry (EPIMAD). *Dig. Liver Dis.* **2013**, *45*, 89–94. [CrossRef] [PubMed]

25. Ananthakrishnan, A.N.; Binion, D.G. Treatment of ulcerative colitis in the elderly. *Dig. Dis.* **2009**, *27*, 327–334. [CrossRef]

26. Loftus, E.V. A matter of life or death: Mortality in Crohn's disease. *Inflamm. Bowel Dis.* **2002**, *8*, 428–429. [CrossRef]

27. Wolters, F.L.; Russel, M.G.; Sijbrandij, J.; Ambergen, T.; Odes, S.; Riis, L.; Langholz, E.; Politi, P.; Qasim, A.; Koutroubakis, I.; et al. Phenotype at diagnosis predicts recurrence rates in Crohn's disease. *Gut* **2006**, *55*, 1124–1130. [CrossRef]

28. Foxworthy, D.M.; Wilson, J.A. Crohn's disease in the elderly. Prolonged delay in diagnosis. *J. Am. Geriatr. Soc.* **1985**, *33*, 492–495. [CrossRef]

29. Farrokhyar, F.; Swarbrick, E.T.; Irvine, E.J. A critical review of epidemiological studies in inflammatory bowel disease. *Scand. J. Gastroenterol.* **2001**, *36*, 2–15. [CrossRef]

30. Stepaniuk, P.; Bernstein, C.N.; Targownik, L.E.; Singh, H. Characterization of inflammatory bowel disease in elderly patients: A review of epidemiology, current practices and outcomes of current management strategies. *Can. J. Gastroenterol. Hepatol.* **2015**, *29*, 327–333. [CrossRef]

31. MacLaughlin, E.J.; Raehl, C.L.; Treadway, A.K.; Sterling, T.L.; Zoller, D.P.; Bond, C.A. Assessing medication adherence in the elderly: Which tools to use in clinical practice? *Drugs Aging* **2005**, *22*, 231–255. [CrossRef] [PubMed]

32. Hanauer, S.B. Clinical perspectives in Crohn's disease. Turning traditional treatment strategies on their heads: Current evidence for "step-up" versus "top-down". *Rev. Gastroenterol. Disord.* **2007**, *7*, 17–22.

33. Prelipcean, C.C.; Mihai, C.; Gogalniceanu, P.; Mihai, B. What is the impact of age on adult patients with inflammatory bowel disease? *Clujul. Med.* **2013**, *86*, 3–9. [PubMed]

34. Greenwald, D.A.; Brandt, L.J. Inflammatory Bowel Disease After Age 60. *Curr. Treat Options Gastroenterol.* **2003**, *6*, 213–225. [CrossRef] [PubMed]

35. De Boer, N.K.; Wong, D.R.; Jharap, B.; de Graaf, P.; Hooymans, P.M.; Mulder, C.J.; Rijmen, F.; Engels, L.G.; van Bodegraven, A.A. Dose-dependent influence of 5-aminosalicylates on thiopurine metabolism. *Am. J. Gastroenterol.* **2007**, *102*, 2747–2753. [CrossRef] [PubMed]

36. Gisbert, J.P.; Gomollón, F. Thiopurine-induced myelotoxicity in patients with inflammatory bowel disease: A review. *Am. J. Gastroenterol.* **2008**, *103*, 1783–1800. [CrossRef]

37. Wells, P.S.; Holbrook, A.M.; Crowther, N.R.; Hirsh, J. Interactions of warfarin with drugs and food. *Ann. Intern. Med.* **1994**, *121*, 676–683. [CrossRef] [PubMed]

38. Thomas, T.P. The complications of systemic corticosteroid therapy in the elderly. A retrospective study. *Gerontology* **1984**, *30*, 60–65. [CrossRef] [PubMed]

39. Akerkar, G.A.; Peppercorn, M.A.; Hamel, M.B.; Parker, R.A. Corticosteroid-associated complications in elderly Crohn's disease patients. *Am. J. Gastroenterol.* **1997**, *92*, 461–464.

40. Stallmach, A.; Hagel, S.; Gharbi, A.; Settmacher, U.; Hartmann, M.; Schmidt, C.; Bruns, T. Medical and surgical therapy of inflammatory bowel disease in the elderly-prospects and complications. *J. Crohns Colitis* **2011**, *5*, 177–188. [CrossRef]

41. Frey, B.M.; Frey, F.J. Clinical pharmacokinetics of prednisone and prednisolone. *Clin. Pharmacokinet.* **1990**, *19*, 126–146. [CrossRef] [PubMed]

42. Govani, S.M.; Higgins, P.D. Combination of thiopurines and allopurinol: Adverse events and clinical benefit in IBD. *J. Crohns Colitis* **2010**, *4*, 444–449. [CrossRef] [PubMed]

43. Present, D.H.; Meltzer, S.J.; Krumholz, M.P.; Wolke, A.; Korelitz, B.I. 6-Mercaptopurine in the management of inflammatory bowel disease: Short- and long-term toxicity. *Ann. Intern. Med.* **1989**, *111*, 641–649. [CrossRef] [PubMed]

44. Black, A.J.; McLeod, H.L.; Capell, H.A.; Powrie, R.H.; Matowe, L.K.; Pritchard, S.C.; Collie-Duguid, E.S.; Reid, D.M. Thiopurine methyltransferase genotype predicts therapy-limiting severe toxicity from azathioprine. *Ann. Intern. Med.* **1998**, *129*, 716–718. [CrossRef]

45. Cuffari, C.; Dassopoulos, T.; Turnbough, L.; Thompson, R.E.; Bayless, T.M. Thiopurine methyltransferase activity influences clinical response to azathioprine in inflammatory bowel disease. *Clin. Gastroenterol. Hepatol.* **2004**, *2*, 410–417. [CrossRef]

46. Siegel, C.A.; Marden, S.M.; Persing, S.M.; Larson, R.J.; Sands, B.E. Risk of lymphoma associated with combination anti-tumor necrosis factor and immunomodulator therapy for the treatment of Crohn's disease: A meta-analysis. *Clin. Gastroenterol. Hepatol.* **2009**, *7*, 874–881. [CrossRef]

47. Khan, N.; Abbas, A.M.; Lichtenstein, G.R.; Loftus, E.V.; Bazzano, L.A. Risk of lymphoma in patients with ulcerative colitis treated with thiopurines: A nationwide retrospective cohort study. *Gastroenterology* **2013**, *145*, 1007–1015. [CrossRef]

48. Beaugerie, L.; Brousse, N.; Bouvier, A.M.; Colombel, J.F.; Lémann, M.; Cosnes, J.; Hébuterne, X.; Cortot, A.; Bouhnik, Y.; Gendre, J.P.; et al. Lymphoproliferative disorders in patients receiving thiopurines for inflammatory bowel disease: A prospective observational cohort study. *Lancet* **2009**, *374*, 1617–1625. [CrossRef]

49. Cottone, M.; Kohn, A.; Daperno, M.; Armuzzi, A.; Guidi, L.; D'Inca, R.; Bossa, F.; Angelucci, E.; Biancone, L.; Gionchetti, P.; et al. Advanced age is an independent risk factor for severe infections and mortality in patients given anti-tumor necrosis factor therapy for inflammatory bowel disease. *Clin. Gastroenterol. Hepatol.* **2011**, *9*, 30–35. [CrossRef]

50. Colombel, J.F.; Loftus, E.V.; Tremaine, W.J.; Egan, L.J.; Harmsen, W.S.; Schleck, C.D.; Zinsmeister, A.R.; Sandborn, W.J. The safety profile of infliximab in patients with Crohn's disease: The Mayo clinic experience in 500 patients. *Gastroenterology* **2004**, *126*, 19–31. [CrossRef]

51. Fidder, H.; Schnitzler, F.; Ferrante, M.; Noman, M.; Katsanos, K.; Segaert, S.; Henckaerts, L.; Van Assche, G.; Vermeire, S.; Rutgeerts, P. Long-term safety of infliximab for the treatment of inflammatory bowel disease: A single-centre cohort study. *Gut* **2009**, *58*, 501–508. [CrossRef] [PubMed]

52. O'Meara, S.; Nanda, K.S.; Moss, A.C. Antibodies to infliximab and risk of infusion reactions in patients with inflammatory bowel disease: A systematic review and meta-analysis. *Inflamm. Bowel Dis.* **2014**, *20*, 1–6. [CrossRef] [PubMed]

53. Denadai, R.; Teixeira, F.V.; Saad-Hossne, R. Management of psoriatic lesions associated with anti-TNF therapy in patients with IBD. *Nat. Rev. Gastroenterol. Hepatol.* **2012**, *9*, 744. [CrossRef] [PubMed]

54. Singh, J.A.; Wells, G.A.; Christensen, R.; Tanjong Ghogomu, E.; Maxwell, L.; Macdonald, J.K.; Filippini, G.; Skoetz, N.; Francis, D.; Lopes, L.C.; et al. Adverse effects of biologics: A network meta-analysis and Cochrane overview. *Cochrane Database Syst. Rev.* **2011**, *2*, CD008794. [CrossRef] [PubMed]

55. Kaplan, G.G.; Hubbard, J.; Panaccione, R.; Shaheen, A.A.; Quan, H.; Nguyen, G.C.; Dixon, E.; Ghosh, S.; Myers, R.P. Risk of comorbidities on postoperative outcomes in patients with inflammatory bowel disease. *Arch Surg.* **2011**, *146*, 959–964. [CrossRef]

56. Bollegala, N.; Jackson, T.D.; Nguyen, G.C. Increased postoperative mortality and complications among elderly patients with inflammatory bowel diseases: An analysis of the national surgical quality improvement program cohort. *Clin. Gastroenterol. Hepatol.* **2016**, *14*, 1274–1281. [CrossRef] [PubMed]

57. Nguyen, G.C.; Bernstein, C.N.; Benchimol, E.I. Risk of Surgery and Mortality in Elderly-onset Inflammatory Bowel Disease: A Population-based Cohort Study. *Inflamm. Bowel Dis.* **2017**, *23*, 218–223. [CrossRef]

58. Cintolo, M.; Costantino, G.; Pallio, S.; Fries, W. Mucosal healing in inflammatory bowel disease: Maintain or de-escaleta therapy. *World J. Gastrointest. Pathophysiol.* **2016**, *7*, 1–16. [CrossRef]

59. Vrabie, R.; Kane, S. Noninvasive markers of disease activity in inflammatory bowel disease. *Gastroenterol. Hepatol.* **2014**, *10*, 576–584.

60. Kucharzik, T.; Kannengiesser, K.; Petersen, F. The use of ultrasound in inflammatory bowel disease. *Ann. Gastroenterol.* **2017**, *30*, 135–144. [CrossRef]

61. De La Montana, J.; Miguez, M. Suitability of the short-form Mini Nutritional Assessment in free-living elderly people in the northwest of Spain. *J. Nutr. Health Aging* **2011**, *15*, 187–191. [CrossRef] [PubMed]

62. Guigoz, Y.; Vellas, B.; Garry, P.J. Mini Nutritional Assessment: A practical assessment tool for grading the nutritional state of elderly patients. *Facts Res. Gerontol.* **1994**, *2*, 15–59.

63. Kozakova, R.; Jarosova, D.; Zelenikova, R. Comparison of three screening tools for nutritional status assessment of the elderly in their homes. *Biomed. Pap. Med. Fac. Univ. Palacky Olomouc. Czech Repub.* **2012**, *156*, 371–376. [CrossRef] [PubMed]

64. Cederholm, T.; Barazzoni, R.; Austin, P.; Ballmer, P.; Biolo, G.; Bischoff, S.C.; Compher, C.; Correia, I.; Higashiguchi, T.; Kolst, M.; et al. ESPEN guidelines on definitions and terminology of clinical nutrition. *Clin. Nutr.* **2017**, *36*, 49–64. [CrossRef] [PubMed]

65. Fávaro-Moreira, N.C.; Krausch-Hofmann, S.; Matthys, C.; Vereecken, C.; Vanhauwaert, E.; Declercq, A.; Bekkering, G.E.; Duyck, J. Risk Factors for Malnutrition in Older Adults: A Systematic Review of the Literature Based on Longitudinal Data. *Adv. Nutr.* **2016**, *7*, 507–522. [CrossRef] [PubMed]

66. Burks, C.E.; Jones, C.W.; Braz, V.A.; Swor, R.A.; Richmond, N.L.; Hwang, K.S.; Hollowell, A.G.; Weaver, M.A.; Platts-Mills, T.F. Risk Factors for Malnutrition among Older Adults in the Emergency Department: A Multicenter Study. *J. Am. Geriatr. Soc.* **2017**, *65*, 1741–1747. [CrossRef] [PubMed]

67. Mangels, A.R. Malnutrition in Older Adults. *Am. J. Nurs.* **2018**, *118*, 34–41. [CrossRef] [PubMed]

68. Kossioni, A.E. The Association of Poor Oral Health Parameters with Malnutrition in Older Adults: A Review Considering the Potential Implications for Cognitive Impairment. *Nutrients* **2018**, *10*, 1709. [CrossRef]

69. Kazemi, S.; Savabi, G.; Khazaei, S.; Savabi, O.; Esmaillzadeh, A.; Hassanzadeh Keshteli, A.; Adibi, P. Association between food intake and oral health in elderly: SEPAHAN systematic review no. 8. *Dent. Res. J.* **2011**, *8*, 15–20.

70. Prell, T.; Perner, C. Disease Specific Aspects of Malnutrition in Neurogeriatric Patients. *Front Aging Neurosci.* **2018**, *10*, 80. [CrossRef]

71. Al-Rasheed, R.; Alrasheedi, R.; Johani, R.; Alrashidi, H.; Almaimany, B.; Alshalawi, B.; Kelantan, A.; Banjar, G.; Alzaher, A.; Alqadheb, A. Malnutrition in elderly and its relation to depression. *Int. J. Community Med. Public Health* **2018**, *5*, 2156–2160. [CrossRef]

72. Miranda, D.; Cardoso, R.; Gomes, R.; Guimarães, I.; de Abreu, D.; Godinho, C.; Pereira, P.; Domingos, J.; Pona, N.; Ferreira, J.J. Undernutrition in institutionalized elderly patients with neurological diseases: Comparison between different diagnostic criteria. *J. Nursing Home Res.* **2016**, *2*, 76–82.

73. Corish, C.A.; Bardon, L.A. Malnutrition in older adults: Screening and determinants. *Proc. Nutr. Soc.* **2018**, *3*, 1–8. [CrossRef] [PubMed]

74. Jain, M.; Khushboo, G. Physiological Determinants of Malnutrition in Elderly. *Nov. Tech. Nutri. Food Sci.* **2018**, *2*, 1–4. [CrossRef]

75. Artemissia-Phoebe, N. Appetite, Metabolism and Hormonal Regulation in Normal Ageing and Dementia. *Diseases* **2018**, *6*, 66.

76. Morley, J.E. Undernutrition in older adults. *Family Practice* **2012**, *29*, 89–93. [CrossRef] [PubMed]

77. Rizzi, M.; Mazzuoli, S.; Regano, N.; Inguaggiato, R.; Bianco, M.; Leandro, G.; Bugianesi, E.; Noè, D.; Orzes, N.; Pallini, P.; et al. Undernutrition, risk of malnutrition and obesity in gastroenterological patients: A multicenter study. *World J. Gastrointest. Oncol.* **2016**, *8*, 563–572. [CrossRef]

78. Roubenoff, R.; Heymsfield, S.B.; Kehayias, J.J.; Cannon, J.G.; Rosenberg, I.H. Standardization of nomenclature of body composition in weight loss. *Am. J. Clin. Nutr.* **1997**, *66*, 192–196. [CrossRef]

79. Roubenoff, R. Sarcopenia: Effects on Body Composition and Function. *J. Geront.* **2003**, *58*, 1012–1017. [CrossRef]

80. Roubenoff, R. The Pathophysiology of Wasting in the Elderly. *J. Nutr.* **1999**, *129*, 256–259. [CrossRef]

81. Roubenoff, R. Inflammatory and hormonal mediators of cachexia. *J. Nutr.* **1997**, *127*, 1014–1016. [CrossRef] [PubMed]

82. Roubenoff, R. Hormones, cytokines and body composition: Can lessons from illness be applied to aging? *J. Nutr.* **1993**, *123*, 469–473. [CrossRef] [PubMed]

83. Morley, J.E. Hormones and Sarcopenia. *Curr. Pharm. Des.* **2017**, *23*, 4484–4492. [CrossRef] [PubMed]

84. Myung, J.S.; Yun Kyung, J.; In Joo, K. Testosterone and Sarcopenia. *World J. Mens Health* **2018**, *36*, 192–198.

85. Scaldaferri, F.; Pizzoferrato, M.; Lopetuso, L.; Musca, T.; Ingravalle, F.; Sicignano, L.; Mentella, M.; Miggiano, G.; Mele, M.; Gaetani, E.; et al. Nutrition and IBD: Malnutrition and/or sarcopenia? A practical guide. *Gastroenterol. Res. Pract.* **2017**, 8646495.

86. Bryant, R.; Trott, M.; Bartholomeusz, F.; Andrews, J.M. Systematic review: Body composition in adults with inflammatory bowel disease. *Aliment. Pharmacol. Ther.* **2013**, *38*, 213–225. [PubMed]

87. Lucendo, A.; De Rezende, L. Importance of nutrition in inflammatory bowel disease. *World J. Gastroenterol.* **2009**, *15*, 2081–2088.

88. Hwang, C.; Ross, V.; Mahadevan, U. Micronutrient deficiencies in inflammatory bowel disease. *Inflamm. Bowel Dis.* **2012**, *18*, 1961–1981. [CrossRef]

89. Chen, X.; Maguire, B.; Brodaty, H.; O'Leary, F. Dietary Patterns and Cognitive Health in Older Adults: A Systematic Review. *J. Alzheimers Dis.* **2019**, *67*, 583–619. [CrossRef]

90. Bauer, J.; Biolo, G.; Cederholm, T.; Cesari, M.; Cruz-Jentoft, A.J.; Morley, J.E.; Phillips, S.; Sieber, C.; Stehle, P.; Teta, D.; et al. Evidence-based recommendations for optimal dietary protein intake in older people: A position paper from the PROT-AGE Study Group. *J. Am. Med. Dir. Assoc.* **2013**, *14*, 542–559. [CrossRef]

91. Pludowski, P.; Holick, M.F.; Grant, W.B.; Konstantynowicz, J.; Mascarenhas, M.; Hag, A.; Povoroznyuk, V.; Balatska, N.; Barbosa, A.P.; Karonova, T.; et al. Vitamin D supplementation guidelines. *J. Steroid. Biochem. Mol. Biol.* **2018**, *175*, 125–135. [CrossRef] [PubMed]

92. EFSA Panel on Dietetic Products, Nutrition, and Allergies (NDA), Scientific Opinion on Dietary reference values for water. *EFSA J.* **2010**, *8*, 1459.

93. Manz, F. Hydration and disease. *J. Am. Coll. Nutr.* **2007**, *26*, 535–541. [CrossRef]

94. Stover, J.P. Vitamin B12 and older adults. *Curr. Opin. Clin. Nutr. Metab. Care* **2010**, *13*, 24–27. [CrossRef] [PubMed]

95. Hughes, C.F.; Ward, W.; Hoey, L.; McNulty, H. Vitamin B12 and ageing: Current issues and interaction with folate. *Ann. Clin. Biochem.* **2013**, *50*, 315–329. [CrossRef] [PubMed]

96. Owczarek, D.; Rodacki, T.; Domagala-Rodacka, R.; Cibor, D.; Mach, T. Diet and nutritional factors in inflammatory bowel diseases. *World J. Gastroenterol.* **2016**, *22*, 895–905. [CrossRef]

97. Van Gossum, A.; Cabre, E. ESPEN Guidelines on Parenetral Nutrition: Gastroenterology. *Clin. Nutr.* **2009**, *28*, 415–427. [CrossRef]

98. Sasaki, M.; Johtatsu, T. Energy metabolism in Japanese Patients with Crohn's disease. *J. Clin. Biochem. Nutr.* **2010**, *46*, 68–72. [CrossRef]

99. Kłęk, S.; Jankowski, M.; Kruszewski, W.J.; Fijuth, J.; Kapała, A.; Kabata, P.; Wysocki, P.; Krzakowski, M.; Rutkowski, P. Clinical nutrition in oncology: Polish recommendations. *Oncol. Clin. Pract.* **2015**, *11*, 172–188.

100. Claesson, M.J.; Jeffery, I.B.; Conde, S.; Power, S.E.; O'Connor, E.M.; Cusack, S.; Harris, H.M.B.; Coakley, M.; Lakshminarayanan, B.; O'Sullivan, O.; et al. Gut microbiota composition correlates with diet and health in the elderly. *Nature* **2012**, *488*, 178–184. [CrossRef]

101. Brussow, H. Microbiota and healthy ageing: Observational and nutritional intervantion studies. *Microb. Biotechnol.* **2013**, *6*, 326–334. [CrossRef] [PubMed]

102. Lee, D.; Albenberg, L.; Compher, C.; Baldassano, R.; Piccoli, D.; Lewis, J.D.; Wu, G.D. Diet in the Pathogenesis and Treatment of Inflammatory Bowel Diseases. *Gastroenterology* **2015**, *148*, 1087–1106. [CrossRef] [PubMed]

103. Wędrychowicz, A.; Zając, A.; Tomasik, P. Advances in nutritional therapy in inflammatory bowel diseases: Review. *World J. Gastroenterol.* **2016**, *21*, 1045–1066. [CrossRef] [PubMed]

104. Knight-Sepulveda, K.; Kais, S.; Santaolalla, R.; Abreu, M.T. Diet and Inflammatory Bowel Disease. *Gastroenterol. Hepatol.* **2015**, *11*, 511–520.

105. Sanches Machado d'Almeida, K.; Ronchi Spillere, S.; Zuchinali, P.; Corrêa Souza, G. Mediterranean Diet and Other Dietary Patterns in Primary Prevention of Heart Failure and Changes in Cardiac Function Markers: A Systematic Review. *Nutrients* **2018**, *10*, 58. [CrossRef]

106. Casas, R.; Sacanella, E.; Estruch, R. The Immune Protective Effect of the Mediterranean Diet against Chronic Low-grade Inflammatory Diseases. *Endocr. Metab. Immune Disord. Drug Targets* **2016**, *14*, 245–254. [CrossRef]

107. Bischoff, S.C.; Barbara, G.; Buurman, W.; Ockhuizen, T.; Schulzke, J.D.; Serino, M.; Tilg, H.; Watson, A.; Wells, J.M. Intestinal permeability–a new target for disease prevention and therapy. *BMC Gastroenterol.* **2014**, *14*, 189. [CrossRef]

108. Harper, A.; Naghibi, M.M.; Garcha, D. The Role of Bacteria, Probiotics and Diet in Irritable Bowel Syndrome. *Foods* **2018**, *7*, 13. [CrossRef]

109. Shepherd, S.J.; Gibson, P.R. Fructose malabsorption and symptoms of irritable bowel syndrome: Guidelines for effective dietary management. *J. Am. Diet. Assoc* **2006**, *106*, 1631–1639. [CrossRef]

110. Ong, D.K.; Mitchell, S.B.; Barrett, J.S.; Shepherd, S.; Irving, P.; Biesiekierski, J.; Smith, S.; Gibson, P.; Muir, J.G. Manipulation of dietary short chain carbohydrates alters the pattern of gas production and genesis of symptoms in irritable bowel syndrome. *J. Gastroenterol. Hepatol.* **2010**, *25*, 1366–1373. [CrossRef]

111. Biesiekierski, J.R.; Peters, S.L.; Newnham, E.D.; Rosella, O.; Muir, J.; Gibson, P. No effects of gluten in patients with self-reported non-celiac gluten sensitivity after dietary reduction of fermentable, poorly absorbed, short-chain carbohydrates. *Gastroenterology* **2013**, *145*, 320–328. [CrossRef] [PubMed]

112. Gibson, P.R.; Newnham, E.; Barrett, J.S.; Shepherd, S.J.; Muir, J.G. Review article: Fructose malabsorption and the bigger picture. *Aliment. Pharmacol. Ther.* **2007**, *25*, 349–363. [CrossRef] [PubMed]

113. Gibson, P.R.; Shepherd, S.J. Personal view: Food for thought—Western lifestyle and susceptibility to Crohn's disease. The FODMAP hypothesis. *Aliment. Pharmacol. Ther.* **2005**, *21*, 1399–1409. [CrossRef] [PubMed]

114. Gibson, P.R.; Shepherd, S.J. Evidence-based dietary management of functional gastrointestinal symptoms: The FODMAP approach. *J. Gastroenterol. Hepatol.* **2010**, *25*, 252–258. [CrossRef] [PubMed]

115. Gearry, R.B.; Irving, P.M.; Barrett, J.S.; Nathan, D.M.; Shepherd, S.J.; Gibson, P.R. Reduction of dietary poorly absorbed short-chain carbohydrates (FODMAPs) improves abdominal symptoms in patients with inflammatory bowel disease-a pilot study. *J. Crohns Colitis* **2009**, *3*, 8–14. [CrossRef] [PubMed]

116. Olendzki, B.C.; Silverstein, T.D.; Persuitte, G.M.; Ma, Y.; Baldwin, K.R.; Cave, D. An anti-inflammatory diet as treatment for inflammatory bowel disease: A case series report. *Nutr. J.* **2014**, *13*, 5. [CrossRef] [PubMed]

117. Lowering Your BloodPressure With DASH. Available online: www.nhlbi.nih.gov/files/docs/public/heart/new_dash.pdf (accessed on 10 December 2018).

118. Whelton, P.K.; Carey, R.M.; Aronow, W.S.; Casey, D.E.; Collins, K.J.; Dennison Himmelfarm, C.; DePalma, S.M.; Gidding, S.; Jamerson, K.A.; Jones, D.W.; et al. 2017 ACC/AHA/AAPA/ABC/ACPM/AGS/APhA/ASH/ASPC/NMA/PCNA Guideline for the Prevention, Detection, Evaluation, and Management of High Blood Pressure in Adults. *Hypertension* **2018**, *71*, 1269–1324. [CrossRef] [PubMed]

119. Chiavaroli, L.; Viguiliouk, E.; Nishi, S.K.; Blanco Mejia, S.; Rahelić, D.; Kahleová, H.; Salas-Salvadó, J.; Kendall, C.W.; Sievenpiper, J.L. DASH Dietary Pattern and Cardiometabolic Outcomes: An Umbrella Review of Systematic Reviews and Meta-Analyses. *Nutrients* **2019**, *11*, 338. [CrossRef] [PubMed]

120. Hummel, S.L.; Mitchell Seymour, E.; Brook, R.D.; Sheth, S.S.; Ghosh, E.; Zhu, S.; Weder, A.B.; Kovacs, S.J.; Kolias, T.J. Low-Sodium DASH Diet Improves Diastolic Function and Ventricular-Arterial Coupling in Hypertensive Heart Failure with Preserved Ejection Fraction. *Circ. Heart Fail.* **2013**, *6*, 1165–1171. [CrossRef] [PubMed]

121. Azadbakht, L.; Rashidi Pour Fard, N.; Karimi, M.; Hassan Baghaei, M.; Surkan, P.J.; Rahimi, M.; Esmaillzadeh, A.; Willett, W.C. Effects of the Dietary Approaches to Stop Hypertension (DASH) Eating Plan on Cardiovascular Risks Among Type 2 Diabetic Patients. *Diabetes Care* **2011**, *34*, 55–57. [CrossRef]

122. Nilsson, A.; Halvardsson, P.; Kadi, F. Adherence to DASH-Style Dietary Pattern Impacts on Adiponectin and Clustered Metabolic Risk in Older Women. *Nutrients* **2019**, *11*, 805. [CrossRef] [PubMed]

123. Sofi, F.; Abbate, R.; Gensini, G.F.; Casini, A. Accruing evidence on benefits of adherence to the Mediterranean diet on health: An updated systematic review and meta-analysis. *Am. J. Clin. Nutr.* **2010**, *92*, 1189–1196. [CrossRef] [PubMed]

124. Make Each Day Mediterranean. Available online: https://oldwayspt.org/system/files/atoms/files/NewMedKit_0.pdf (accessed on 6 December 2018).

125. Marlow, G.; Ellett, S.; Ferguson, I.R.; Zhu, S.; Karunasinghe, N.; Jesuthasan, A.C.; Yeo Han, D.; Fraser, A.G.; Ferguson, L.R. Transcriptomics to study the effect of a Mediterranean-inspired diet on inflammation in Crohn's disease patients. *Hum. Genomics* **2013**, *7*, 24. [CrossRef] [PubMed]

126. Godny, L.; Pfeffer-Gik, T.; Goren, I.; Tulchinsky, H.; Dotan, I. Adherence to Mediterranean diet is associated with decreased faecal calprotectin in patients after pouch surgery. In Proceedings of the 13th Congress of the European Crohn's and Colitis Organisation, Vienna, Austria, 14–17 February 2018.

127. Molendijk, I.; Martens, J.; van Lingen, E.; van der Marel, S.; van Veen-Lievaart, M.; van der Meulen, A.; Barnhoorn, M.; Ernst-Stegeman, A.; Maljaars, J. Towards a Food Pharmacy: Increased dietary quality reduces CRP and improves quality of life in IBD patients in remission. In Proceedings of the 14th Congress of the European Crohn's and Colitis Organisation, Copenhagen, Denmark, 6–9 March 2019.

128. Ananthakrishnan, A.N.; Khalili, H.; Konijeti, G.G.; Higuchi, L.M.; de Silva, P.; Fuchs, C.S.; Willett, W.C.; Richter, J.M.; Chan, A.T. Long-term intake of dietary fat and risk of ulcerative colitis and Crohn's disease. *Gut* **2014**, *63*, 776–784. [CrossRef] [PubMed]

129. Hou, J.K.; Abraham, B.; El-Serag, H. Dietary intake and risk of developing inflammatory bowel disease: A systematic review of the literature. *Am. J. Gastroenterol.* **2011**, *106*, 563–573. [CrossRef] [PubMed]

130. Tyagi, A.; Kumar, U.; Reddy, S.; Santosh, V.S.; Mohammed, S.B.; Ehtesham, N.Z.; Ibrahim, A. Attenuation of colonic inflammation by partial replacement of dietary linoleic acid with α-linolenic acid in a rat model of inflammatory bowel disease. *Br. J. Nutr.* **2012**, *108*, 1612–1622. [CrossRef] [PubMed]

131. Pearl, D.S.; Masoodi, M.; Eiden, M.; Brümmer, J.; Gullick, D.; McKeever, T.M.; Whittaker, M.A.; Nitch-Smith, H.; Brown, J.F.; Shute, J.K.; et al. Altered colonic mucosal availability of n-3 and n-6 polyunsaturated fatty acids in ulcerative colitis and the relationship to disease activity. *J. Crohns Colitis* **2014**, *8*, 70–79. [CrossRef]

132. Uchiyama, K.; Nakamura, M.; Odahara, S.; Koido, S.; Katahira, K.; Shiraishi, H.; Shiraishi, H.; Ohkusa, T.; Fujise, K.; Tajiri, H. N-3 polyunsaturated fatty acid diet therapy for patients with inflammatory bowel disease. *Inflamm. Bowel Dis.* **2010**, *16*, 1696–1707. [CrossRef]

133. Charpentier, C.; Chan, R.; Salameh, E.; Mbodji, K.; Ueno, A.; Guérin, C.; Ghosh, S.; Savoye, G.; Marion-Letellier, R. Dietary n-3 PUFA may attenuate experimental colitis. *Mediators Inflamm.* **2018**, 8430614. [CrossRef]

134. Han, M.; Wang, C.; Liu, P.; Li, D.; Li, Y.; Ma, X. Dietary Fiber Gap and Host Gut Microbiota. *Protein Pept. Lett.* **2017**, *24*, 388–396. [CrossRef]

135. Liu, B.; Lin, Q.; Yang, T.; Zeng, L.; Shi, L.; Chen, Y.; Luo, F. Oat β-glucan ameliorates dextran sulfate sodium (DSS)—Induced ulcerative colitis in mice. *Food Funct.* **2015**, *6*, 3454–3463. [CrossRef] [PubMed]

136. Ananthakrishnan, A.N.; Khalili, H.; Konijeti, G.G.; Higuchi, L.M.; de Silva, P.; Korzenik, J.R.; Fuchs, C.S.; Willett, W.C.; Richter, J.M.; Chan, A.T. A prospective study of long-term intake of dietary fiber and risk of Crohn's disease and ulcerative colitis. *Gastroenterology* **2013**, *145*, 970–977. [CrossRef] [PubMed]

137. Liu, X.; Wu, Y.; Li, F.; Zhang, D. Dietary fiber intake reduces risk of inflammatory bowel disease: Result from a meta-analysis. *Nutr. Res.* **2015**, *35*, 753–758. [CrossRef] [PubMed]

138. Juneja, M.; Baidoo, L.; Marc, B.; Schwartz, A.B.; Regueiro, M.; Dunn, M.; Binion, D.G. Geriatric inflammatory bowel disease: Phenotypic presentation, treatment patterns, nutritional status, outcomes, and comorbidity. *Dig. Dis. Sci.* **2012**, *57*, 2408–2415. [CrossRef] [PubMed]

13

Dietary Factors in Sulfur Metabolism and Pathogenesis of Ulcerative Colitis

Levi M. Teigen [1], Zhuo Geng [1], Michael J. Sadowsky [2], Byron P. Vaughn [1], Matthew J. Hamilton [2] and Alexander Khoruts [1,2,*]

[1] Division of Gastroenterology, Hepatology and Nutrition, Department of Medicine, University of Minnesota, Minneapolis, MN 55455, USA; teige027@umn.edu (L.M.T.); geng0053@umn.edu (Z.G.); bvaughn@umn.edu (B.P.V.)

[2] BioTechnology Insititute, Department of Soil, Water & Climate, and Department of Plant & Microbial Biology, University of Minnesota, St. Paul, MN 55108, USA; sadowsky@umn.edu (M.J.S.); hami0192@umn.edu (M.J.H.)

[*] Correspondence: khoru001@umn.edu

Abstract: The biogeography of inflammation in ulcerative colitis (UC) suggests a proximal to distal concentration gradient of a toxin. Hydrogen sulfide (H_2S) has long been considered one such toxin candidate, and dietary sulfur along with the abundance of sulfate reducing bacteria (SRB) were considered the primary determinants of H_2S production and clinical course of UC. The metabolic milieu in the lumen of the colon, however, is the result of a multitude of factors beyond dietary sulfur intake and SRB abundance. Here we present an updated formulation of the H_2S toxin hypothesis for UC pathogenesis, which strives to incorporate the interdependency of diet composition and the metabolic activity of the *entire* colon microbial community. Specifically, we suggest that the increasing severity of inflammation along the proximal-to-distal axis in UC is due to the dilution of beneficial factors, concentration of toxic factors, and changing detoxification capacity of the host, all of which are intimately linked to the nutrient flow from the diet.

Keywords: colon; high-sulfur foods; inflammation; metagenomics; microbiota; sulfur reducing

1. Introduction

Inflammatory bowel disease (IBD), which includes both Crohn's disease and ulcerative colitis (UC), is estimated to affect ~3 million individuals in the U.S. alone and continues to increase in incidence and prevalence worldwide [1]. Epidemiological evidence implicates industrialization, an increasingly western lifestyle, and associated changes in the microbiome with the development of IBD [2–4]. Diet is a major determinant of intestinal microbiota composition and activity [4,5]; therefore, it is a focus of intense interest for the mechanistic understanding of IBD pathogenesis.

The risk of IBD development increases in immigrant children from developing countries [6] and substantial changes in the intestinal microbiome, including loss of diversity and displacement of *Prevotella* by *Bacteroides* strains, which can be observed following immigration from developing countries to the United States [7]. These findings lend strong support to the notion that changes in the gut microbiota, driven in part by diet, contribute to the pathogenesis of UC. Although attempts to identify consistent, specific 'trigger' foods that predict the development of UC have been unsuccessful, there appears to be an overall trend for an association between an animal-based diet and UC development and activity, while a plant-based diet may be protective against UC [8]. Conceptually, the epidemiological data that demonstrates an increasing prevalence of IBD with westernization lend support to this notion as westernization generally results in a transition from a plant-based to an animal-based diet [9].

The unique distribution of gut inflammation seen with UC, typically greatest in the rectum and extending continuously towards the proximal colon, supports the notion that a directionally concentrated toxic substance(s) may be involved in its pathogenesis. While the nature of this compound remains unknown, several lines of evidence, both observational and mechanistic, implicate hydrogen sulfide (H_2S) as a possible candidate. The H_2S toxin hypothesis, however, is complicated by the fact that H_2S at low levels can be anti-inflammatory [10]. Consequently, the H_2S toxin hypothesis may be better viewed in a concentration dependent manner where each individual host likely has a varied tolerance to a specific concentration of H_2S above which intestinal damage occurs [11].

To date, attempts to examine the role of diet in the H_2S toxin hypothesis have focused primarily on the intake of sulfur-containing foods, without regard for the overall diet composition [12–15]. It is important to consider, however, that outside of a laboratory setting diets are far more complex than can be captured by the measurement of a single or a few nutrients. Therefore, rather than focus on the specific intake of a single dietary component (e.g., sulfur) in the pathogenesis of UC, an emphasis should be placed on overall diet patterns (e.g., animal- vs plant-based diet). This approach has been the focus of a number of recent reviews [16,17], and preliminary data suggest that these types of compositional dietary changes may be beneficial in IBD [18].

The high protein content of animal-based diets provides a greater amount of sulfur that becomes available to distal gut microbiota [19]. Additionally, the higher fat content of a typical animal-based diet may lead to an increase in taurine conjugation to bile acids and a corresponding increase in the quantity of sulfur in the colonic lumen through an endogenous source [20]. Importantly, an animal-based diet pattern will also tend to be low in fiber, which may drive a metabolic shift of microbiota away from carbohydrate and towards protein fermentation and increased mucin degradation (Figure 1) [21,22].

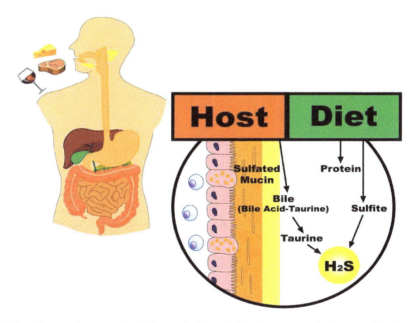

Figure 1. Contributions of an animal-based diet to hydrogen sulfide production. Legend: An animal-based diet results in a greater amount of dietary sulfur available to distal gut microbiota, both directly through sulfur-containing amino acids and indirectly through an increase in taurine conjugated bile acids and mucin degradation.

A complimentary hypothesis to explain the directional biogeography of UC may be the dilution of beneficial microbial metabolites along the luminal flow in the intestine. One such set of products is the short-chain fatty acids (SCFA), which are generated as a result of complex polysaccharide fermentation and play essential roles in colon physiology and mucosal homeostasis. Thus, butyrate (a SCFA), in addition to being a preferred energy source for the colonocytes [23,24], also promotes the presence of regulatory T cells in the colon [25,26], strengthens the gut barrier function [27], decreases epithelial oxygenation [28,29], and inhibits excessive colonic stem cell proliferation [30]. Furthermore, the chemical milieu established by microbial metabolites impact the overall microbial community structure through feedback loops affecting the relative abundances of different microbial trophic groups. Lower pH, driven by higher concentrations of SCFA, favors the growth of methanogens over that of sulfate reducing bacteria (SRB) [31], whereas H_2S may increase the oxygenation in colonocytes by inhibiting β-oxidation [32] and lead to the inhibition of obligate anaerobes that produce SCFA.

Therefore, the updated understanding of the H_2S toxin hypothesis for UC pathogenesis presented here strives to account for the activity of the *entire* microbial community rather than individual microbial subgroups working in isolation (e.g., *Desulfovibrio*) and appreciates the interdependency of diet composition on both the structure and function of the microbial community. In many respects, this is a synecological approach to study of the relationship between gut microbiota and the development of UC.

1.1. Toxic Effects of Hydrogen Sulfide

Although H_2S is generated by the host and is increasingly recognized to have a multitude of important beneficial physiologic functions [33], it becomes a potent toxin once its concentration exceeds the detoxifying capacity in the tissue. Specifically, higher amounts of H_2S generated in the intestine have the potential to disrupt the gut barrier function, which may be an early and critical initiating event in triggering the onset of UC and the perpetuation of its activity [34]. Traditionally, the H_2S toxin hypothesis has focused on the potential injurious effects of sulfide gas on the cellular metabolism of colonocytes, mainly the inhibition of cytochrome *c* oxidase activity in mitochondria, which induces oxidative stress in a fashion similar to cyanide [35]. Roediger and colleagues demonstrated that H_2S inhibits β-oxidation of butyrate by colonocytes, their preferred energy source [36]. Notably, UC mucosa has lower rates of butyrate uptake and oxidation relative to healthy controls [37]. In summary, oxidative stress and energy starvation caused by excessive H_2S concentrations may lead to colonocyte death, penetration of the epithelial barrier by the intestinal microbes and their direct interaction with the mucosal immune system. Resulting inflammation leads to further disruption of the gut barrier, decreased butyrate oxidation [37], and decreased mucosal sulfide detoxification and the subsequent perpetuation of inflammation [38].

In recent years, considerable attention has also been focused on mucus integrity in UC. The mucus layer of the colon consists of an outer (loose) and an inner (dense) layer, the latter being largely impenetrable to the resident intestinal microbiota [39,40]. The inner mucus layer in UC patients and in some animal models of IBD is more penetrable to bacteria relative to healthy controls [41]. Mucin glycoproteins form the major building blocks of mucus. The dominant mucin secreted by the goblet cells in the colon is MUC2, which contains cysteine-rich domains that mediate its multimerization through disulfide bonds. H_2S can directly break the sulfide bonds in the mucus and disrupt the MUC2 network leading to a loss of mucus viscosity and greater permeability [42].

1.2. Pre-Clinical Models

Some of the strongest support for the H_2S toxin hypothesis in the literature comes from pre-clinical models. The most commonly used animal model of IBD uses dextran sodium sulfate (DSS) to induce damage to the epithelium [43]. This allows for bacterial translocation from the lumen of the intestine resulting in inflammation [43]. This model is renowned for its simplicity and consistency in producing epithelial damage similar to that seen in IBD and also lends support to a role of sulfur in the pathogenesis of UC in humans.

In IL-10 knockout mice, a common murine model of IBD, a diet high in saturated fat increases the presence of taurine-conjugated bile acids, leading to an expansion of the sulphite-reducing pathobiont *Bilophila wadsworthia* and a greater severity of inflammation [20]. High fat diets also promote intestinal inflammation in rats as well as adenoma formation in the presence of a mutagen [44]. A high protein diet in a similar model increases SRB abundance and sulfide production and decreases the abundance of bacterial taxa associated with SCFA production and the amount of butyrate in stool [45]. Similarly, a high protein diet has been associated with post-weaning diarrhea in piglets [46]. Taken together, a high protein and saturated fat diet (characteristic of a western, animal-based diet) seems to result in an increased capacity for H_2S production, decreased capacity for butyrate production, and a potential to cause intestinal inflammation.

1.3. Clinical Observations

Mesalamine, a first-line agent in treatment of mild-to-moderate ulcerative colitis, inhibits sulfide production in a dose-dependent manner when added to a fecal slurry *in vitro* [47]. Furthermore, UC patients taking mesalamine have reduced fecal sulfide relative to patients who do not [47]. It is noteworthy that mesalamine and butyrate are both peroxisome proliferator activated receptor gamma (PPAR-γ) agonists [48,49]. Stimulation of PPAR-γ promotes β oxidation of fatty acids and epithelial hypoxia in the colon, which favors obligate anaerobes and lowers the abundance of Proteobacteria [50]. Interestingly, some antibiotics (e.g., aminoglycosides) which target Proteobacteria (including SRB) have short-term benefits in UC patients [13,51].

Few studies have attempted to link dietary interventions targeting the updated H_2S toxin hypothesis (i.e., transition from a western-style diet) with UC. The available handful of reports is limited to small case series or individual case studies (Table 1) [52–56]. These low dietary sulfur interventions generally emphasize transitions to a plant-based, semi-vegetarian diet. While all these experiences describe positive outcomes, conclusions are limited given the small patient numbers. The earliest case series conducted by Roediger et al. included only four patients and relied on symptom and histological criteria [52]. These patients sustained improvement in the activity of UC over 18 months of follow-up, while being maintained on the low sulfur diet. Chiba et al. reported a decreased relapse rate of UC relative to historical expectations among 60 patients instructed to follow a plant-based diet and followed for up to five years [56].

Table 1. Summary of reports detailing dietary interventions in the treatment of ulcerative colitis (UC) targeting the updated H_2S hypothesis.

Author Year	Location	Study Design	Intervention	Outcomes
Roediger 1998 [52]	Australia	Prospective pilot, Single-arm, 12 months duration ($n = 4$)	Reduction of sulfur amino acid intake for 12 months following an acute attack of UC	Histological improvement at 12 months. Decreased number of daily bowel movements and stool more formed. Two patients noted worsening symptoms when off diet.
Kashyap et al. 2013 [53]	United States	Case Report 26-year-old male with notable history of migration to Canada at the age of 10 from Southeast Asia and transition to western diet	Eliminated dairy, refined sugar, pork, beef, and fried food. Emphasized vegetables, fruit, chicken, and fish.	Majority of UC symptoms alleviated at 12 months. Prospectively, symptoms worsened when off diet and improved when returned to diet.
Chiba et al. 2016 [54]	Japan	Case Report 38-year-old male who began an Atkins-type diet that emphasized meat and animal fat 2-years prior to UC diagnosis	Transitioned to plant-based, semi-vegetarian diet	Achieved remission without medication. Qualitative comment that symptoms returned with worsening diet compliance over time.
Chiba et al. 2018 [55]	Japan	Case Report 36-year-old female diagnosed with UC at 21 weeks gestation who experienced notable diet changes with onset of emesis	Transitioned to a plant-based, lacto-ovo-vegetarian diet	Remission achieved and maintained through pregnancy

Table 1. *Cont.*

Author Year	Location	Study Design	Intervention	Outcomes
Chiba et al. 2018 [56]	Japan	Prospective, single-arm (n = 60)	Individuals with mild UC or UC in remission were provided with plant-based diet education	Relapse rates extending to follow-up at 5 years ≤19%, which the authors purport is better than those previously reported. Diet adherence decreased over time.

2. Sources of Sulfur in the Colon

2.1. Dietary Intake

While sulfur is ubiquitous in the food supply [57], and the fifth most abundant element on earth, its dietary linkage is not well characterized. For example, the USDA Food Composition Database does not include sulfur as a searchable nutrient. The sulfur content of food can be estimated using the sulfur-containing amino acids (methionine and cysteine) as surrogates, but this fails to account for sulfur-containing food modifiers or additives, such as sulfiting agents (e.g., potassium bisulfate, sodium bisulfate), sulfuric acid, or carrageenan [58]. Therefore, the most robust method of estimating dietary sulfur intake, including an estimate for inorganic sulfur, is through a 24–48 hour urine collection [59,60]. Because the primary dietary sources of sulfur are the sulfur-containing amino acids, in practice, quantification of sulfur-containing amino acid content has been used to create low- and high-sulfur diets [52,61].

Dietary input and small intestinal absorption are considered the main determinants of sulfur delivery to the colon [19]. The small intestine has an efficient but saturable dietary sulfate absorptive capacity of ~5–7 mmol/day [62]. Once dietary sulfate intake exceeds ~5–7 mmol/day the amount reaching the colon increases linearly with intake. Therefore, the amount of dietary sulfur that reaches the colon, particularly with increasing levels, can be generally assumed to parallel dietary intake. A number of additional factors, however, such as food preparation (e.g., cooked versus uncooked, cooking temperature and method, ground versus whole), meal consumption habits (e.g., chewing), and transit time have been shown to influence small intestinal absorption of sulfur-containing molecules and the total amount of sulfur reaching the colon [63–67].

2.2. Endogenous Sources

The main endogenous sources of sulfur are taurine-conjugated bile acids and mucin. Taurine is a sulfur-containing amino acid that is synthesized in the liver from methionine and cysteine. Diet can influence the rate of taurine conjugation and subsequent presence of taurine conjugated bile acids in the colon [68]. Although the majority of bile acids are re-absorbed in the distal small intestine into the enterohepatic circulation, a small percentage will spill into the colon [69]. Deconjugation of bile acids is an early step in secondary bile metabolism and is mediated by gut microbiota.

Intestinal mucins are glycoproteins that form a mucus barrier along the epithelial surface of the gastrointestinal tract. The primary intestinal mucin MUC2 contains cysteine amino acids as core components of its structure [39,70]. Glycosylation of mucin proteins makes up a substantial portion of their size and provides protection of the peptide backbone and the gel-forming capacity [70]. The glycosylation pattern of mucin varies along the intestinal tract with increasing sulfation moving distally through the small intestine and into the colon [71,72]. The colonic mucus barrier is predominately composed of sulfomucins with a trend toward slightly diminished sulfation moving distally (100% sulfation in the right colon and 86% in the rectum) [73]. The normal sulfation pattern is altered in UC and is associated with the concentration of SRB [73].

2.3. H_2S Measurement

The ideal experimental system to test the role of H_2S in UC pathogenesis would be able to measure its intraluminal concentration at different segments in the intestine. Unfortunately, technology to do that does not yet exist; therefore, studies that measure H_2S have focused on ex-vivo determination of its production from fecal samples. Fecal concentrations of hydrogen sulfide, however, are notoriously difficult due to the volatility of the gas, low intestinal concentrations, and instrumentation issues. Historically, the majority of work assessing stool sulfide concentrations in UC relied on colorimetric assays [62,74,75]. This method requires 'trapping' H_2S in fresh fecal samples for measurement and is associated with a number of inherent limitations [76,77]. Ion-exchange chromatography has also been used to measure H_2S in feces [78].

H_2S gas measurements, done using gas chromatography (GC) with sulfur chemiluminescence detection, are considered the reference standard for H_2S measurement [79]. These measures, however, cannot be obtained in real time and require *in vitro* incubation of the fecal sample. Only one study of UC has used GC as the measurement method and found that H_2S production was elevated substantially in UC compared to controls over a 24 hour period [80]. Although this method does not capture the H_2S content of fresh fecal samples, *in vitro* incubation may reflect *in vivo* H_2S production capacity of the microbiota, providing a *functional* measure of the microbiota metabolic capacity. Furthermore, this method allows for interrogation of the capacity of various dietary components to affect H_2S production (e.g., more H_2S production with cysteine or mucin vs sulfate) [80,81].

3. Colonic Microbiota and H_2S Production

3.1. Sulfate-Reducing Bacteria

Microbial production of H_2S is generally thought to be carried out by a limited number of bacteria and archael species. Sulfate-reducing bacteria (SRB) and the dissimilatory sulfur cycle, a form of anaerobic respiration that uses sulfate as the terminal electron acceptor, have been the primary focus of the H_2S toxin hypothesis in UC [14]. This pathway generates H_2S as an end-product of sulfate reduction. The pathway consists of three enzymatic steps involving ATP sulfurylase, adenosine 5'-phosphosulfate reductase, and sulfite reductase [82]. The final step in the pathway, sulfite reduction, is considered the rate limiting step. The genus *Desulfovibrio* is regarded as the most abundant SRB in humans [83]. Despite the focus on *Desulfovibrio* spp. as the primary producer of H_2S in the human gut, the number of microbial groups known to be capable of dissimilatory sulfate reduction continues to expand [82,84]. Many of these microbes can also reduce sulfite, dithionite, thiosulfate, elemental sulfur, and several thionates. The three sulfite reductase genes which catalyze the production of hydrogen sulfide are dissimilatory sulfite reductase (dsr), anaerobic sulfite reductase (asr), and cytochrome *c* sulfite reductase (*mccA*) [82].

In humans, the measurement of key enzymes involved in the sulfate reduction pathway is a more specific method for measurement of SRB than measurement of bacterial genera such as *Desulfovibrio* [85]. This approach identified a unique capacity of SRB genera in UC to generate H_2S and induce epithelial apoptosis, compared with healthy controls [74,86]. Recent multiomics data in colon cancer lends additional support to the importance of accounting for the functional capacity of microbes (e.g., via measurement of key enzymes) in addition to their community composition [87].

Despite their importance and usefulness, there is a dearth of literature that relies on the quantification of sulfite reductase genes to characterize SRBs in large UC cohorts. Use of this technique in healthy subjects demonstrated that an animal-based diet increases sulfite reductase gene expression [5]. Recent work by Jia et al. used a semi-nested PCR method to detect *dsrB* DNA, but failed to find a difference in abundance between healthy and UC cohorts ($n = 18$ and $n = 14$, respectively) [88]. The agar shake dilution method, which measures SRB growth over a specified incubation period, has often been employed to measure SRB in individuals with UC. Studies done using this methodology found elevated SRB abundance in individuals with UC compared to those without [47,74,89].

3.2. Cysteine Degraders

Although sulfate intake and quantity of SRB has been the primary focus of the H_2S toxin hypothesis, there is a growing appreciation for the contribution of protein intake to H_2S production. The efficiency of protein degradation is greatest in the distal colon and at neutral to alkaline pH, which suggests a possible relationship with the pathogenesis of UC [90]. A cross-over diet study conducted by Magee and colleagues demonstrated that dietary protein intake positively correlates with fecal sulfide concentrations in healthy individuals [78].

A recent *in vitro* study that profiled gas production from incubated fecal samples implicated cysteine specifically as a primary driver of H_2S production—conversely, the effect of sulfate was small [81]. Cysteine degradation to H_2S is catalyzed by enzymes with cysteine desulfhydrase activity. Although the enzymes with cysteine desulfhydrase activity are well characterized in humans [91], identifying enzymes with this activity in microorganisms has proven far more challenging. *Escherichia coli* possess several enzymes with cysteine desulfhydrase activity, including *O*-acetylserine sulfhydrylase-A, *O*-acetylserine sulfhydrylase-B, MalY, tryptophanase and cystathionine β-lyase [92]. Because cysteine likely makes a substantial contribution to H_2S production in the colonic lumen, there is a critical need to detail cysteine desulfhydrase activity within the colonic microbiome.

Prevention of excessive cysteine degradation to H_2S may underlie the possible protective role of appendectomy for appendicitis in UC [93]. Although the mechanism underlying the purported beneficial effect of appendectomy in UC has yet to be elucidated, one possibility is related to the potential role of the appendix as a reservoir for gut microbes [93]. Specifically, the appendix contains *Fusobacterium* spp. in its healthy state [94] and appendicitis is associated with an abundance of this bacteria [95]. *Fusobacterium* spp. contain a number of proteins necessary to metabolize L-cysteine to H_2S [96,97]. Therefore, removal of the appendix, and subsequently a source of H_2S production, may contribute to its possible therapeutic role in the prevention of UC.

3.3. Interplay Between Functional Microbial Groups

A number of physicochemical factors shape the composition and functional output of microbial communities, which need to be integrated in order to fully account for the inter-individual differences. One such factor is the availability of hydrogen (H_2), which is essential as a substrate for anaerobic respiration in the colonic lumen. The groups of bacteria that rely on and compete for H_2 for anaerobic respiration are acetogens, methanogens, and SRB (Figure 2) [98]. H_2 production results from microbial fermentation of carbohydrates in the lumen of the intestine. Therefore, the balance between H_2 production and consumption is often referred to as the 'hydrogen economy' [99]. An imbalance of H_2 consumption and production may result in a metabolic environment that consumes NADH for H_2 production at the expense of butyrate production [100]. In the context of the H_2S toxin hypothesis, it is important to consider possible imbalances in H_2 consumption (e.g., altered SRB concentration) or production (e.g., low dietary intake of fermentable carbohydrate) that could create a metabolic environment leading to UC—namely, excessive H_2S production [80], mucin degradation [22,41], and diminished butyrate production [5].

Other physical (e.g., intestinal transit time) and chemical factors (e.g., pH and oxygen tension), also contribute to the microbial community structure in the colon by favoring some groups of microbes over others. Accelerated colon motility is likely to benefit fast-growing microorganisms and disfavor slow growing microorganisms, and constipation is associated with higher carriage of methanogenic archaea and increased methane production [101]. Fermentation of digestible carbohydrate results in the production of SCFA and a drop in luminal pH in the colon relative to the small intestine [102–104]. Increased dietary fiber also results in faster intestinal transit [105]. Indeed, the colon pH is lowest proximally and increases distally, which is likely driven by the decreasing availability of digestible carbohydrate [102]. Mildly acidic pH, characteristic of the proximal colon, is inhibitory to the growth of SRB, but favors the growth of methanogens and some butyrate producers [30,106,107]. In contrast, sulfate reduction and H_2S production are optimal at an alkaline pH [108].

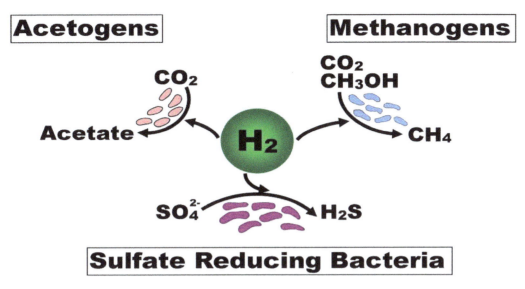

Figure 2. Bacterial competition for hydrogen for anaerobic respiration in the lumen of the intestine. Legend: Acetogens, methanogens, and sulfate reducing bacteria are the microbial groups that compete for H_2 in anaerobic respiration in the lumen of the colon. The availability of hydrogen can shape the composition and functional output of microbial communities.

3.4. H_2S Clearance

Clearance of hydrogen sulfide in the gut can be viewed as the final component of the H_2S toxin hypothesis. Due to its potential deleterious effects, H_2S is highly regulated in the cell. As H_2S is freely permeable across membranes, luminal concentration in the colon would be expected to correlate with intracellular concentrations [10]. Recent work in animal models demonstrates the relationship between luminal H_2S and intracellular regulation [109]. Although a small amount of H_2S present in the lumen of the colon is able to be cleared through flatus [110], the primary pathway for H_2S clearance is via intracellular sulfide oxidation. Interestingly, this pathway may be facilitated by cyanide, which has been proposed by Levitt and colleagues to explain the well-documented beneficial role of smoking in UC [111].

Colonic mucosa possesses a very efficient system for H_2S detoxification, and defects in these pathways are hypothesized to contribute to pathogenesis of colitis [111,112]. In earlier work, thiol methyltransferase and rhodanese were thought to have a major role in the detoxification of intestinal H_2S [113]. However, the investigators found conflicting results when using these enzymes to estimate the H_2S detoxification capacity in UC [38,114]. Around the time this work was being conducted, however, a more detailed and comprehensive understanding of H_2S detoxification was being developed that implicates sulfide quinone oxidoreductase (SQR) as the rate-limiting enzyme in sulfur oxidation [115,116].

The SQR enzyme is located within the inner mitochondrial membrane [117]. The reaction of H_2S with SQR results in oxidation of H_2S to a small-molecule persulfide and reduction of coenzyme Q (CoQ), which links H_2S oxidation with complex III of the electron transport chain [117]. The sulfur transfer from H_2S to a small molecule acceptor occurs via a cysteine intermediate within the SQR enzyme. Therefore, the availability of a small molecule acceptor is believed to be the rate-limiting step in the SQR reaction [118]. The antioxidant glutathione (GSH) is also believed to be the primary acceptor in a physiological setting, but sulfite has also been proposed as an alternative acceptor [118]. If GSH is utilized as the acceptor, the result is formation of glutathione persulfide (GSSH), which is then utilized by persulfide dioxygenase (ETHE1) or rhodanese to form sulfite or thiosulfate, respectively [117,119]. If sulfite is used as the acceptor, thiosulfate is produced, and rhodanese instead converts thiosulfate to GSSH, which is then converted to sulfite by ETHE1 [117,119]. In a steady state, GSH has been estimated to be favored ~5:1 over sulfite [118], but elevated intracellular sulfite concentrations or depletion of

GSH have been suggested to inhibit SQR [116,118,119]. Furthermore, although H$_2$S oxidation appears to be a robust pathway for intracellular control of H$_2$S levels, an excess of H$_2$S may paradoxically result in feedback inhibition of SQR from the electron transport chain as a result of its deleterious effect on cytochrome *c* oxidase activity [119].

The H$_2$S detoxification capacity and expression of enzymes involved in the H$_2$S detoxification pathway (SQR, ETHE1, and thiosulfate sulfurtransferase) have been shown to follow a general trend of highest in the proximal colon to lowest in the rectum [120]. This expression pattern lends further support to the H$_2$S toxin hypothesis as the progression of UC progresses from the lowest to the highest H$_2$S detoxification capacity and enzyme expression (Figure 3). In addition, GSH synthesis has been demonstrated to be impaired in IBD [121].

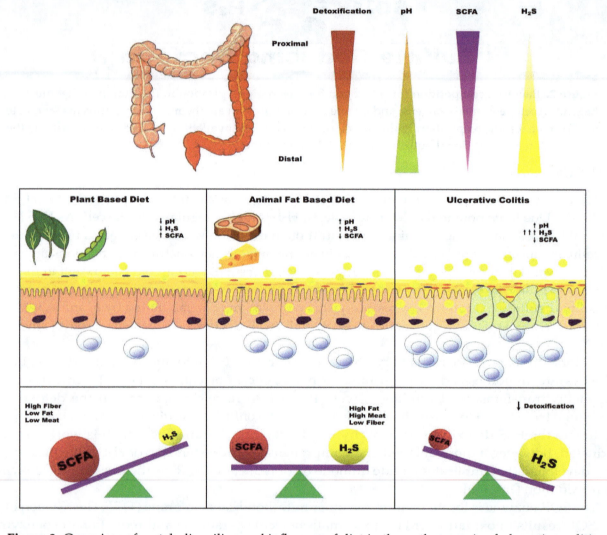

Figure 3. Overview of metabolic milieu and influence of diet in the pathogenesis of ulcerative colitis. Legend: The distribution of inflammation seen with ulcerative colitis is typically greatest in the rectum and extends continuously towards the proximal colon with varying severity. This pattern of inflammation parallels decreasing expression of the host H$_2$S detoxifying enzymes, rising pH, and decreasing concentrations of short-chain fatty acids (SCFA). A plant-based diet promotes greater production of SCFA, but not H$_2$S. SCFA production decreases in an animal-based diet, while H$_2$S production increases; however, there is a sufficient capacity for H$_2$S detoxification to prevent epithelial cell damage. Nonetheless, a decreased capacity for H$_2$S detoxification results in inflammation, which in turn further exacerbates the gradients of SCFA and H$_2$S concentrations along the proximal-to-distal colon axis.

4. Dietary Factors Influencing Colonic H$_2$S Production

4.1. Protein

Dietary protein has been shown to be a robust driver of *in vitro* and *in vivo* H$_2$S production [78,81]. Furthermore, the efficiency of protein degradation is inverse to that of carbohydrate fermentation (and SCFA production) and parallels that of UC pathogenesis (highest in the distal colon and decreasing proximally) [90]. Dietary protein is efficiently absorbed in the small intestine, but the amount reaching the colon is thought to be positively correlated with the amount consumed [90].

In both human and animal studies, a high protein diet results in fecal microbiota changes that increase H$_2$S production and decrease SCFA production [5,45]. Increases in SRB and *Bacteroidetes* sp. observed in UC also occur in a high protein diet [5,45,122] and observed decreases in specific butyrate producing species within a high protein diet (*F. Prausnitzii, Akkermansia, and Ruminococcus*) mirror those seen in UC [45,122–124].

Sulfur-containing amino acids are the primary source of dietary sulfur. Because of limited information on the sulfur content of food, outside of a metabolic unit, a 'high' or 'low' sulfur diet is defined according to cysteine and methionine concentration [52]. Therefore, a 'low sulfur' diet is actually a 'sulfur-containing amino acid-controlled diet', rather than a true 'sulfur-controlled diet' [52]. In general, a sulfur-containing amino acid-controlled diet results in a shift from a more traditional western diet (high in animal protein and fat, and low in fiber) to more of a plant-based diet (high in fiber, low in animal protein and fat). Recently published diet composition data from a small sulfur-containing amino acid diet intervention study ($n = 4$) conducted in the U.S. suggests that a typical U.S. diet is already high in sulfur-containing amino acids; a transition from a baseline diet to a 'high sulfur' diet results in minor diet composition changes, while a transition from a baseline to a 'low sulfur' diet results in a substantial transition from an animal-based to a plant-based diet (resulting in increased fiber, and decreased protein and fat intake) [61].

As described above, H$_2$S production capacity is often characterized by quantifying SRB, but cysteine desulfhydrase activity provides another route of H$_2$S production for the colonic microbiota that is often left unassessed. In fact, *in vitro* modeling using healthy human feces suggests that the contribution of cysteine to H$_2$S production is substantially more than that from sulfate [81].

4.2. Carbohydrate and Fiber

High carbohydrate availability in the colon, as noted above, promotes microbial groups able to utilize carbohydrate substrates, but also affects other aspects of microbial metabolism and especially impacts protein degradation. The addition of fermentable fiber to healthy human feces in an *in vitro* setting drastically reduces H$_2$S production from any source (e.g., cysteine, sulfate) [81]. Lower pH associated with microbial carbohydrate fermentation also leads to inhibition of dissimilatory aromatic amino acid metabolism [125]. Interestingly, stool pH is lower in vegan and vegetarian individuals relative to omnivores, consistent with greater abundance of carbohydrates in the proximal colon, faster colon transit, and higher delivery of SCFA to the distal colon [126]. This finding underscores the importance of overall diet composition when considering the relative proportions of different end-products of microbial metabolism.

4.3. Dietary Fat

Although there is little data supporting a direct role of dietary fat in the H$_2$S toxin hypothesis, animal fat was shown in a murine model to result in increased production of taurine-conjugated bile acids and a bloom of the sulfite-reducer *Bilophila wadsworthia* in the colonic microenvironment [127]. A high fat diet in mice is associated with lesser production of SCFA and greater production of H$_2$S, even when the protein content of high fat chow is lower relative to regular chow [128]. It is obvious that a relative contribution of macronutrients to H$_2$S production is difficult to isolate in a single comparison, given that an increase in one will correspondingly necessitate reduction in at least one other to maintain the same caloric intake.

4.4. Endogenous Sulfur

The most significant source of endogenous sulfur (both as sulfate and cysteine) is intestinal mucin. The mucous layer of the colon is composed of two layers [40], the microbiota is abundant in the outer loose mucous layer, while the inner dense mucous layer—largely devoid of bacteria—maintains a barrier between the colonic microbiota and colonocytes [39,40]. The composition of the colon microbiota has been shown to influence mucin secretion, breakdown, structure, and the glycosylation pattern [22,42,129–131]. Conversely, mucin glycosylation patterns have been shown to influence the colonic microbiota [132]. Therefore, the H_2S toxin hypothesis must consider these complex relationships between the mucin, microbiota, and diet. A characteristically high sulfur diet (high in animal protein and fat, and low in fiber) leads to nutrient deprivation for the microbiota and results in increased mucin desulfating sulfatase activity and mucin degradation [5,22,131,133]. This pattern is remarkably similar to that seen in UC [134–136]. The phenotypic changes resulting in increased mucin breakdown (e.g., low fiber) and H_2S production (e.g., high protein/sulfur intake) [5,22,45,78] may produce H_2S concentrations that overwhelm the detoxification capacity of colonocytes and contribute to H_2S toxicity.

4.5. Miscellaneous Dietary Factors

Finally, it is also important to consider factors that may correlate with sulfur content in the diet but are not related to sulfur metabolism. An increased intake of heme, present in its highest concentrations in red meat, can have cytotoxic effects on colonocytes [42]. Consumption of processed foods expose individuals to additives such as phosphates, nitrates, and emulsifiers, which have been shown to influence the composition of microbiota, mucin layer thickness, and intestinal inflammation [137–140]. Even specific cooking methods may alter the potential of diet to impact the intestinal microbiome and microbiota-host interactions. Both enzymatic and non-enzymatic mechanisms of protein modification may also influence intestinal H_2S production. Thus, glycation of dietary protein can to shift the colonic microbiota towards greater abundance of SRB and lesser production of butyrate [64]. Conversely, there are likely undiscovered or underappreciated components of a plant-based diet that may be protective in UC [141].

4.6. Inflammatory Factors

Onset of inflammation triggers a number of positive feedback loops that amplify the detrimental effects of H_2S on the homeostasis of colonic mucosa. Increased synthesis of inducible nitric oxide synthetase (iNOS) results in increased release of nitrate, which contributes to dysbiosis by encouraging the expansion of facultative anaerobic Proteobacteria [28]. Nitric oxide also impairs H_2S detoxification [109], thus lowering the threshold concentration where H_2S becomes toxic to epithelial cells. Epithelial injury results in crypt hyperplasia and loss of epithelial hypoxia, which are detrimental to butyrate-producing obligate anaerobes. In animal models and human studies, SCFA (and specifically butyrate) production is inhibited in the presence of inflammation [122–124,142]. Inflammation is also correlated with a lower BcoAT gene content of fecal microbiota, consistent with lower butyrate production capacity [143]. Collectively, these changes hasten the collapse of the gut barrier to intestinal microbes and inhibit regulatory immune circuits, such as regulatory T cells, which further augment the inflammatory response.

4.7. Interventions Targeting the Colon Microbiota

The underlying mechanisms that make up the H_2S toxin hypothesis are supported by changes produced with fermentable fiber supplementation in individuals with UC (increased butyrate production) [144] and findings from a recent fecal microbial transplantation (FMT) trial that demonstrated a correlation between sustained remission and increased butyrate production, while increased abundances of Bacteroidetes and Proteobacteria correlated with no response or relapse [122]. Notably, members of the Bacteroidetes phylum contain mucin desulfating sulfatase enzymes [122,145,146]. The FMT in UC findings have also been recently expanded upon by Wei et al. who demonstrated a role for fiber in maintaining the gut microbiota composition in individuals with UC following FMT [147].

The role of carbohydrate, and more specifically fermentable carbohydrate, intake within the H_2S toxin hypothesis may be its overall impact on protein degradation by colonic bacteria. These findings are supported by a diet study in healthy volunteers [148], where administration of metronidazole effectively reduced SRB counts, but fecal concentration of H_2S remained unchanged. In contrast, consumption of fermentable fiber (oligofructose) resulted in a decrease in fecal H_2S, concomitant increase in SCFA concentrations, but failure to influence SRB counts. The impact of fiber on microbial H_2S production is further supported by recent data demonstrating a decrease in SRB with a high brassica diet (sulfur-containing vegetables) [149]. Although brassica vegetables are technically considered to be high sulfate foods, they also have a high fiber content. These findings underscore the beneficial role for the latter within the H_2S toxin hypothesis and support a clinical approach focusing on plant versus animal-based diets rather than high- and low-sulfur diets.

It is important to consider that while short-term changes in diet can affect activities of different microbial groups in the intestine, they do not change the overall individual-specific taxonomic composition of microbiota [61,150]. Short-term low carbohydrate, high protein diets are among the most popular approaches used to achieve weight loss. Such diets do result in decreases in relative abundance of some butyrate producing bacteria, as well as altered fecal metabolite profiles, including lower content of SCFA and fiber-derived antioxidant phenolic acids [151]. It is possible that such dietary changes can even trigger the onset of UC, which may be reversed with increasing plant-derived dietary components [54,56]. However, long-term diets low in microbiota-accessible carbohydrates can lead to complete extinctions of microbial taxa [152]. Therefore, it is possible that most consistent benefits of dietary therapies will also require transplantation of relevant microbiota, optimized in capacity for the individual patients.

5. Conclusions

There is an intriguing body of literature supporting a relationship between dietary sulfur intake and the H_2S toxin hypothesis in the development of UC. To date, the focus of the H_2S toxin hypothesis in UC has primarily been focused on the abundance and activity of SRB (e.g., *Desulfovibrio*) and dietary sulfur intake. However, this provides only a partial window on the total activity of the microbiota that is relevant to UC pathogenesis. An updated approach to the H_2S hypothesis has to incorporate interactions between different microbial groups as well as multiple components of the diet. A compelling case does exist that a typical western diet, which tends to be high in protein and low in fermentable fiber, may promote the accumulation of harmful products such as H_2S and even increase their toxicity, and is also associated with a lower production of beneficial products such as butyrate. Patients are intensely interested in adjunctive dietary therapies for UC. Multiple technological developments that allow compositional and functional measurements of entire microbial communities should facilitate the development and testing of novel microbiota-targeting interventions that include the dietary management of IBD.

Author Contributions: Conceptulization, L.M.T, A.K.; writing—original draft preparation, L.M.T.; writing—review and editing, L.M.T, M.J.S., B.P.V., M.J.H., Z.G., A.K.; supervision, A.K.

Acknowledgments: This work was partially supported by grants from the Healthy Foods Healthy Lives Institute, the Allen Foundation, and Achieving Cures Together.

References

1. Kaplan, G.G. The global burden of IBD: From 2015 to 2025. *Nat. Rev. Gastroenterol. Hepatol.* **2015**, *12*, 720–727. [CrossRef]

2. Ng, S.C.; Shi, H.Y.; Hamidi, N.; Underwood, F.E.; Tang, W.; Benchimol, E.I.; Panaccione, R.; Ghosh, S.; Wu, J.C.Y.; Chan, F.K.L.; et al. Worldwide incidence and prevalence of inflammatory bowel disease in the 21st century: A systematic review of population-based studies. *Lancet* **2017**, *390*, 2769–2778. [CrossRef]

3. Ng, S.C.; Kaplan, G.G.; Tang, W.; Banerjee, R.; Adigopula, B.; Underwood, F.E.; Tanyingoh, D.; Wei, S.C.; Lin, W.C.; Lin, H.H.; et al. Population Density and Risk of Inflammatory Bowel Disease: A Prospective Population-Based Study in 13 Countries or Regions in Asia-Pacific. *Am. J. Gastroenterol.* **2019**, *114*, 107–115. [CrossRef]

4. Rothschild, D.; Weissbrod, O.; Barkan, E.; Kurilshikov, A.; Korem, T.; Zeevi, D.; Costea, P.I.; Godneva, A.; Kalka, I.N.; Bar, N.; et al. Environment dominates over host genetics in shaping human gut microbiota. *Nature* **2018**, *555*, 210–215. [CrossRef] [PubMed]

5. David, L.A.; Maurice, C.F.; Carmody, R.N.; Gootenberg, D.B.; Button, J.E.; Wolfe, B.E.; Ling, A.V.; Devlin, A.S.; Varma, Y.; Fischbach, M.A.; et al. Diet rapidly and reproducibly alters the human gut microbiome. *Nature* **2014**, *505*, 559–563. [CrossRef] [PubMed]

6. Benchimol, E.I.; Mack, D.R.; Guttmann, A.; Nguyen, G.C.; To, T.; Mojaverian, N.; Quach, P.; Manuel, D.G. Inflammatory bowel disease in immigrants to Canada and their children: A population-based cohort study. *Am. J. Gastroenterol.* **2015**, *110*, 553–563. [CrossRef] [PubMed]

7. Vangay, P.; Johnson, A.J.; Ward, T.L.; Al-Ghalith, G.A.; Shields-Cutler, R.R.; Hillmann, B.M.; Lucas, S.K.; Beura, L.K.; Thompson, E.A.; Till, L.M.; et al. US Immigration Westernizes the Human Gut Microbiome. *Cell* **2018**, *175*, 962–972.e10. [CrossRef]

8. Hou, J.K.; Abraham, B.; El-Serag, H. Dietary intake and risk of developing inflammatory bowel disease: A systematic review of the literature. *Am. J. Gastroenterol.* **2011**, *106*, 563–573. [CrossRef] [PubMed]

9. Kaplan, G.G.; Ng, S.C. Understanding and Preventing the Global Increase of Inflammatory Bowel Disease. *Gastroenterology* **2017**, *152*, 313–321.e2. [CrossRef] [PubMed]

10. Yang, G. Hydrogen sulfide in cell survival: A double-edged sword. *Expert Rev. Clin. Pharmacol.* **2011**, *4*, 33–47. [CrossRef]

11. Barton, L.L.; Ritz, N.L.; Fauque, G.D.; Lin, H.C. Sulfur Cycling and the Intestinal Microbiome. *Dig. Dis. Sci.* **2017**, *62*, 2241–2257. [CrossRef]

12. Pitcher, M.C.L.; Cummings, J.H. Hydrogen sulphide: A bacterial toxin in ulcerative colitis? *Gut* **1996**, *39*, 1–4. [CrossRef] [PubMed]

13. Roediger, W.E.W.; Moore, J.; Babidge, W. Colonic sulfide in pathogenesis and treatment of ulcerative colitis. *Dig. Dis. Sci.* **1997**, *42*, 1571–1579. [CrossRef] [PubMed]

14. Rowan, F.E.; Docherty, N.G.; Coffey, J.C.; O'Connell, P.R. Sulphate-reducing bacteria and hydrogen sulphide in the aetiology of ulcerative colitis. *Br. J. Surg.* **2009**, *96*, 151–158. [CrossRef] [PubMed]

15. Blachier, F.; Davila, A.M.; Mimoun, S.; Benetti, P.H.; Atanasiu, C.; Andriamihaja, M.; Benamouzig, R.; Bouillaud, F.; Tome, D. Luminal sulfide and large intestine mucosa: Friend or foe? *Amino Acids* **2010**, *39*, 335–347. [CrossRef]

16. Blachier, F.; Beaumont, M.; Andriamihaja, M.; Davila, A.M.; Lan, A.; Grauso, M.; Armand, L.; Benamouzig, R.; Tome, D. Changes in the Luminal Environment of the Colonic Epithelial Cells and Physiopathological Consequences. *Am. J. Pathol.* **2017**, *187*, 476–486. [CrossRef]

17. Levine, A.; Sigall Boneh, R.; Wine, E. Evolving role of diet in the pathogenesis and treatment of inflammatory bowel diseases. *Gut* **2018**, *67*, 1726–1738. [CrossRef]

18. Chiba, M.; Abe, T.; Tsuda, H.; Sugawara, T.; Tsuda, S.; Tozawa, H.; Fujiwara, K.; Imai, H. Lifestyle-related disease in Crohn's disease: Relapse prevention by a semi-vegetarian diet. *World J. Gastroenterol.* **2010**, *16*, 2484–2495. [CrossRef]

19. Florin, T.; Neale, G.; Gibson, G.R.; Christl, S.U.; Cummings, J.H. Metabolism of dietary sulphate: Absorption and excretion in humans. *Gut* **1991**, *32*, 766–773. [CrossRef]

20. Devkota, S.; Wang, Y.; Musch, M.W.; Leone, V.; Fehlner-Peach, H.; Nadimpalli, A.; Antonopoulos, D.A.; Jabri, B.; Chang, E.B. Dietary-fat-induced taurocholic acid promotes pathobiont expansion and colitis in Il10-/- mice. *Nature* **2012**, *487*, 104–108. [CrossRef]

21. Holmes, A.J.; Chew, Y.V.; Colakoglu, F.; Cliff, J.B.; Klaassens, E.; Read, M.N.; Solon-Biet, S.M.; McMahon, A.C.; Cogger, V.C.; Ruohonen, K.; et al. Diet-Microbiome Interactions in Health Are Controlled by Intestinal Nitrogen Source Constraints. *Cell Metab.* **2017**, *25*, 140–151. [CrossRef] [PubMed]

22. Desai, M.S.; Seekatz, A.M.; Koropatkin, N.M.; Kamada, N.; Hickey, C.A.; Wolter, M.; Pudlo, N.A.; Kitamoto, S.; Terrapon, N.; Muller, A.; et al. A Dietary Fiber-Deprived Gut Microbiota Degrades the Colonic Mucus Barrier and Enhances Pathogen Susceptibility. *Cell* **2016**, *167*, 1339–1353.e1321. [CrossRef]

23. Wong, J.M.; de Souza, R.; Kendall, C.W.; Emam, A.; Jenkins, D.J. Colonic health: Fermentation and short chain fatty acids. *J. Clin. Gastroenterol.* **2006**, *40*, 235–243. [CrossRef] [PubMed]

24. Roediger, W.E. Role of anaerobic bacteria in the metabolic welfare of the colonic mucosa in man. *Gut* **1980**, *21*, 793–798. [CrossRef] [PubMed]

25. Furusawa, Y.; Obata, Y.; Fukuda, S.; Endo, T.A.; Nakato, G.; Takahashi, D.; Nakanishi, Y.; Uetake, C.; Kato, K.; Kato, T.; et al. Commensal microbe-derived butyrate induces the differentiation of colonic regulatory T cells. *Nature* **2013**, *504*, 446–450. [CrossRef] [PubMed]

26. Arpaia, N.; Campbell, C.; Fan, X.; Dikiy, S.; van der Veeken, J.; deRoos, P.; Liu, H.; Cross, J.R.; Pfeffer, K.; Coffer, P.J.; et al. Metabolites produced by commensal bacteria promote peripheral regulatory T-cell generation. *Nature* **2013**, *504*, 451–455. [CrossRef] [PubMed]

27. Finnie, I.A.; Dwarakanath, A.D.; Taylor, B.A.; Rhodes, J.M. Colonic mucin synthesis is increased by sodium butyrate. *Gut* **1995**, *36*, 93–99. [CrossRef]

28. Byndloss, M.X.; Olsan, E.E.; Rivera-Chavez, F.; Tiffany, C.R.; Cevallos, S.A.; Lokken, K.L.; Torres, T.P.; Byndloss, A.J.; Faber, F.; Gao, Y.; et al. Microbiota-activated PPAR-gamma signaling inhibits dysbiotic Enterobacteriaceae expansion. *Science* **2017**, *357*, 570–575. [CrossRef]

29. Litvak, Y.; Byndloss, M.X.; Tsolis, R.M.; Baumler, A.J. Dysbiotic Proteobacteria expansion: A microbial signature of epithelial dysfunction. *Curr. Opin. Microbiol.* **2017**, *39*, 1–6. [CrossRef] [PubMed]

30. Christl, S.U.; Eisner, H.D.; Dusel, G.; Kasper, H.; Scheppach, W. Antagonistic effects of sulfide and butyrate on proliferation of colonic mucosa: A potential role for these agents in the pathogenesis of ulcerative colitis. *Dig. Dis. Sci.* **1996**, *41*, 2477–2481. [CrossRef]

31. O'Flaherty, V.; Mahony, T.; O'Kennedy, R.; Colleran, E. Effect of pH on growth kinetics and sulphide toxicity thresholds of a range of methanogeic, syntrophic and sulphate-reducing bacteria. *Process Biochem.* **1998**, *33*, 555–569. [CrossRef]

32. Babidge, W.; Millard, S.; Roediger, W. Sulfides impair short chain fatty acid beta-oxidation at acyl-CoA dehydrogenase level in colonocytes: Implications for ulcerative colitis. *Mol. Cell. Biochem.* **1998**, *181*, 117–124. [CrossRef]

33. Wallace, J.L.; Blackler, R.W.; Chan, M.V.; Da Silva, G.J.; Elsheikh, W.; Flannigan, K.L.; Gamaniek, I.; Manko, A.; Wang, L.; Motta, J.P.; et al. Anti-inflammatory and cytoprotective actions of hydrogen sulfide: Translation to therapeutics. *Antioxid. Redox Signal.* **2015**, *22*, 398–410. [CrossRef] [PubMed]

34. Odenwald, M.A.; Turner, J.R. The intestinal epithelial barrier: A therapeutic target? *Nat. Rev. Gastroenterol. Hepatol.* **2017**, *14*, 9–21. [CrossRef]

35. Jiang, J.; Chan, A.; Ali, S.; Saha, A.; Haushalter, K.J.; Lam, W.L.; Glasheen, M.; Parker, J.; Brenner, M.; Mahon, S.B.; et al. Hydrogen Sulfide–Mechanisms of Toxicity and Development of an Antidote. *Sci. Rep.* **2016**, *6*, 20831. [CrossRef]

36. Roediger, W.E.; Duncan, A.; Kapaniris, O.; Millard, S. Reducing sulfur compounds of the colon impair colonocyte nutrition: Implications for ulcerative colitis. *Gastroenterology* **1993**, *104*, 802–809. [CrossRef]

37. De Preter, V.; Arijs, I.; Windey, K.; Vanhove, W.; Vermeire, S.; Schuit, F.; Rutgeerts, P.; Verbeke, K. Impaired butyrate oxidation in ulcerative colitis is due to decreased butyrate uptake and a defect in the oxidation pathway. *Inflamm. Bowel Dis.* **2012**, *18*, 1127–1136. [CrossRef] [PubMed]

38. De Preter, V.; Arijs, I.; Windey, K.; Vanhove, W.; Vermeire, S.; Schuit, F.; Rutgeerts, P.; Verbeke, K. Decreased mucosal sulfide detoxification is related to an impaired butyrate oxidation in ulcerative colitis. *Inflamm. Bowel Dis.* **2012**, *18*, 2371–2380. [CrossRef] [PubMed]

39. Johansson, M.E.; Hansson, G.C. Immunological aspects of intestinal mucus and mucins. *Nat. Rev. Immunol.* **2016**, *16*, 639–649. [CrossRef] [PubMed]

40. Johansson, M.E.; Phillipson, M.; Petersson, J.; Velcich, A.; Holm, L.; Hansson, G.C. The inner of the two Muc2 mucin-dependent mucus layers in colon is devoid of bacteria. *Proc. Natl. Acad. Sci. USA* **2008**, *105*, 15064–15069. [CrossRef] [PubMed]

41. Johansson, M.E.; Gustafsson, J.K.; Holmen-Larsson, J.; Jabbar, K.S.; Xia, L.; Xu, H.; Ghishan, F.K.; Carvalho, F.A.; Gewirtz, A.T.; Sjovall, H.; et al. Bacteria penetrate the normally impenetrable inner

colon mucus layer in both murine colitis models and patients with ulcerative colitis. *Gut* **2014**, *63*, 281–291. [CrossRef]

42. Ijssennagger, N.; Belzer, C.; Hooiveld, G.J.; Dekker, J.; van Mil, S.W.; Muller, M.; Kleerebezem, M.; van der Meer, R. Gut microbiota facilitates dietary heme-induced epithelial hyperproliferation by opening the mucus barrier in colon. *Proc. Natl. Acad. Sci. USA* **2015**, *112*, 10038–10043. [CrossRef]

43. Eichele, D.D.; Kharbanda, K.K. Dextran sodium sulfate colitis murine model: An indispensable tool for advancing our understanding of inflammatory bowel diseases pathogenesis. *World J. Gastroenterol.* **2017**, *23*, 6016–6029. [CrossRef]

44. Zhu, Q.C.; Gao, R.Y.; Wu, W.; Guo, B.M.; Peng, J.Y.; Qin, H.L. Effect of a high-fat diet in development of colonic adenoma in an animal model. *World J. Gastroenterol.* **2014**, *20*, 8119–8129. [CrossRef]

45. Mu, C.; Yang, Y.; Luo, Z.; Guan, L.; Zhu, W. The Colonic Microbiome and Epithelial Transcriptome Are Altered in Rats Fed a High-Protein Diet Compared with a Normal-Protein Diet. *J. Nutr.* **2016**, *146*, 474–483. [CrossRef]

46. Heo, J.M.; Kim, J.C.; Hansen, C.F.; Mullan, B.P.; Hampson, D.J.; Pluske, J.R. Effects of feeding low protein diets to piglets on plasma urea nitrogen, faecal ammonia nitrogen, the incidence of diarrhoea and performance after weaning. *Arch. Anim. Nutr.* **2008**, *62*, 343–358. [CrossRef]

47. Pitcher, M.C.; Beatty, E.R.; Cummings, J.H. The contribution of sulphate reducing bacteria and 5-aminosalicylic acid to faecal sulphide in patients with ulcerative colitis. *Gut* **2000**, *46*, 64–72. [CrossRef] [PubMed]

48. Dubuquoy, L.; Rousseaux, C.; Thuru, X.; Peyrin-Biroulet, L.; Romano, O.; Chavatte, P.; Chamaillard, M.; Desreumaux, P. PPARgamma as a new therapeutic target in inflammatory bowel diseases. *Gut* **2006**, *55*, 1341–1349. [CrossRef]

49. Alex, S.; Lange, K.; Amolo, T.; Grinstead, J.S.; Haakonsson, A.K.; Szalowska, E.; Koppen, A.; Mudde, K.; Haenen, D.; Al-Lahham, S.; et al. Short-chain fatty acids stimulate angiopoietin-like 4 synthesis in human colon adenocarcinoma cells by activating peroxisome proliferator-activated receptor gamma. *Mol. Cell. Biol.* **2013**, *33*, 1303–1316. [CrossRef]

50. Xu, J.; Chen, N.; Wu, Z.; Song, Y.; Zhang, Y.; Wu, N.; Zhang, F.; Ren, X.; Liu, Y. 5-Aminosalicylic Acid Alters the Gut Bacterial Microbiota in Patients with Ulcerative Colitis. *Front. Microbiol.* **2018**, *9*, 1274. [CrossRef]

51. Burke, D.A.; Axon, A.T.; Clayden, S.A.; Dixon, M.F.; Johnston, D.; Lacey, R.W. The efficacy of tobramycin in the treatment of ulcerative colitis. *Aliment. Pharmacol. Ther.* **1990**, *4*, 123–129. [CrossRef]

52. Roediger, W.E.W. Decreased sulphur aminoacid intake in ulcerative colitis. *Lancet* **1998**, *351*. [CrossRef]

53. Kashyap, P.C.; Reigstad, C.S.; Loftus, E.V., Jr. Role of diet and gut microbiota in management of inflammatory bowel disease in an Asian migrant. *J. Allergy Clin. Immunol.* **2013**, *132*, 250–250.e255. [CrossRef] [PubMed]

54. Chiba, M.; Tsuda, S.; Komatsu, M.; Tozawa, H.; Takayama, Y. Onset of Ulcerative Colitis during a Low-Carbohydrate Weight-Loss Diet and Treatment with a Plant-Based Diet: A Case Report. *Perm. J.* **2016**, *20*, 80–84. [CrossRef] [PubMed]

55. Chiba, M.; Sugawara, T.; Komatsu, M.; Tozawa, H. Onset of Ulcerative Colitis in the Second Trimester after Emesis Gravidarum: Treatment with Plant-based Diet. *Inflamm. Bowel Dis.* **2018**, *24*, e8–e9. [CrossRef]

56. Chiba, M.; Nakane, K.; Tsuji, T.; Tsuda, S.; Ishii, H.; Ohno, H.; Watanabe, K.; Ito, M.; Komatsu, M.; Yamada, K.; et al. Relapse Prevention in Ulcerative Colitis by Plant-Based Diet Through Educational Hospitalization: A Single-Group Trial. *Perm. J.* **2018**, *22*. [CrossRef] [PubMed]

57. Florin, T.H.J.; Neale, G.; Goretski, S.; Cummings, J.H. The sulfate content of foods and beverages. *J. Food Compos. Anal.* **1993**, *6*, 140–151. [CrossRef]

58. U.S. Food and Drug Administration. Food Additive Status List. Available online: https://www.fda.gov/food/ingredientspackaginglabeling/foodadditivesingredients/ucm091048.htm (accessed on 15 August 2018).

59. Curno, R.; Magee, E.A.; Edmond, L.M.; Cummings, J.H. Studies of a urinary biomarker of dietary inorganic sulphur in subjects on diets containing 1–38 mmol sulphur/day and of the half-life of ingested 34SO4(2-). *Eur. J. Clin. Nutr.* **2008**, *62*, 1106–1115. [CrossRef]

60. Magee, E.A.; Curno, R.; Edmond, L.M.; Cummings, J.H. Contribution of dietary protein and inorganic sulfur to urinary sulfate: Toward a biomarker of inorganic sulfur intake. *Am. J. Clin. Nutr.* **2004**, *80*, 137–142. [CrossRef]

61. Dostal Webster, A.; Staley, C.; Hamilton, M.J.; Huang, M.; Fryxell, K.; Erickson, R.; Kabage, A.J.; Sadowsky, M.J.; Khoruts, A. Influence of short-term changes in dietary sulfur on the relative abundances of intestinal sulfate-reducing bacteria. *Gut Microbes* **2019**, 1–11. [CrossRef]

62. Florin, T.H. Hydrogen sulphide and total acid-volatile sulphide in faeces, determined with a direct spectrophotometric method. *Clin. Chim. Acta* **1991**, *196*, 127–134. [CrossRef]

63. Buffiere, C.; Gaudichon, C.; Hafnaoui, N.; Migne, C.; Scislowsky, V.; Khodorova, N.; Mosoni, L.; Blot, A.; Boirie, Y.; Dardevet, D.; et al. In the elderly, meat protein assimilation from rare meat is lower than that from meat that is well done. *Am. J. Clin. Nutr.* **2017**, *106*, 1257–1266. [CrossRef]

64. Mills, D.J.; Tuohy, K.M.; Booth, J.; Buck, M.; Crabbe, M.J.; Gibson, G.R.; Ames, J.M. Dietary glycated protein modulates the colonic microbiota towards a more detrimental composition in ulcerative colitis patients and non-ulcerative colitis subjects. *J. Appl. Microbiol.* **2008**, *105*, 706–714. [CrossRef] [PubMed]

65. Oberli, M.; Marsset-Baglieri, A.; Airinei, G.; Sante-Lhoutellier, V.; Khodorova, N.; Remond, D.; Foucault-Simonin, A.; Piedcoq, J.; Tome, D.; Fromentin, G.; et al. High True Ileal Digestibility but Not Postprandial Utilization of Nitrogen from Bovine Meat Protein in Humans Is Moderately Decreased by High-Temperature, Long-Duration Cooking. *J. Nutr.* **2015**, *145*, 2221–2228. [CrossRef]

66. Pennings, B.; Groen, B.B.; van Dijk, J.W.; de Lange, A.; Kiskini, A.; Kuklinski, M.; Senden, J.M.; van Loon, L.J. Minced beef is more rapidly digested and absorbed than beef steak, resulting in greater postprandial protein retention in older men. *Am. J. Clin. Nutr.* **2013**, *98*, 121–128. [CrossRef] [PubMed]

67. Remond, D.; Machebeuf, M.; Yven, C.; Buffiere, C.; Mioche, L.; Mosoni, L.; Mirand, P.P. Postprandial whole-body protein metabolism after a meat meal is influenced by chewing efficiency in elderly subjects. *Am. J. Clin. Nutr.* **2007**, *85*, 1286–1292. [CrossRef] [PubMed]

68. Ridlon, J.M.; Wolf, P.G.; Gaskins, H.R. Taurocholic acid metabolism by gut microbes and colon cancer. *Gut Microbes* **2016**, *7*, 201–215. [CrossRef] [PubMed]

69. Di Ciaula, A.; Garruti, G.; Lunardi Baccetto, R.; Molina-Molina, E.; Bonfrate, L.; Wang, D.Q.; Portincasa, P. Bile Acid Physiology. *Ann. Hepatol.* **2017**, *16*, s4–s14. [CrossRef]

70. Johansson, M.E.; Larsson, J.M.; Hansson, G.C. The two mucus layers of colon are organized by the MUC2 mucin, whereas the outer layer is a legislator of host-microbial interactions. *Proc. Natl. Acad. Sci. USA* **2011**, *108* (Suppl. 1), 4659–4665. [CrossRef]

71. Holmen Larsson, J.M.; Thomsson, K.A.; Rodriguez-Pineiro, A.M.; Karlsson, H.; Hansson, G.C. Studies of mucus in mouse stomach, small intestine, and colon. III. Gastrointestinal Muc5ac and Muc2 mucin O-glycan patterns reveal a regiospecific distribution. *Am. J. Physiol. Gastrointest. Liver Physiol.* **2013**, *305*, G357–G363. [CrossRef] [PubMed]

72. Robbe, C.; Capon, C.; Coddeville, B.; Michalski, J.-C. Structural diversity and specific distribution of O-glycans in normal human mucins along the intestinal tract. *Biochem. J.* **2004**, *384*, 307–316. [CrossRef] [PubMed]

73. Lennon, G.; Balfe, A.; Bambury, N.; Lavelle, A.; Maguire, A.; Docherty, N.G.; Coffey, J.C.; Winter, D.C.; Sheahan, K.; O'Connell, P.R. Correlations between colonic crypt mucin chemotype, inflammatory grade and Desulfovibrio species in ulcerative colitis. *Colorectal Dis.* **2014**, *16*, O161–O169. [CrossRef] [PubMed]

74. Gibson, G.R.; Cummings, J.H.; Macfarlane, G.T. Growth and activities of sulphate-reducing bacteria in gut contents of healthy subjects and patients with ulcerative colitis. *FEMS Microbiol. Ecol.* **1991**, *86*, 103–112. [CrossRef]

75. Moore, J.; Babidge, W.; Millard, S.; Roediger, W. Colonic luminal hydrogen sulfide is not elevated in ulcerative colitis. *Dig. Dis. Sci.* **1998**, *43*, 162–165. [CrossRef]

76. Hughes, M.N.; Centelles, M.N.; Moore, K.P. Making and working with hydrogen sulfide: The chemistry and generation of hydrogen sulfide in vitro and its measurement in vivo: A review. *Free Radic. Biol. Med.* **2009**, *47*, 1346–1353. [CrossRef]

77. Kolluru, G.K.; Shen, X.; Bir, S.C.; Kevil, C.G. Hydrogen sulfide chemical biology: Pathophysiological roles and detection. *Nitric Oxide* **2013**, *35*, 5–20. [CrossRef] [PubMed]

78. Magee, E.A.; Richardson, C.J.; Hughes, R.; Cummings, J.H. Contribution of dietary protein to sulfide production in the large intestine: An in vitro and a controlled feeding study in humans. *Am. J. Clin. Nutr.* **2000**, *72*, 1488–1494. [CrossRef] [PubMed]

79. Vitvitsky, V.; Banerjee, R. H_2S analysis in biological samples using gas chromatography with sulfur chemiluminescence detection. *Methods Enzymol.* **2015**, *554*, 111–123. [CrossRef] [PubMed]

80. Levine, J.; Ellis, C.J.; Furne, J.K.; Springfield, J.; Levitt, M.D. Fecal hydrogen sulfide production in ulcerative colitis. *Am. J. Gastroenterol.* **1998**, *93*, 83–87. [CrossRef]

81. Yao, C.K.; Rotbart, A.; Ou, J.Z.; Kalantar-Zadeh, K.; Muir, J.G.; Gibson, P.R. Modulation of colonic hydrogen sulfide production by diet and mesalazine utilizing a novel gas-profiling technology. *Gut Microbes* **2018**, 1–13. [CrossRef]

82. Anantharaman, K.; Hausmann, B.; Jungbluth, S.P.; Kantor, R.S.; Lavy, A.; Warren, L.A.; Rappe, M.S.; Pester, M.; Loy, A.; Thomas, B.C.; et al. Expanded diversity of microbial groups that shape the dissimilatory sulfur cycle. *ISME J.* **2018**, *12*, 1715–1728. [CrossRef]

83. Scanlan, P.D.; Shanahan, F.; Marchesi, J.R. Culture-independent analysis of desulfovibrios in the human distal colon of healthy, colorectal cancer and polypectomized individuals. *FEMS Microbiol. Ecol.* **2009**, *69*, 213–221. [CrossRef]

84. Muller, A.L.; Kjeldsen, K.U.; Rattei, T.; Pester, M.; Loy, A. Phylogenetic and environmental diversity of DsrAB-type dissimilatory (bi)sulfite reductases. *ISME J.* **2015**, *9*, 1152–1165. [CrossRef] [PubMed]

85. Christophersen, C.T.; Morrison, M.; Conlon, M.A. Overestimation of the abundance of sulfate-reducing bacteria in human feces by quantitative PCR targeting the Desulfovibrio 16S rRNA gene. *Appl. Environ. Microbiol.* **2011**, *77*, 3544–3546. [CrossRef] [PubMed]

86. Coutinho, C.; Coutinho-Silva, R.; Zinkevich, V.; Pearce, C.B.; Ojcius, D.M.; Beech, I. Sulphate-reducing bacteria from ulcerative colitis patients induce apoptosis of gastrointestinal epithelial cells. *Microb. Pathog.* **2017**, *112*, 126–134. [CrossRef] [PubMed]

87. Hale, V.L.; Jeraldo, P.; Mundy, M.; Yao, J.; Keeney, G.; Scott, N.; Cheek, E.H.; Davidson, J.; Green, M.; Martinez, C.; et al. Synthesis of multi-omic data and community metabolic models reveals insights into the role of hydrogen sulfide in colon cancer. *Methods* **2018**. [CrossRef] [PubMed]

88. Jia, W.; Whitehead, R.N.; Griffiths, L.; Dawson, C.; Bai, H.; Waring, R.H.; Ramsden, D.B.; Hunter, J.O.; Cauchi, M.; Bessant, C.; et al. Diversity and distribution of sulphate-reducing bacteria in human faeces from healthy subjects and patients with inflammatory bowel disease. *FEMS Immunol. Med. Microbiol.* **2012**, *65*, 55–68. [CrossRef] [PubMed]

89. Duffy, M.; O'Mahony, L.; Coffey, J.C.; Collins, J.K.; Shanahan, F.; Redmond, H.P.; Kirwan, W.O. Sulfate-Reducing Bacteria Colonize Pouches Formed for Ulcerative Colitis but Not for Familial Adenomatous Polyposis. *Dis. Colon Rectum* **2002**, *45*, 384–388. [CrossRef]

90. Windey, K.; De Preter, V.; Verbeke, K. Relevance of protein fermentation to gut health. *Mol. Nutr. Food Res.* **2012**, *56*, 184–196. [CrossRef] [PubMed]

91. Kimura, H. Metabolic turnover of hydrogen sulfide. *Front. Physiol.* **2012**, *3*, 101. [CrossRef]

92. Awano, N.; Wada, M.; Mori, H.; Nakamori, S.; Takagi, H. Identification and functional analysis of Escherichia coli cysteine desulfhydrases. *Appl. Environ. Microbiol.* **2005**, *71*, 4149–4152. [CrossRef]

93. Sahami, S.; Kooij, I.A.; Meijer, S.L.; Van den Brink, G.R.; Buskens, C.J.; Te Velde, A.A. The Link between the Appendix and Ulcerative Colitis: Clinical Relevance and Potential Immunological Mechanisms. *Am. J. Gastroenterol.* **2016**, *111*, 163–169. [CrossRef] [PubMed]

94. Rogers, M.B.; Brower-Sinning, R.; Firek, B.; Zhong, D.; Morowitz, M.J. Acute Appendicitis in Children Is Associated with a Local Expansion of Fusobacteria. *Clin. Infect. Dis.* **2016**, *63*, 71–78. [CrossRef] [PubMed]

95. Zhong, D.; Brower-Sinning, R.; Firek, B.; Morowitz, M.J. Acute appendicitis in children is associated with an abundance of bacteria from the phylum Fusobacteria. *J. Pediatr. Surg.* **2014**, *49*, 441–446. [CrossRef]

96. Basic, A.; Blomqvist, M.; Dahlen, G.; Svensater, G. The proteins of Fusobacterium spp. involved in hydrogen sulfide production from L-cysteine. *BMC Microbiol.* **2017**, *17*, 61. [CrossRef] [PubMed]

97. Basic, A.; Blomqvist, S.; Carlen, A.; Dahlen, G. Estimation of bacterial hydrogen sulfide production in vitro. *J. Oral Microbiol.* **2015**, *7*, 28166. [CrossRef] [PubMed]

98. Wolf, P.G.; Biswas, A.; Morales, S.E.; Greening, C.; Gaskins, H.R. H_2 metabolism is widespread and diverse among human colonic microbes. *Gut Microbes* **2016**, *7*, 235–245. [CrossRef]

99. Carbonero, F.; Benefiel, A.C.; Gaskins, H.R. Contributions of the microbial hydrogen economy to colonic homeostasis. *Nat. Rev. Gastroenterol. Hepatol.* **2012**, *9*, 504–518. [CrossRef]

100. Macfarlane, S.; Macfarlane, G.T. Regulation of short-chain fatty acid production. *Proc. Nutr. Soc.* **2003**, *62*, 67–72. [CrossRef]

101. Kunkel, D.; Basseri, R.J.; Makhani, M.D.; Chong, K.; Chang, C.; Pimentel, M. Methane on breath testing is associated with constipation: A systematic review and meta-analysis. *Dig. Dis. Sci.* **2011**, *56*, 1612–1618. [CrossRef]

102. Macfarlane, G.T.; Gibson, G.R.; Cummings, J.H. Comparison of fermentation reactions in different regions of the human colon. *J. Appl. Bacteriol.* **1992**, *72*, 57–64.

103. Rao, S.S.; Kuo, B.; McCallum, R.W.; Chey, W.D.; DiBaise, J.K.; Hasler, W.L.; Koch, K.L.; Lackner, J.M.; Miller, C.; Saad, R.; et al. Investigation of colonic and whole-gut transit with wireless motility capsule and radiopaque markers in constipation. *Clin. Gastroenterol. Hepatol.* **2009**, *7*, 537–544. [CrossRef]

104. Videla, S.; Vilaseca, J.; Antolin, M.; Garcia-Lafuente, A.; Guarner, F.; Crespo, E.; Casalots, J.; Salas, A.; Malagelada, J.R. Dietary inulin improves distal colitis induced by dextran sodium sulfate in the rat. *Am. J. Gastroenterol.* **2001**, *96*, 1486–1493. [CrossRef] [PubMed]

105. de Vries, J.; Miller, P.E.; Verbeke, K. Effects of cereal fiber on bowel function: A systematic review of intervention trials. *World J. Gastroenterol.* **2015**, *21*, 8952–8963. [CrossRef]

106. Walker, A.W.; Duncan, S.H.; McWilliam Leitch, E.C.; Child, M.W.; Flint, H.J. pH and peptide supply can radically alter bacterial populations and short-chain fatty acid ratios within microbial communities from the human colon. *Appl. Environ. Microbiol.* **2005**, *71*, 3692–3700. [CrossRef] [PubMed]

107. Duncan, S.H.; Louis, P.; Thomson, J.M.; Flint, H.J. The role of pH in determining the species composition of the human colonic microbiota. *Environ. Microbiol.* **2009**, *11*, 2112–2122. [CrossRef]

108. Gibson, G.R.; Cummings, J.H.; Macfarlane, G.T.; Allison, C.; Segal, I.; Vorster, H.H.; Walker, A.R.P. Alternative pathways for hydrogen disposal during fermentation in the human colon. *Gut* **1990**, *31*, 679–683. [CrossRef]

109. Beaumont, M.; Andriamihaja, M.; Lan, A.; Khodorova, N.; Audebert, M.; Blouin, J.M.; Grauso, M.; Lancha, L.; Benetti, P.H.; Benamouzig, R.; et al. Detrimental effects for colonocytes of an increased exposure to luminal hydrogen sulfide: The adaptive response. *Free Radic. Biol. Med.* **2016**, *93*, 155–164. [CrossRef] [PubMed]

110. Suarez, F.; Furne, J.; Springfield, J.; Levitt, M. Insights into human colonic physiology obtained from the study of flatus composition. *Am. Physiol. Soc.* **1997**, *272*, G1028–G1033. [CrossRef] [PubMed]

111. Levitt, M.D.; Furne, J.; Springfield, J.; Suarez, F.; DeMaster, E. Detoxification of hydrogen sulfide and methanethiol in the cecal mucosa. *J. Clin. Investig.* **1999**, *104*, 1107–1114. [CrossRef] [PubMed]

112. Furne, J.; Springfield, J.; Koenig, T.; DeMaster, E.; Levitt, M.D. Oxidation of hydrogen sulfide and methanethiol to thiosulfate by rat tissues: A specialized function of the colonic mucosa. *Biochem. Pharmacol.* **2001**, *62*, 255–259. [CrossRef]

113. Picton, R.; Eggo, M.C.; Merrill, G.A.; Langman, M.J.S.; Singh, S. Mucosal protection against sulphide: Importance of the enzyme rhodanese. *Gut* **2002**, *50*, 201–205. [CrossRef] [PubMed]

114. Picton, R.; Eggo, M.C.; Langman, M.J.; Singh, S. Impaired detoxication of hydrogen sulfide in ulcerative colitis? *Dig. Dis. Sci.* **2007**, *52*, 373–378. [CrossRef]

115. Wilson, K.; Mudra, M.; Furne, J.; Levitt, M. Differentiation of the roles of sulfide oxidase and rhodanese in the detoxification of sulfide by the colonic mucosa. *Dig. Dis. Sci.* **2008**, *53*, 277–283. [CrossRef]

116. Landry, A.P.; Ballou, D.P.; Banerjee, R. Modulation of Catalytic Promiscuity during Hydrogen Sulfide Oxidation. *ACS Chem. Biol.* **2018**, *13*, 1651–1658. [CrossRef]

117. Filipovic, M.R.; Zivanovic, J.; Alvarez, B.; Banerjee, R. Chemical Biology of H_2S Signaling through Persulfidation. *Chem. Rev.* **2018**, *118*, 1253–1337. [CrossRef]

118. Landry, A.P.; Ballou, D.P.; Banerjee, R. H_2S oxidation by nanodisc-embedded human sulfide quinone oxidoreductase. *J. Biol. Chem.* **2017**, *292*, 11641–11649. [CrossRef] [PubMed]

119. Libiad, M.; Yadav, P.K.; Vitvitsky, V.; Martinov, M.; Banerjee, R. Organization of the human mitochondrial hydrogen sulfide oxidation pathway. *J. Biol. Chem.* **2014**, *289*, 30901–30910. [CrossRef] [PubMed]

120. Mimoun, S.; Andriamihaja, M.; Chaumontet, C.; Atanasiu, C.; Benamouzig, R.; Blouin, J.M.; Tome, D.; Bouillaud, F.; Blachier, F. Detoxification of H(2)S by differentiated colonic epithelial cells: Implication of the sulfide oxidizing unit and of the cell respiratory capacity. *Antioxid. Redox Signal.* **2012**, *17*, 1–10. [CrossRef] [PubMed]

121. Sido, B.; Hack, V.; Hochlehnert, A.; Lipps, H.; Herfarth, C.; Droge, W. Impairment of intestinal glutathione synthesis in patients with inflammatory bowel disease. *Gut* **1998**, *42*, 485–492. [CrossRef]

122. Fuentes, S.; Rossen, N.G.; van der Spek, M.J.; Hartman, J.H.; Huuskonen, L.; Korpela, K.; Salojarvi, J.; Aalvink, S.; de Vos, W.M.; D'Haens, G.R.; et al. Microbial shifts and signatures of long-term remission in ulcerative colitis after faecal microbiota transplantation. *ISME J.* **2017**, *11*, 1877–1889. [CrossRef]

123. Bajer, L.; Kverka, M.; Kostovcik, M.; Macinga, P.; Dvorak, J.; Stehlikova, Z.; Brezina, J.; Wohl, P.; Spicak, J.; Drastich, P. Distinct gut microbiota profiles in patients with primary sclerosing cholangitis and ulcerative colitis. *World J. Gastroenterol.* **2017**, *23*, 4548–4558. [CrossRef]

124. Vermeire, S.; Joossens, M.; Verbeke, K.; Wang, J.; Machiels, K.; Sabino, J.; Ferrante, M.; Van Assche, G.; Rutgeerts, P.; Raes, J. Donor Species Richness Determines Faecal Microbiota Transplantation Success in Inflammatory Bowel Disease. *J. Crohn's Colitis* **2016**, *10*, 387–394. [CrossRef]

125. Smith, E.A.; Macfarlane, G.T. Enumeration of human colonic bacteria producing phenolic and indolic compounds: Effects of pH, carbohydrate availability and retention time on dissimilatory aromatic amino acid metabolism. *J. Appl. Bacteriol.* **1996**, *81*, 288–302. [CrossRef]

126. Zimmer, J.; Lange, B.; Frick, J.S.; Sauer, H.; Zimmermann, K.; Schwiertz, A.; Rusch, K.; Klosterhalfen, S.; Enck, P. A vegan or vegetarian diet substantially alters the human colonic faecal microbiota. *Eur. J. Clin. Nutr.* **2012**, *66*, 53–60. [CrossRef]

127. Devkota, S.; Chang, E.B. Interactions between Diet, Bile Acid Metabolism, Gut Microbiota, and Inflammatory Bowel Diseases. *Dig. Dis.* **2015**, *33*, 351–356. [CrossRef]

128. Leone, V.; Gibbons, S.M.; Martinez, K.; Hutchison, A.L.; Huang, E.Y.; Cham, C.M.; Pierre, J.F.; Heneghan, A.F.; Nadimpalli, A.; Hubert, N.; et al. Effects of diurnal variation of gut microbes and high-fat feeding on host circadian clock function and metabolism. *Cell Host Microbe* **2015**, *17*, 681–689. [CrossRef]

129. Barcelo, A.; Claustre, J.; Moro, F.; Chayvialle, J.-A.; Cuber, J.-C. Plaisancia. Mucin secretion is modulated by luminal factors in the isolated vascularly perfused rat colon. *Gut* **2000**, *46*, 218–224. [CrossRef] [PubMed]

130. Deplancke, B.; Finster, K.; Vallen Graham, W.; Collier, C.T.; Thurmond, J.E.; Gaskins, H.R. Gastrointestinal and Microbial Responses to Sulfate-Supplemented Drinking Water in Mice. *Exp. Biol. Med.* **2003**, *228*, 424–433. [CrossRef]

131. Schroeder, B.O.; Birchenough, G.M.H.; Stahlman, M.; Arike, L.; Johansson, M.E.V.; Hansson, G.C.; Backhed, F. Bifidobacteria or Fiber Protects against Diet-Induced Microbiota-Mediated Colonic Mucus Deterioration. *Cell Host Microbe* **2018**, *23*, 27–40.e27. [CrossRef] [PubMed]

132. Croix, J.A.; Carbonero, F.; Nava, G.M.; Russell, M.; Greenberg, E.; Gaskins, H.R. On the relationship between sialomucin and sulfomucin expression and hydrogenotrophic microbes in the human colonic mucosa. *PLoS ONE* **2011**, *6*, e24447. [CrossRef] [PubMed]

133. Rey, F.E.; Gonzalez, M.D.; Cheng, J.; Wu, M.; Ahern, P.P.; Gordon, J.I. Metabolic niche of a prominent sulfate-reducing human gut bacterium. *Proc. Natl. Acad. Sci. USA* **2013**, *110*, 13582–13587. [CrossRef]

134. Dwarakanath, A.D.; Campbell, B.J.; Tsai, H.H.; Sunderland, D.; Hart, C.A.; Rhodes, J.M. Faecal mucinase activity assessed in inflammatory bowel disease using 14C threonine labelled mucin substrate. *Gut* **1995**, *37*, 58–62. [CrossRef] [PubMed]

135. Press, A.G.; Hauptmann, I.A.; Hauptmann, L.; Fuchs, B.; Fuchs, M.; Ewe, K.; Ramadori, G. Gastrointestinal pH profiles in patients with inflammatory bowel disease. *Aliment Pharmacol. Ther.* **1998**, *12*, 673–678. [CrossRef] [PubMed]

136. Tsai, H.H.; Dwarakanath, A.D.; Hart, C.A.; Milton, J.D.; Rhodes, J.M. Increased faecal mucin sulphatase activity in ulcerative colitis: A potential target for treatment. *Gut* **1995**, *36*, 570–576. [CrossRef] [PubMed]

137. Chassaing, B.; Koren, O.; Goodrich, J.K.; Poole, A.C.; Srinivasan, S.; Ley, R.E.; Gewirtz, A.T. Dietary emulsifiers impact the mouse gut microbiota promoting colitis and metabolic syndrome. *Nature* **2015**, *519*, 92–96. [CrossRef]

138. Roberts, C.L.; Keita, A.V.; Duncan, S.H.; O'Kennedy, N.; Soderholm, J.D.; Rhodes, J.M.; Campbell, B.J. Translocation of Crohn's disease Escherichia coli across M-cells: Contrasting effects of soluble plant fibres and emulsifiers. *Gut* **2010**, *59*, 1331–1339. [CrossRef] [PubMed]

139. Sugihara, K.; Masuda, M.; Nakao, M.; Abuduli, M.; Imi, Y.; Oda, N.; Okahisa, T.; Yamamoto, H.; Takeda, E.; Taketani, Y. Dietary phosphate exacerbates intestinal inflammation in experimental colitis. *J. Clin. Biochem. Nutr.* **2017**, *61*, 91–99. [CrossRef]

140. Swidsinski, A.; Ung, V.; Sydora, B.C.; Loening-Baucke, V.; Doerffel, Y.; Verstraelen, H.; Fedorak, R.N. Bacterial overgrowth and inflammation of small intestine after carboxymethylcellulose ingestion in genetically susceptible mice. *Inflamm. Bowel Dis.* **2009**, *15*, 359–364. [CrossRef]

141. Sadar, S.S.; Vyawahare, N.S.; Bodhankar, S.L. Ferulic acid ameliorates TNBS-induced ulcerative colitis through modulation of cytokines, oxidative stress, iNOs, COX-2, and apoptosis in laboratory rats. *EXCLI J.* **2016**, *15*, 482–499. [CrossRef]

142. Zheng, H.; Chen, M.; Li, Y.; Wang, Y.; Wei, L.; Liao, Z.; Wang, M.; Ma, F.; Liao, Q.; Xie, Z. Modulation of Gut Microbiome Composition and Function in Experimental Colitis Treated with Sulfasalazine. *Front. Microbiol.* **2017**, *8*, 1703. [CrossRef] [PubMed]

143. Laserna-Mendieta, E.J.; Clooney, A.G.; Carretero-Gomez, J.F.; Moran, C.; Sheehan, D.; Nolan, J.A.; Hill, C.; Gahan, C.G.M.; Joyce, S.A.; Shanahan, F.; et al. Determinants of Reduced Genetic Capacity for Butyrate Synthesis by the Gut Microbiome in Crohn's Disease and Ulcerative Colitis. *J. Crohn's Colitis* **2018**, *12*, 204–216. [CrossRef] [PubMed]

144. Valcheva, R.; Koleva, P.; Martinez, I.; Walter, J.; Ganzle, M.G.; Dieleman, L.A. Inulin-type fructans improve active ulcerative colitis associated with microbiota changes and increased short-chain fatty acids levels. *Gut Microbes* **2018**, 1–24. [CrossRef]

145. Earley, H.; Lennon, G.; Balfe, A.; Kilcoyne, M.; Clyne, M.; Joshi, L.; Carrington, S.; Martin, S.T.; Coffey, J.C.; Winter, D.C.; et al. A Preliminary Study Examining the Binding Capacity of *Akkermansia muciniphila* and *Desulfovibrio* spp., to Colonic Mucin in Health and Ulcerative Colitis. *PLoS ONE* **2015**, *10*, e0135280. [CrossRef]

146. Tsai, H.H.; Sunderland, D.; Gibson, G.R.; Hart, C.A.; Rhodes, J.M. A novel mucin sulphatase from human faeces: Its identification, purification and characterization. *Clin. Sci.* **1992**, *82*, 447–454. [CrossRef]

147. Wei, Y.; Gong, J.; Zhu, W.; Tian, H.; Ding, C.; Gu, L.; Li, N.; Li, J. Pectin enhances the effect of fecal microbiota transplantation in ulcerative colitis by delaying the loss of diversity of gut flora. *BMC Microbiol.* **2016**, *16*, 255. [CrossRef]

148. Lewis, S.; Brazier, J.; Beard, D.; Nazem, N.; Proctor, D. Effects of metronidazole and oligofructose on faecal concentrations of sulphate-reducing bacteria and their activity in human volunteers. *Scand. J. Gastroenterol.* **2009**, *40*, 1296–1303. [CrossRef]

149. Kellingray, L.; Tapp, H.S.; Saha, S.; Doleman, J.F.; Narbad, A.; Mithen, R.F. Consumption of a diet rich in Brassica vegetables is associated with a reduced abundance of sulphate-reducing bacteria: A randomised crossover study. *Mol. Nutr. Food Res.* **2017**, *61*. [CrossRef]

150. Wu, G.D.; Chen, J.; Hoffmann, C.; Bittinger, K.; Chen, Y.Y.; Keilbaugh, S.A.; Bewtra, M.; Knights, D.; Walters, W.A.; Knight, R.; et al. Linking long-term dietary patterns with gut microbial enterotypes. *Science* **2011**, *334*, 105–108. [CrossRef]

151. Russell, W.R.; Gratz, S.W.; Duncan, S.H.; Holtrop, G.; Ince, J.; Scobbie, L.; Duncan, G.; Johnstone, A.M.; Lobley, G.E.; Wallace, R.J.; et al. High-protein, reduced-carbohydrate weight-loss diets promote metabolite profiles likely to be detrimental to colonic health. *Am. J. Clin. Nutr.* **2011**, *93*, 1062–1072. [CrossRef]

152. Sonnenburg, E.D.; Smits, S.A.; Tikhonov, M.; Higginbottom, S.K.; Wingreen, N.S.; Sonnenburg, J.L. Diet-induced extinctions in the gut microbiota compound over generations. *Nature* **2016**, *529*, 212–215. [CrossRef] [PubMed]

Permissions

All chapters in this book were first published by MDPI; hereby published with permission under the Creative Commons Attribution License or equivalent. Every chapter published in this book has been scrutinized by our experts. Their significance has been extensively debated. The topics covered herein carry significant findings which will fuel the growth of the discipline. They may even be implemented as practical applications or may be referred to as a beginning point for another development.

The contributors of this book come from diverse backgrounds, making this book a truly international effort. This book will bring forth new frontiers with its revolutionizing research information and detailed analysis of the nascent developments around the world.

We would like to thank all the contributing authors for lending their expertise to make the book truly unique. They have played a crucial role in the development of this book. Without their invaluable contributions this book wouldn't have been possible. They have made vital efforts to compile up to date information on the varied aspects of this subject to make this book a valuable addition to the collection of many professionals and students.

This book was conceptualized with the vision of imparting up-to-date information and advanced data in this field. To ensure the same, a matchless editorial board was set up. Every individual on the board went through rigorous rounds of assessment to prove their worth. After which they invested a large part of their time researching and compiling the most relevant data for our readers.

The editorial board has been involved in producing this book since its inception. They have spent rigorous hours researching and exploring the diverse topics which have resulted in the successful publishing of this book. They have passed on their knowledge of decades through this book. To expedite this challenging task, the publisher supported the team at every step. A small team of assistant editors was also appointed to further simplify the editing procedure and attain best results for the readers.

Apart from the editorial board, the designing team has also invested a significant amount of their time in understanding the subject and creating the most relevant covers. They scrutinized every image to scout for the most suitable representation of the subject and create an appropriate cover for the book.

The publishing team has been an ardent support to the editorial, designing and production team. Their endless efforts to recruit the best for this project, has resulted in the accomplishment of this book. They are a veteran in the field of academics and their pool of knowledge is as vast as their experience in printing. Their expertise and guidance has proved useful at every step. Their uncompromising quality standards have made this book an exceptional effort. Their encouragement from time to time has been an inspiration for everyone.

The publisher and the editorial board hope that this book will prove to be a valuable piece of knowledge for researchers, students, practitioners and scholars across the globe.

List of Contributors

Francesca Penagini, Dario Dilillo, Barbara Borsani, Lucia Cococcioni, Erica Galli, Giovanna Zuin and Gian Vincenzo Zuccotti
Pediatric Department, "V. Buzzi" Children's Hospital, University of Milan, Via Castelvetro 32, 20154 Milan, Italy

Giorgio Bedogni
Clinical Epidemiology Unit, Liver Research Center, Basovizza, 34012 Trieste, Italy

Natasha Haskey and Deanna L. Gibson
Department of Biology, The Irving K. Barber School of Arts and Sciences, University of British Columbia, Room, ASC 368, 3187 University Way, Okanagan campus, Kelowna, BC V1V 1V7, Canada

Vibeke Andersen
Focused Research Unit for Molecular Diagnostic and Clinical Research, IRS-Centre Sonderjylland, Hospital of Southern Jutland, Åbenrå 6200, Denmark
Institute of Molecular Medicine, University of Southern Denmark, Odense 5000, Denmark

Axel Kornerup Hansen
Department of Veterinary and Animal Sciences, University of Copenhagen, Frederiksberg 1871, Denmark

Berit Lilienthal Heitmann
Research Unit for Dietary Studies, Parker Institute, Frederiksberg 2000, Denmark
Section for General Medicine, Department of Public Health, University of Copenhagen, Copenhagen 1353, Denmark
National Institute of Public Health, University of Southern Denmark, Odense 5000, Denmark

Gian Carlo Tenore, Ester Pagano, Francesco Merlino, Francesca Borrelli, Ettore Novellino and Maria Maisto
Department of Pharmacy, School of Medicine and Surgery, University of Naples Federico II, Via D. Montesano 49, 80131 Naples, Italy

Stefania Lama, Daniela Vanacore and Paola Stiuso
Department of Precision Medicine, University of Campania "Luigi Vanvitelli", Via De Crecchio 7, 80138 Naples, Italy

Salvatore Di Maro
DiSTABiF, Università degli Studi della Campania "Luigi Vanvitelli", via Vivaldi 43, 81100 Caserta, Italy

Raffaele Capasso
Department of Agricultural Sciences, University of Naples Federico II, 80055 Portici, Italy

Jane Fletcher
Nutrition Nurses, University Hospitals Birmingham NHS Trust, Queen Elizabeth Hospital Birmingham, Mindelsohn Way, Edgbaston, Birmingham B15 2TH 1, UK

Sheldon C. Cooper
Gastroenterology Department, University Hospitals Birmingham NHS Trust, Queen Elizabeth Hospital Birmingham, Mindelsohn Way, Edgbaston, Birmingham B15 2WB 2, UK

Subrata Ghosh
NIHR Biomedical Research Centre, University Hospitals Birmingham NHS Foundation Trust, Queen Elizabeth Hospital Birmingham, Mindelsohn Way, Edgbaston, Birmingham B15 2TH, UK
Institute of Translational Medicine, University of Birmingham, Birmingham B15 2TH, UK

Martin Hewison
Institute of Metabolism and Systems Research, The University of Birmingham, Birmingham B15 2TT, UK

Tong Chen and Ni Shi
Division of Medical Oncology, Department of Internal Medicine, The Ohio State University, Columbus, OH 43210, USA
Comprehensive Cancer Center, The Ohio State University, Columbus, OH 43210, USA

Anita Afzali
Division of Gastroenterology, Hepatology and Nutrition, The Ohio State University, Columbus, OH 43210, USA
Inflammatory Bowel Disease Center, Wexner Medical Center, The Ohio State University, Columbus, OH 43210, USA

Anecita Gigi Lim and Lynnette R Ferguson
Faculty of Medical and Health Sciences, University of Auckland, Auckland 1023, New Zealand

Bobbi B Laing
Faculty of Medical and Health Sciences, University of Auckland, Auckland 1023, New Zealand
Nutrition Society of New Zealand, Palmerston North 4444, New Zealand

Lorian Taylor, Abdulelah Almutairdi, Nusrat Shommu, Remo Panaccione and Maitreyi Raman
Department of Medicine, University of Calgary, Calgary, AB T2N 4N1, Canada

Richard Fedorak
Faculty of Medicine & Dentistry, University of Alberta, Edmonton, AB T6G 2R7, Canada

Raylene A. Reimer
Faculty of Kinesiology, University of Calgary, Calgary, AB T2N 4N1, Canada

Pedro López-Muñoz
IBD Unit, Department of Gastroenterology, Hospital Universitari i Politècnic la Fe, 46026 Valencia, Spain

Esteban Sáez-González
IBD Unit, Department of Gastroenterology, Hospital Universitari i Politècnic la Fe, 46026 Valencia, Spain
IBD Research Group, Medical Research Institute Hospital la Fe (IIS La Fe), 46026 Valencia, Spain

Belén Beltrán, Pilar Nos and Marisa Iborra
IBD Unit, Department of Gastroenterology, Hospital Universitari i Politècnic la Fe, 46026 Valencia, Spain
IBD Research Group, Medical Research Institute Hospital la Fe (IIS La Fe), 46026 Valencia, Spain
Networked Biomedical Research Center for Hepatic and Digestive Diseases (CIBEREHD), Institute of Health Carlos III, 28029 Madrid, Spain

Amparo Alba
Department of Clinical Analysis, Hospital Universitari i Politècnic la Fe, 46026 Valencia, Spain

Sandra Vidal-Lletjós, Mireille Andriamihaja, Anne Blais, Marta Grauso, Anne-Marie Davila, Claire Gaudichon, François Blachier and Annaïg Lan
UMR PNCA, AgroParisTech, INRA, Université Paris-Saclay, 75005 Paris, France

Patricia Lepage and Marion Leclerc
UMR MICALIS, AgroParisTech, INRA, Université Paris-Saclay, 78350 Jouy-en-Josas, France

Roselyne Viel
H2P2, Biosit-Biogenouest, Université de Rennes 1, 35005 Rennes, France

Rachel Marion-Letellier and Asma Amamou
INSERM unit 1073, Normandie University, UNIROUEN, 22 boulevard Gambetta, F-76183 Rouen, France
Institute for Research and Innovation in Biomedicine (IRIB), Normandie University, UNIROUEN, F-76183 Rouen, France

Guillaume Savoye
INSERM unit 1073, Normandie University, UNIROUEN, 22 boulevard Gambetta, F-76183 Rouen, France
Institute for Research and Innovation in Biomedicine (IRIB), Normandie University, UNIROUEN, F-76183 Rouen, France
Department of Gastroenterology, Rouen University Hospital, 1 rue de Germont, F-76031 Rouen, France

Piotr Eder, Alina Niezgódka, Iwona Krela-Kaźmierczak, Kamila Stawczyk-Eder, Estera Banasik and Agnieszka Dobrowolska
Department of Gastroenterology, Dietetics and Internal Medicine, Poznan University of Medical Sciences, Heliodor Święcicki Hospital, 60-355 Poznań, Poland

Levi M. Teigen, Zhuo Geng and Byron P. Vaughn
Division of Gastroenterology, Hepatology and Nutrition, Department of Medicine, University of Minnesota, Minneapolis, MN 55455, USA

Michael J. Sadowsky and Matthew J. Hamilton
BioTechnology Insititute, Department of Soil, Water & Climate and Department of Plant & Microbial Biology, University of Minnesota, St. Paul, MN 55108, USA

Alexander Khoruts
Division of Gastroenterology, Hepatology and Nutrition, Department of Medicine, University of Minnesota, Minneapolis, MN 55455, USA
BioTechnology Insititute, Department of Soil, Water & Climate and Department of Plant & Microbial Biology, University of Minnesota, St. Paul, MN 55108, USA

Index

A
Abdominal Pain, 28, 35-38, 78, 120, 122-124, 194, 201, 203-204
Adenoma, 85, 96, 218, 230
Anaemia, 116-117, 201
Anthocyanins, 95, 101-102, 105-107, 111-113
Apoptosis, 26, 51, 64, 98-102, 106, 110-112, 119, 158, 221, 232, 234

C
Carcinogenesis, 77, 94, 96-99, 106-113, 119, 132-133, 140, 191-192, 197
Chemoprevention, 94-96, 98-99, 105, 107-108, 111-113
Chronic Disease, 41, 115, 143
Clinical Activity, 6, 14, 37, 39, 158, 160, 168, 207
Colon, 6, 10, 46, 57, 60, 65-68, 71-72, 74, 76, 78, 95-96, 99, 102, 105-107, 109-113, 119-120, 128, 132, 137, 140-141, 158, 170, 172-178, 180, 183-186, 191-192, 197, 207, 216-226, 229-234
Colorectal Cancer, 56, 61-62, 75-76, 87, 94-96, 98-99, 108-112, 126, 133, 140, 160, 204, 232
Crohn's Disease, 1, 4, 7, 16, 22-28, 38, 41-48, 52, 57-60, 62-63, 78, 80, 87-92, 94-96, 110, 115-116, 125, 129-131, 133-135, 137-140, 142, 153-154, 156, 158, 163, 169-171, 188, 195-200, 209-211, 213-216, 228, 234-235
Cytokines, 32, 50-51, 54, 64, 80, 97-100, 105-107, 110-111, 143, 157, 172, 175, 177, 190, 192, 198, 202-204, 212, 234

D
Dendritic Cells, 82, 97, 110, 158, 170, 204
Diarrhea, 15, 28, 35-38, 78, 96, 105, 143, 174, 201, 203-204, 219
Dietary Assessment, 115, 151, 190
Dietary Fiber Intake, 29, 142, 145, 151, 215
Dietary Intake, 18, 22, 24, 29, 33, 42, 49, 54, 59, 80, 83-84, 91, 116, 130, 142-144, 150-152, 189-190, 199, 202, 215, 220, 222, 228
Dietary Protein Level, 172-173, 176
Distal Colon, 66, 175, 222, 224-225, 232
Dysbiosis, 34, 41, 46, 53, 121, 124, 138, 181, 186, 190-191, 193, 196, 198, 205, 226
Dysplasia, 94-97, 109-110

E
Emulsifiers, 122, 131, 136, 188, 191-192, 197, 226, 234
Epidemiological Studies, 1, 34, 143, 188, 190, 210
Epithelial Hypoxia, 219, 226
Epithelial Repair, 172-174, 178-179, 183-184
Epithelium, 48-50, 53, 55-56, 62-64, 71, 73, 75, 81, 95, 99, 105, 119, 124, 135, 141, 158, 173, 183-184, 186, 190, 218
Escalating Treatment, 156, 159-161, 163, 167-168

F
Fat Intake, 33, 133, 142, 145, 225
Fatigue, 78, 85, 128, 140, 203
Fermentation, 5, 61, 118-119, 130, 137, 186, 205, 217, 222, 225, 229, 232-233
Food Additive, 188-189, 191-194, 196, 230
Food Intake, 33, 114-115, 129, 132, 136, 143, 150-151, 202-203, 212
Food Intolerance, 42, 114, 138, 140
Fructose, 35, 114, 120-124, 133-135, 205, 213-214

G
Genotypes, 114-115, 123-124, 126, 128, 139
Gluten, 12, 57, 60, 114, 119, 123-125, 139, 194, 204-205, 214
Gluten Sensitivity, 124-125, 139, 194, 214

H
High Salt Diet, 54, 188, 196
Hypermotility, 67, 74-76
Hypersensitivity, 28, 192-193, 197, 205

I
Immune Pathway, 91, 169
Immune System, 26, 50, 57, 61, 74, 79, 81, 87, 98, 117, 119, 121-122, 150, 157, 169, 218
Inflammation, 1, 5, 7, 11-12, 18, 26, 32, 36, 38, 40, 43-44, 48-49, 53-57, 59, 61-64, 68, 71, 74-78, 80-82, 86, 89-90, 94-100, 105-109, 112-114, 135, 142-144, 150, 153, 156-158, 161, 167-177, 183-184, 187, 189-193, 196-198, 204-207, 214-219, 224, 226, 234
Inflammatory Bowel Diseases, 23, 26, 42, 44-48, 58, 60-61, 78, 87-90, 92, 108, 129-131, 137-138, 140, 153, 171-172, 185-186, 188, 195, 197, 209-211, 213, 228, 230, 234
Intestinal Inflammation, 5, 12, 44, 54, 59, 63-64, 74-76, 90, 132, 156, 161, 168-170, 189-191, 196-197, 204, 206, 218-219, 226, 234
Intestinal Transit, 75, 222
Irritable Bowel Syndrome, 35, 46, 80, 121, 124, 134, 138, 189, 192, 205, 213-214

L
Lactose, 35-36, 114, 123, 125, 134, 137-139, 190, 194, 199, 204
Lesions, 46, 106, 108-109, 116, 118, 197, 211
Logistic Regression, 160, 167

M
Macronutrients, 143, 184, 203, 225
Macrophages, 50-51, 53, 77, 96-97, 99, 106, 109-110, 113, 117, 130, 135, 157-158, 192, 204

Malnutrition, 7, 18, 27, 114-116, 128, 142-143, 151, 153, 194-195, 198, 200-205, 212

Mediterranean Diet, 30, 33, 38, 43, 45, 47, 142-144, 153-154, 200, 205-208, 213-214

Methanogens, 218, 222-223

Microbial Community, 123, 138, 216, 218, 222

Microbiota, 32, 34, 38, 41, 43, 53, 59-62, 78-79, 81-82, 86-87, 90, 98, 110, 114, 119, 121-124, 128-130, 132, 135-139, 142, 158, 170, 172-173, 176, 181-189, 191, 193-194, 197-198, 204-206, 213, 215-218, 220-221, 225-231, 233-235

Mucosa, 5, 28, 36, 46, 48-50, 55-56, 61, 99, 116, 119-120, 122, 135, 137-138, 142, 172-173, 175-176, 178, 181, 183-186, 197, 206, 218, 223, 226, 228-229, 233-234

Mucosa-adherent Microbiota, 172, 176, 181, 183-184

N
Neutrophils, 96-99, 106, 119, 132

Nutrient Deficiency, 114, 116-117, 152

O
Older Age, 200-201, 208-209

Outpatients, 44, 115, 125-126

P
Pathogenesis, 5, 18, 23, 28, 34, 36, 41, 45, 47, 58, 61, 70, 75, 78, 91, 110, 130-131, 140, 142, 151, 188, 204, 213, 216-218, 221-225, 227-230

Pelargonidin, 101-102, 105-106

Peptides, 54-55, 63-64, 76, 126, 158, 186

Peripheral Blood, 56, 85, 92, 157

Plant-based Diet, 41, 194, 216-217, 219, 224-226, 230

Plasma Concentration, 175

Protein Degradation, 222, 225, 227

Proteobacteria, 124, 181, 191, 196, 219, 226-227, 229

R
Risk Factor, 3-4, 32-34, 38, 40, 45, 80, 139, 188, 194, 211

S
Steroids, 16, 156, 159-161, 163, 167-168, 203

Sulfide Production, 186, 217-219, 231-232

Surgical Intervention, 85, 201

T
Tumor Necrosis Factor, 6, 59-60, 64, 76, 92, 97, 144-145, 151, 201-202, 211

Tumor Suppressor, 97, 99, 101, 106, 109, 111

U
Ulceration, 78, 99-100, 177

Ulcerative Colitis, 4, 12, 16, 22-23, 25-26, 28, 41-42, 44-48, 52, 57-63, 76, 78, 80, 88, 90, 94-96, 99, 106, 108-112, 115, 129-130, 135, 139-141, 143, 150, 153, 156, 158, 163, 169-171, 185-188, 195-197, 199-200, 209-211, 215-216, 219, 224, 228-235

W
Weight Loss, 14, 18, 29, 54, 78, 96, 124, 174, 189, 201-202, 207, 212, 227

Westernisation, 114, 118, 121